Human Diseases

Second Edition

by

John H. Dirckx, M.D.

Health Professions Institute

Modesto, California

2003

Human Diseases
Second Edition

by John H. Dirckx, M.D.

Copyright ©2003, Health Professions Institute

First Edition, Health Professions Institute, 1997

Cover design by Lori Raven Smith

Published by
Health Professions Institute
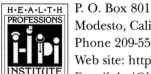 P. O. Box 801
Modesto, California 95353
Phone 209-551-2112; Fax 209-551-0404
Web site: http://www.hpisum.com
E-mail: hpi@hpisum.com
Sally Crenshaw Pitman, Editor & Publisher

Printed by
Parks Printing & Lithograph
Modesto, California

ISBN: 0-934385-38-6

Last digit is the print number: 9 8 7 6 5 4 3 2 1

For my

daughter Patricia

with love

Preface

Human Diseases is intended to provide students and practitioners of medical transcription with a grasp of basic information about the causes, symptoms, diagnosis, and treatment of common diseases. It should also prove useful to workers in the allied health professions, health information management, insurance, law, and other fields who need clear, concise data about these topics. Rare diseases and arcane, trivial, and controversial issues have been carefully avoided throughout.

Discussions of specific diseases are self-contained and can be profitably consulted in isolation from adjacent material. However, topics are presented in an orderly sequence (proceeding from the general to the particular and from the known to the unknown) so as to make *Human Diseases* useful as a textbook. The earlier chapters set forth basic principles, and the later ones discuss, one by one, the bodily systems and important disorders to which they are subject. Preliminary discussions in each of the later chapters review relevant anatomy and physiology and describe symptoms, signs, and diagnostic measures.

This book presupposes some familiarity with the basic concepts and terminology of human biology and healthcare. Most of the less common terms presented in the text are defined in parenthesis when they first occur. A Glossary of concise definitions for these and many other terms can be found at the end of the book. Terms that cannot be found in the Glossary should be sought in the Index, and vice versa.

About the Case Studies. The exercises based on case studies have been designed to impart an element of reality and immediacy to this introduction to clinical medicine. The diagnostic process is frequently a series of fumbles and often enough the problem goes away (or the patient dies) before any clear diagnosis can be made. Efforts at treatment go awry, confuse the clinical picture, aggravate the condition under treatment. Social and psychological issues are ever-present to complicate diagnosis and therapy. The patient's personality, beliefs, and lifestyle may present insurmountable obstacles to a satisfactory outcome.

A puzzle is much harder to solve when pieces are missing, and some pieces are virtually always missing in clinical diagnosis. The history as presented to the physician may be incomplete or inaccurate, diagnostic maneuvers may yield equivocal or enigmatic results, and the physician may simply be unaware or ignorant of the information essential to correct diagnosis and appropriate treatment. To reproduce this ambience of uncertainty and ambiguity, the cases as presented may not accurately or fully represent the underlying reality, and some of the information needed to answer the questions is not in this book. And some of the questions simply have no answers.

John H. Dirckx, M.D.

Contents

Art Acknowledgments

Illustrations of karyotype, immunoglobulins, cardiovascular system, coronary circulation, electrocardiogram, pharynx, menstrual cycle, cranial nerves, and autonomic nervous system are reprinted with permission from *Melloni's Illustrated Medical Dictionary*, 4th ed. (London: The Parthenon Publishing Group, 2002).

Illustrations of digestive system, urinary tract, cerebrum, and spinal cord are reprinted by permission of Pearson Education, Inc., Upper Saddle River, NJ, from Bonnie F. Fremgen, *Essentials of Medical Assisting* (Prentice Hall, 1998).

Illustrations of skin, ear, portal circulation, pancreas, male genitourinary system, female genitourinary system, sagittal section, female genitourinary system, anterior view, placental and fetal circulation, fetal membranes, stages of labor, composition of blood, eye, nerve cell, and meninges are reprinted by permission of Pearson Education, Inc., Upper Saddle River, NJ, from Martini & Bartholomew, *Structure & Function of the Human Body* (Prentice Hall, 1999).

Illustrations

About the Exercises

To the Student: Whether you are an independent study student or enrolled in a traditional classroom, you will find *Human Diseases* an interesting and engaging text. You will get the most from your study efforts if you first familiarize yourself with the entire book, reading all the introductory material and examining closely the Contents and the Index. Review the last section of Chapter 1 where the author describes how the material is presented and explains key terms. Before reading a chapter, review the Chapter Outline and Learning Objectives. Then look ahead to the "Questions for Study and Review" at the end of the chapter. This "preview" sets the stage for what you are about to read and will improve your understanding and retention. Complete the exercises at the end of each chapter or as assigned by your teacher. When doing the "Case Study: You're the Doctor" sections, don't read ahead until you have completed all the questions for that segment. It helps to cover up the remainder of the page with a sheet of paper so you don't accidentally see what happens next! The "Suggestions for Additional Learning Activities" are for all students. Some require you to do research outside of this textbook while others may require the assistance of classmates, friends, or family members, especially for learning games. Even though these exercises may seem more like fun than actual work, they promote "whole brain learning" and will aid your mastery of the study of human diseases. Answers to objective questions appear in the back of the book. Some questions are more subjective and will not have a single right answer.

To the Teacher: This second edition of *Human Diseases* contains an expanded and multi-faceted selection of exercises to help your students master the material and build essential critical thinking skills that will help them excel in school and in the workplace. "Questions for Study and Review" can be assigned as self-graded homework and discussed in class or be completed in the classroom as a test of reading comprehension. In "Case Study: You're the Doctor," students are asked to render their opinions on both clinical and ethical dilemmas. Have students complete the first case study in the classroom, working together or in small groups, reviewing Dr. Dirckx's Preface before they begin. The case studies are presented in segments, each appearing in a shaded box followed by a series of questions. Encourage students to answer all the questions for each segment, without looking ahead to the next segment. Covering the remainder of the page with a sheet of paper is suggested. In "Suggestions for Additional Learning Activities," you'll find ideas for creative classroom activities and homework assignments that will add interest and variety to your course. Some activities require students to go outside the text for more information. Others require interaction with others in learning groups. And virtually all of the individual Learning Activities can be adapted for the classroom by asking students to work together, compare their work with others, or present their findings to the class. The answers to objective questions are contained in the back of the book for easy access. An exhaustive Index is also included as an indispensable study aid.

Georgia Green, CMT
Director of Education
Health Professions Institute

1

The Nature of Disease

LEARNING OBJECTIVES

Upon completion of this chapter, you should be able to

• explain the nature of disease;

• describe how diseases are named and classified;

• give the meanings of terms referring to various features of diseases;

• assess the diagnostic process;

• use the terminology of diagnosis and treatment.

THE NATURE OF DISEASE

Disease is a broad general concept, encompassing every imaginable impairment of normal bodily structure and function, and every imaginable threat to health and well-being, from genetic disorders affecting all of the cells in the body to highly localized, even microscopic, lesions; from conditions causing lifelong symptoms to mere passing indispositions; from severely disabling conditions to trivial aberrations detectable only by laboratory testing or statistical measurement.

A disease is not a "thing." Even though physicians and laity alike find it convenient to talk about diseases as if they were self-subsisting entities, a disease is actually just a state, condition, or process occurring in a living body.

Hence every case of disease is unique. No two persons with pneumococcal pneumonia or myocardial infarction have exactly the same symptoms, signs, and outcomes. On the other hand, all cases of these diseases have enough in common that it is reasonable and expedient to group them together under a single concept and give them a single name.

When we speak of the transmission of a disease from one person to another, we really mean the transmission of the germs that cause that disease. Similarly, expressions about diseases "going away" or "coming back" are purely metaphorical.

Disease is a complex notion, including not only biological alterations of normal structure and function but also psychological, social, and economic factors. In addition, in our culture disease is regarded as something to be treated and perhaps cured by a physician.

The discussion of diseases that follows is based on the beliefs and traditions of Western scientific medicine. Although this system of medicine is rational and coherent, and gives satisfactory explanations or interpretations of facts and, often, acceptable results in treatment, it is far from perfect. In our understanding of the causes of various diseases, their prevention, diagnosis, and treatment, we have a long way to go.

Radically different views on the cause, nature, and treatment of disease are held by adherents of some religions or philosophies, by members of other cultures, and by some within our own culture. Many of these alternative systems—Christian Science, the folk medicine of various ethnic groups, chiropractic, acupuncture—contain valid and useful elements, as well as other elements that conflict with basic facts and principles of scientific medicine.

A disease is a recognizable pattern of symptoms or abnormalities. What constitutes a disease? A single migraine headache is not a disease, but a lifelong tendency to get migraine headaches is considered a disease state. Is a sprained ankle a disease? A hangover? Pregnancy? There can be no precise or "official" answer to these questions. Some physicians and psychologists have objected to the classification of alcoholism as a disease on the grounds that this diminishes patients' sense of personal accountability and responsiveness to counseling. Fibrocystic disease of the breast has been renamed fibrocystic condition (or disorder) of the breast because the word "disease" was perceived as having negative and ominous connotations in this context. Legislation or regulations regarding health insurance coverage often require that pregnancy be treated "the same as any other disease."

NAMING AND CLASSIFYING DISEASES

Diseases can be, and have been, named and classified in many different ways, but no system of naming or classification in present use is entirely consistent or satisfactory. Many names attached long ago to diseases remain in use today even though they have been shown to be inaccurate or misleading (see box).

Influenza, a disease causing fever, headache, muscle aches, and cough, was so named because it was blamed on the influence (Italian *influenza*) of the stars and planets. We retain the name even though we know that the disease is caused by a virus.

Malaria got its name because it was more prevalent in swampy areas, and was believed to be due to the damp, malodorous air in such places (Italian *mal'aria* 'bad air'). We now know that it is caused by a parasite, which is transmitted by mosquitoes that breed in shallow, stagnant water, but we still retain the old name.

Cholera, a bacterial infection of the intestine, was formerly thought to be due to an excess of bile (Greek *chole*).

Some disease names go back to classical Greek (asthma, coryza, dysentery, nephritis) or Latin (fistula, impetigo, scabies, vertigo). Before the era of modern science, diseases were often named for some obvious symptom or characteristic (diabetes 'a flowing through [of urine]', chlorosis 'greenness', jaundice 'yellowness'). Many older disease names are metaphorical in origin: cancer 'crab', chalazion 'hailstone', lupus 'wolf', tinea 'moth'. Nowadays we are more likely to name diseases according to their causes, if we know them (ehrlichiosis, trichomoniasis). Numerous disease names are eponymic (based on proper names), usually honoring the person or persons who first discovered or described them (Hodgkin disease, Osgood-Schlatter disease, parkinsonism), but sometimes referring to persons so afflicted (Christmas disease, Hartnup disease, Lou Gehrig disease) or geographic areas where they were first noted or where they are endemic (California encephalitis, Lyme disease, Rocky Mountain spotted fever).

A disease name may denote a single, very specific disorder, such as otitis media or typhoid fever, or it may stand for a whole group of different conditions with one thing in common, such as anemia (a general term for any disorder characterized by a deficiency of circulating red blood cells) or salmonellosis (an infection caused by any of hundreds of species or varieties of *Salmonella*). The term hyperthyroidism means a condition in which excessive thyroid hormone causes symptoms. This is not one single disease, but an abnormal state that can have various causes. It may be appropriate for a physician to diagnose hyperthyroidism on the basis of an initial evaluation of the patient, but with further investigation a more precise diagnosis, such as Graves disease, will usually be possible.

A **syndrome** is a combination of symptoms that consistently occur together (Cushing syndrome, irritable bowel syndrome, toxic shock syndrome). For some syndromes there are several known causes; for others, no cause has been identified. Disease names formed with Greek suffixes have fairly predictable patterns of meaning: *-ia* denotes an abnormal condition (ophthalmia, pneumonia); *-itis* means inflammation (appendicitis, dermatitis); *-osis*, an abnormal condition (cyanosis, nephrosis); *-ism*, habituation or intoxication (alcoholism, atropinism).

Textbooks of medicine contain elaborate classifications of disease. In addition, official systems of naming and classification, particularly the *International Classification of Diseases (ICD)*, are in wide use to standardize the statistical reporting of diseases and billing for medical services. Some of these classificatory systems, such as the *Diagnostic and Statistical Manual of Mental Disorders* published by the American Psychiatric Association, include precise definitions of diseases.

The classification of diseases must constantly change as scientific information increases. What was formerly considered a single disease may come to be recognized as a group of diseases with similar symptoms but different causes, while diseases that were formerly thought to be different may eventually be recognized as different forms or stages of the same disease.

One classification may be appropriate in one setting, and another classification in another setting. For example, anemia can be classified on the basis of its cause as due to:

Deficient formation of red blood cells.
Excessive hemolysis (destruction of red blood cells in the body).
Blood loss.

But for the diagnostician, a more useful classification may be on the basis of the size of the red blood cells:

Normocytic, with normal-sized cells.
Macrocytic, with cells larger than normal.
Microcytic, with cells smaller than normal.

These two classifications overlap but do not match; they cannot be meaningfully combined, and yet each has its place in the theory and practice of medicine.

The discussion of diseases presented in the following chapters is not exhaustive, and the classification used does not necessarily match those used in textbooks of medicine or in the *ICD*. The purpose of these chapters is not to impart a medical education but to give the student an awareness of the range of disorders, diagnostic measures, and treatments, with emphasis on conditions that are encountered daily in medical practice. Material has been selected and arranged so as to be maximally useful for study, review, and reference.

The following are some common ways of describing, characterizing, or classifying diseases. Under each basis of classification, some of the more common terms are defined or explained, and examples are given.

Classification According to Onset, Duration, Severity, or Rapidity of Evolution and Resolution

Acquired: Not congenital (acquired hemolytic anemia, acquired immunodeficiency syndrome).

Acute: Developing relatively suddenly and running its course in a few days or weeks (acute pharyngitis, acute glomerulonephritis).

Asymptomatic: Causing no symptoms; often referring to a disease or condition that is discovered during a routine or screening examination, or in the evaluation of another condition.

Chronic: Having a protracted course, often lifelong (chronic bronchitis, chronic pancreatitis).

Congenital: Present at birth, though not necessarily inherited (congenital cataract, congenital adrenal hyperplasia).

Disabling: Causing impairment of normal functions or capabilities, such as the ability to see, stand, and walk, or earn a living.

End-stage: Referring to a progressively deteriorating condition that has reached the point of lethal (terminal) functional impairment of an organ or organ system (end-stage renal failure, end-stage lung disease).

Fulminant or **fulminating**: Rapidly progressive and severe (fulminant hepatitis, fulminating dysentery).

Hyperacute: Having a very abrupt onset or very brief course (hyperacute purulent conjunctivitis, hyperacute graft rejection).

Infantile: Occurring or becoming evident during infancy (infantile autism, infantile cataract).

Intermittent: Causing symptoms at intervals, with intervening periods without symptoms (intermittent claudication, intermittent acute porphyria).

Juvenile: Occurring in early life (juvenile rheumatoid arthritis, juvenile kyphosis).

Life-threatening: Referring to a disease or injury that may prove lethal, even with aggressive treatment.

Malignant: Tending to cause death (malignant tumor, malignant hypertension).

Neonatal: Affecting newborn infants (neonatal anemia, neonatal hypoglycemia).

Paroxysmal: Occurring in sudden attacks (paroxysmal cold hemoglobinuria, paroxysmal atrial tachycardia).

Progressive: Characterized by increasingly extensive or severe symptoms or signs (progressive cataract, progressive muscular atrophy).

Recurrent: Referring to a condition that reappears after symptoms had largely or entirely resolved (recurrent corneal erosion, recurrent ulcerative stomatitis).

Relapsing: Essentially the same as the preceding (relapsing fever, relapsing polychondritis).

Remissive, remittent: Referring to a condition of which most or all signs and symptoms have resolved, either naturally or as a result of treatment; remission may be temporary or permanent.

Self-limiting (or **self-limited**): Said of a disease such as the common cold that typically runs its course and resolves spontaneously without complications or sequelae, even when left untreated.

Senile: Occurring as a result of aging (senile cataract, senile dementia).

Silent: Asymptomatic; referring to a disease or medical event discovered only by chance (silent gallstones, silent myocardial infarction).

Subacute: Lasting somewhat longer than an acute illness (subacute bacterial endocarditis, subacute granulomatous thyroiditis).

Subclinical: Causing no symptoms or signs; essentially the same as silent.

Terminal: A disease that is expected to cause death within the near future, regardless of treatment.

Etiologic Classification (by Cause)

Deficiency: Due to a lack or insufficiency of some essential chemical substance or property (leukocyte adhesion deficiency, iron deficiency anemia).

Degenerative: Caused by deterioration in the structure or function of cells or tissues, usually with aging (degenerative joint disease, degenerative myopia).

Developmental: Characterized by some abnormality in the development of a tissue, organ, or body part, either before or after birth (rickets, ventricular septal defect).

Essential: Of unknown cause; apparently arising spontaneously (essential hypertension, benign essential tremor).

Familial (heredofamilial): Due to an inherited abnormality expressed in other members of the patient's family (familial hypertrophic cardiomyopathy, heredofamilial tremor).

Functional: Due to a disturbance of function without evidence of structural or chemical abnormality (functional dysmenorrhea, functional heart murmur).

Hereditary: Due to an inherited abnormality or tendency (hereditary cerebellar ataxia, hereditary multiple exostoses).

Idiopathic: Of unknown cause; apparently arising spontaneously (idiopathic cardiomyopathy, idiopathic hypertrophic subaortic stenosis).

Infectious (infective): Caused by the adverse biologic, chemical, or immunologic effects of the growth of microorganisms in the body (infectious mononucleosis, infective embolism).

Molecular: A disease caused by abnormality in the chemical structure or concentration of a single molecule, usually a protein or enzyme; virtually all molecular diseases are inherited (congenital adrenal hyperplasia, sickle cell anemia).

Neoplastic: Involving the formation of one or more growths or tumors, which may be benign or malignant.

Nutritional: Due to insufficient or excessive dietary intake of some nutrient (nutritional anemia, nutritional hemosiderosis).

Organic: Due to some demonstrable abnormality in a bodily structure (organic dementia, organic heart murmur).

Traumatic: Due to injury—physical, chemical, thermal, or psychological (traumatic amnesia, traumatic neuroma).

Diseases can also be classified anatomically, by the organs or tissues principally involved; physiologically, by the body system or function affected; or by the medical specialties concerned with their treatment.

THE DIAGNOSTIC PROCESS

The training of a physician includes an intensive study of diseases and their symptoms from two distinct points of view: (1) the symptoms and signs of each disease, such as pneumonia and pericarditis; and (2) all the diseases that can produce any given symptom or sign, such as dyspnea or chest pain.

Training in diagnostics also includes learning to apply and interpret the basic maneuvers of physical diagnosis as well as the full range of supplementary diagnostic tests available. Equipped with this battery of information and technical skills, the physician takes a history, performs a physical examination, orders diagnostic tests, and coordinates the resulting data to formulate a tentative or working diagnosis.

The **medical history and physical examination** are the cornerstone of all medical practice. For every patient admitted to a hospital, the physician must dictate or write a history and physical examination. Similar documentation of diagnostic findings, though often less extensive, is a part of medical office records and consultations. The history and physical shows the extent of the physician's evaluation of the patient and provides support for the diagnosis made. Conspicuous among the data reported in a history and physical examination are pertinent negatives—listing of symptoms and signs that are not present. Inclusion of these negatives is essential to providing a complete clinical picture and a complete account of the diagnostic procedures performed by the physician.

Sometimes the diagnosis is evident at once: a cut on the hand from a sharp tool; a foreign body in the eye. In other instances, diagnostic procedures may yield negative, normal, ambiguous, or contradictory results, and the tentative diagnosis must be based on a balancing of such probabilities as are suggested by the history. **Differential diagnosis** refers to this consideration and ranking of several alternative explanations of a patient's symptoms and physical findings. For example, the differential diagnosis (often shortened to just "the differential") of chest pain and shortness of breath includes myocardial infarction, spontaneous pneumothorax, rib fracture, pneumonia, and a number of other possibilities.

The diagnostician must always reckon with the possibility that the patient has two or more unrelated diseases, each of which is contributing to the total clinical picture. The likelihood that a patient has more than one disease at the same time increases with age.

HOW DISEASES ARE DESCRIBED IN THIS BOOK

In the remaining chapters, each disease or category of disease chosen for inclusion is treated in a separate section. The more elaborate discussions are divided under some or all of the following headings:

Disease Name and Synonyms
Brief Description
Cause(s)
History
Physical Examination
Diagnostic Tests
Course
Treatment

In the following section, crucial terms and concepts relating to some of these divisions of the material are defined or explained.

Cause

Etiology: Strictly speaking, the study of the causes of disease; universally used by physicians to mean the cause itself.

Multifactorial etiology: Indicates that a given disease has more than one cause operating together (lung cancer may develop because of a genetic predisposition and exposure to carcinogens in cigarette smoke; *Pneumocystis carinii* pneumonia is due to the parasite, *Pneumocystis carinii,* but usually does not develop unless the immune system is impaired, as in AIDS).

Primary: Said of a disease or condition that does not result from some other disease (primary aldosteronism, primary malignancy).

Secondary: Said of a disease or condition that results from some other disease (secondary hypertension, secondary malignancy; tachycardia secondary to congestive heart failure).

History

The medical history is a detailed record of the course of an illness, as perceived and recalled by the patient.

Noncontributory: Information of no help in arriving at a diagnosis; said principally of elements of the patient's history, such as family medical history.

Symptom: Any distress, abnormality, or malfunction experienced by the patient as a result of illness; a symptom may be entirely subjective (headache, vertigo) or it may be partly or entirely evident to others (paralysis, vomiting).

Physical Examination

A formal assessment of bodily structure and function by the physician in an effort to establish a complete clinical picture of the patient's illness. Traditionally, physical examination includes four basic techniques: inspection, palpation, percussion, and auscultation.

Inspection: Visual examination of the external body surface and of the mouth and pharynx, the external ear, the nares, and other orifices and cavities accessible to direct examination without a surgical incision.

Palpation: Feeling superficial and deep structures with the fingers or palm to detect tenderness, spasm, abnormal masses, abnormal texture of tissues, enlargement of abdominal organs, and other departures from the normal or expected.

Percussion: Tapping with a finger on the body wall, usually with a finger of the other hand interposed, to detect variations in sound quality over abnormal cavities, masses, accumulations of gas or air, or effusions of fluid (see box).

Auscultation: Listening to selected body regions with a stethoscope, principally to assess heart sounds, breath sounds, and bowel sounds.

Sign: Any abnormality of bodily structure or function that is observable by the physician, whether evident to the patient or not.

Diagnostic Tests

Under this heading are included all diagnostic procedures not included in the basic physical examination. These include laboratory tests, diagnostic imaging, electrophysiologic measurements, endoscopy, radionuclide procedures, and others.

Culture: The growth of microorganisms from a specimen (blood or other body fluid, secretions, tissue) under controlled laboratory conditions.

Cytology: Microscopic examination of stained cells, usually cells brushed or scraped from a surface such as the uterine cervix or the interior of the stomach; the principal use of cytology is in detecting any malignant or premalignant cellular changes.

Electrodiagnostic procedures: Methods for recording the electrical activity accompanying the function of certain organs or tissues (electrocardiogram, electroencephalogram, electromyogram, and others).

Endoscopy: Examination of the interior of a cavity or hollow organ with an instrument introduced through a natural orifice (cystoscopy, colonoscopy) or a small incision (laparoscopy, arthroscopy).

Histology: Microscopic examination of stained, very thin sections of tissue obtained by biopsy or surgical excision, or at autopsy.

The technique of **percussion**, which has been rendered largely superfluous by x-ray, fluoroscopy, ultrasound, and MRI, is now the least used of the four basic methods of physical diagnosis. Before these imaging procedures became available, however, percussion was at least as important as auscultation in the examination of the chest.

This technique was first described by the Austrian physician Leopold Auenbrugger (1722-1809), who translated to clinical medicine the common practice of tapping on a wine barrel to determine the level of the fluid inside. Auenbrugger made extensive experiments with the method and confirmed its validity by comparing his findings in the living patient with autopsy results.

He published his method in a small book in 1761, which was largely ignored by the medical profession until Corvisart, Napoleon's personal physician, issued a French version in 1808. Auenbrugger was a man of wide interests and broad culture. He played an important role in Viennese society for several decades, and wrote the libretto for an opera, *Der Rauchfangkehrer* (*The Chimney Sweep*, 1781), for which the music was composed by Mozart's rival, Antonio Salieri.

Imaging (diagnostic): Any procedure used to study or visualize internal organs or tissues by application of irradiation or other physical energy: x-ray, CT scan, fluoroscopy, ultrasound, magnetic resonance imaging, and others.

Invasive: Refers to a procedure requiring the introduction of a needle, catheter, or other instrument into the body through a natural orifice, puncture, or incision.

Laboratory test: Any test performed in a laboratory on a specimen of tissue or body fluids removed from the patient; includes physical, chemical, microscopic, microbiologic, immunologic, and other examinations.

Microbiology: The branch of biology and medical laboratory technology concerned with the study of microorganisms (bacteria, fungi), particularly those that are pathogenic for human beings.

Noninvasive: Referring to a diagnostic procedure such as an x-ray examination or electrocardiogram that does not require introduction of instruments into the patient's body.

Radiography: The branch of medical technology concerned with the performance of x-ray and other imaging procedures.

Radiology: The branch of medicine concerned with the diagnosis and treatment of disease through the application of x-rays, ultrasound, magnetic resonance imaging, radioactive materials, and related methods.

Scan: Examination of part or all of the body by a radiographic procedure, particularly one involving radioactive substances, to identify or localize an abnormal condition.

Serology: The branch of medical laboratory technology that employs antigen-antibody reactions to diagnose infections and other diseases, particularly autoimmune diseases.

Smear: A thin film of fluid or semisolid material (blood, stool, nasal secretions, cells scraped from a surface), usually stained (treated with dye), that is examined microscopically for diagnostic purposes.

Course

The course of a disease is the sequence of events from the first appearance of symptoms to the final resolution of all abnormalities. Diseases evolve. The signs and symptoms noted at the beginning of an illness are often entirely different from those noted a few hours, days, or weeks later. In diagnosis and prognosis, the pattern according to which the manifestations of disease change is almost as important as the manifestations themselves.

Complication: A disease or abnormal condition induced by a pre-existing condition, which renders treatment more difficult, recovery more protracted, or death more likely.

Form: Any of several clinical patterns that a disease may manifest (the discoid and systemic forms of lupus erythematosus).

Forme fruste (French): An atypical, prematurely arrested, or incompletely developed form of a disease.

Grade: A measure of the severity of a disease or abnormal condition, particularly a malignant disease.

Life-threatening: A prognostic indication that a disease or injury may prove lethal in spite of aggressive treatment.

Onset: The first appearance of signs or symptoms of a disease.

Present [verb, accented on second syllable]: Refers to the symptoms or signs that are evident when the patient first seeks medical attention. ("Ms. Jones presented to the emergency department at 1:00 a.m. today with acute, diffuse chest pain and dyspnea." "Infectious mononucleosis occasionally presents as painless jaundice or a nonspecific rash.")

Prodrome: A period during which (usually nonspecific) symptoms such as fever or malaise precede the appearance of typical signs and symptoms of a disease.

Prognosis: The probable outcome of a disease, as predicted on the basis of diagnosis and course.

Sequela [plural, sequelae]: An abnormality or impairment, such as scarring or weakness, that persists after a disease has resolved.

Stage: A measure of the extent to which a disease, particularly a malignant disease, has developed.

T-N-M classification: A formal mode of staging that is used for many malignant diseases; T, tumor; N, (lymph) nodes; M, metastases. Arabic numerals are used to indicate the extent of involvement; for example, T1 N2 M0 for a given tumor might mean a tumor that is not locally invasive, with extension to two groups of regional lymph nodes, but no apparent metastases.

Treatment

Under this heading are included all measures undertaken to reduce symptoms, maintain or restore function, eradicate the cause of a disease, and prevent recurrence.

Aggressive: Referring to a prompt, energetic program of treatment.

Benign neglect: A program of doing essentially nothing when a disease is either beyond hope of cure by even the most radical methods, or is expected to resolve without any specific treatment.

Conservative: A mode of treatment, medical or surgical, that has a low risk of causing serious adverse effects, but also less likelihood of effecting a cure than other available methods.

Cosmetic: Referring to physical appearance; said of surgical procedures designed primarily to improve the patient's appearance, such as breast augmentation, revision of scars, and excision of benign skin lesions.

Cure: Complete extinction of a disease, usually by arresting the basic process or removing the cause.

Elective: Referring to a treatment or therapeutic procedure, usually a surgical operation, that is not absolutely required to save the patient's life or restore health, but that is, or may be, performed to improve the prognosis or to correct a minor problem; also, a procedure that is necessary but that is deferred until it is convenient for the patient.

Heroic: Referring to radical or extreme therapeutic measures that are only justified by the desperate condition of the patient.

Inoperable: Referring to a disease, usually malignant, for which surgical treatment is not an option, because of the extent of the disease or the condition of the patient.

Masterly inactivity: Same as *benign neglect*; a phrase first used, in a nonmedical context, by the British political writer Sir James Mackintosh (1765-1832).

Medical: Any form of treatment not involving surgery or physical manipulation.

Monodrug therapy: Treatment of a condition such as hypertension or malignancy with a single drug, rather than a combination of drugs.

Palliative: Referring to treatment of a severe or malignant disease that is intended to relieve pain or conserve function without removing the cause or effecting a cure.

Physical therapy: Treatment involving application of physical modalities (massage, exercise, heat, cold, ultrasound).

Protocol: A therapeutic regimen, usually prescribed for malignant disease, consisting of fixed or proportionate doses of three or more drugs administered concurrently.

Radical: A drastic program of treatment, medical or surgical, with a high risk of adverse effects, justified only by the severity of the patient's condition or the unfavorable prognosis.

Regimen: A program or course of treatment, including diet, exercise, and drug therapy.

Surgical: A mode of treatment involving physical or mechanical manipulation, usually by cutting into the body to repair or remove diseased or injured organs or tissues.

Supportive: Referring to a treatment regimen designed to preserve the patient's comfort, hydration, and nutritional status without affecting the underlying disease.

Symptomatic: Referring to treatment that is intended to relieve symptoms rather than abolish their cause.

Synergism: A positive interaction between two or more drugs in which each boosts the effect of the others.

Therapeutic trial: Experimental administration of a drug in an effort not only to relieve symptoms but also to confirm the working diagnosis.

QUESTIONS FOR STUDY AND REVIEW

1. Define or explain these terms:
   a. acute _Developing suddenly + running its course in a few days or weeks._
   b. chronic _Having a protracted course, often lifelong._
   c. etiology _The study of causes of disease — universally used to mean the cause itself._
   d. sign _an abnormality of bodily structure or function that is evident to physician, whether or not evident to patient (part of physical exam)_
   e. symptom _distress, abnormality, or malfunction experienced by patient as a result of illness_
   f. syndrome _combination of symptoms that consistently occur together._

2. Give two examples of invasive diagnostic procedures: _cystoscopy + biopsy_
   a. _needle or catheter — introduction of instrument into patient's body_
   b. _X-ray or electrocardiogram — no introduction of instrument into patient's body._

3. Give two examples of noninvasive diagnostic procedures:
   a. _____
   b. _____

4. What factors must a physician take into account in choosing what diagnostic tests to perform on a patient, and when to perform them?

   _____
   _____
   _____
   _____
   _____
   _____
   _____
   _____
   _____

5. It is often said that the patient's history provides more useful clues to the diagnosis than the physician's examination, and that the examination is more valuable than laboratory tests. Look through the discussions of genetic diseases in the next chapter and find examples of disorders that can be diagnosed by history alone; those in which physical examination is diagnostic; and those in which only laboratory testing can confirm the presence of genetic disease.

_____

_____

_____

_____

_____

6. If you or a friend or family member has had an illness wrongly diagnosed by a physician, what factors do you think might have played a part in the error?

_____

_____

_____

_____

_____

CASE STUDY: YOU'RE THE DOCTOR   ps. 11-13

Maria Jaspers is a 34-year-old married white woman whose chief complaint is a sore throat of 4 days' duration. She has noted mild nasal congestion and a slight cough, but her dominant symptom is discomfort with swallowing, worse on arising in the morning. She has had some ear discomfort at times, particularly on swallowing, but no hearing loss. She doesn't think she has had any fever. She denies digestive upset, rash, and aching in joints or muscles. She is able to swallow solid food without much difficulty, is not being kept awake at night by throat pain, and has not missed any work because of this illness.

1. Of the various adjectives listed in this chapter that are used to describe or quantify symptoms, choose several that apply to Ms. Jaspers's complaints.

_acquired, acute, intermittent, self-limiting_____

_____

_____

_____

The patient's husband and one of her two school-age children have had similar symptoms. She has been using lozenges and ibuprofen with some relief, but consults you, her family physician, because she feels the problem has gone on too long and that some medical intervention is necessary.

2. Having obtained this history, what basic diagnostic procedures would you use to assess Ms. Jaspers's condition? (Refer to the material on respiratory infections in Chapter 9 for ideas.)

culture, smear

Temperature and other vital signs are normal. The patient is in no distress and is not coughing or hoarse. A careful examination of the throat, nasal passages, and ears reveals no evidence of inflammation. There are no swollen cervical lymph glands and breath sounds are normal on auscultation. Because throat pain is the chief complaint and because the patient has been exposed to her school-age child who also has a sore throat, you perform a rapid strep screen in the office; this is negative. You advise her that she has a viral infection, which is expected to resolve within another few days and for which no specific treatment is available. Ms. Jaspers counters with the remark that this is now her fifth day of illness and that she is not getting any better.

---

3. How important is it for you, as the treating physician, to educate this patient as to the nature of her illness, its prognosis, and appropriate treatment?

Very important, so that appropriate treatment is given. Patient needs to understand that condition will go away in time – no need for antibiotics.

4. Since prescribing an antibiotic will take much less time than persuading her that she doesn't need one, and will be more likely to preserve this patient's goodwill, isn't that the preferable course of action from a purely practical standpoint? Why or why not?

No – overuse of antibiotics is a problem. Symptoms can be treated with OTC meds + aspirin until symptoms go away.

You explain that viral respiratory infections typically take 1-2 weeks to resolve, depending on how quickly and effectively the immune system can produce neutralizing antibodies. You also gently point out that, since Ms. Jaspers first noted soreness in her throat on Monday afternoon and this is Thursday morning, it is still only the third day of illness. You advise her to get extra rest, drink extra fluids, continue symptomatic treatment, and return if symptoms worsen. As she leaves your office she is obviously somewhat dissatisfied.

5. What formal diagnosis will you record in this patient's record?

   Cold Virus - no infections - sore throat, mild cough, mild nasal congestion.

> About 6 weeks later, you see Ms. Jaspers again when she brings her son to the office for a soccer physical. She tells you that on the Saturday following her last visit to you she went to an urgent care clinic for further treatment of her sore throat, on the advice of her neighbor. At the clinic she received an injection and a prescription for ten days of oral antibiotic. No laboratory studies were performed. Her parting shot to you is the remark, "I had pharyngitis. The doctor could tell that just by looking."

6. Define the term *pharyngitis:* _inflamation of pharynx & mucous membrane_

7. Define the term *pharyngitis* as it is understood by this patient: _infection_

8. Would it be prudent for you to point out to her that this is exactly the diagnosis that you entered in her record? Why or why not?

   Yes. Explain overuse of antibiotics & not necessary to give them in this case.

9. Speculate as to why the physician at the clinic treated her with an antibiotic without performing any laboratory studies:

   To make patient happy.

SUGGESTIONS FOR ADDITIONAL LEARNING ACTIVITIES

1. Choose a disease that has been discussed in recent news reports and investigate the origin of its name. If more than one name is associated with the condition, give the origin for each.

2. Obtain a sample report of a history and physical examination. As you read the report, underline the names of diseases the patient has had in the past. Circle the names of diseases the patient is known to have at present. Compare these past and present diagnoses with the working or tentative diagnosis on admission.

3. On 3" x 5" index cards, write each of the entries, including definitions, contained under the headings Cause, History, Physical Examination, Diagnostic Tests, Course, and Treatment. On the back of each card, write the name of each entry's associated heading. Use a pencil and write lightly so the heading doesn't show through to the other side. Make one index card for each of the headings to identify a pile for each. Shuffle the entry cards, then read each entry and place it in the correct pile. Check your work by turning the piles over and examining the headings on the back of the cards.

2

Genetic Disorders

LEARNING OBJECTIVES

Upon completion of this chapter, you should be able to

• differentiate between hereditary and congenital diseases;

• explain the biochemical basis of heredity;

• give examples of procedures diagnostic for hereditary diseases and chromosomal abnormalities;

• describe the features of common inherited diseases;

• discuss the features of common chromosomal abnormalities.

GENETIC DISORDERS

CONGENITAL VS. HEREDITARY

This would be a good place to elaborate on two definitions that were given in the preceding chapter:

Congenital: Beginning, occurring, or first being evident at birth.
Hereditary: Inherited from one or both parents.

The distinction is often poorly understood. A congenital disorder is present at birth, but it is not necessarily transmitted genetically. For example, many congenital disorders result from environmental factors (maternal infections; maternal ingestion of certain medicines, drugs of abuse, or toxins such as dioxin or lead during pregnancy) or from faulty intrauterine development (umbilical cord tightly wrapped around an extremity and shutting off its blood supply). The birth process itself can lead to congenital disease or abnormality, as in the case of infections such as herpes simplex and chlamydia transmitted to the newborn from the birth canal, and cerebral palsy from difficult labor with compromise of blood flow to the baby's brain.

A hereditary disorder is genetically acquired; that is, it is transmitted to the affected individual by the genes of one or both parents. All of the diseases presented in this chapter are hereditary.

The Biochemical Basis of Heredity

The inheritance of physical traits (eye color, hair color, body build) as well as of some diseases and abnormal conditions depends on the transmission of genes from parents to offspring. A gene is a functional unit of heredity; each gene transmits a single trait or function. Every human cell nucleus contains more than 50,000 genes, arranged in bands along coils of protein and deoxyribonucleic acid (DNA) called chromosomes.

There are 46 chromosomes in the nucleus of a human cell, arranged in 23 pairs. One of these pairs, the sex chromosomes, determines the sex of an individual. Women have two X chromosomes (XX), and men have an X and a Y chromosome (XY). In women, one of the X chromosomes is genetically inactive. Hence all persons have one active X chromosome, and in addition men have an active Y chromosome.

The remaining 22 pairs of chromosomes are called autosomes; they are concerned with the transmission of traits having nothing to do with biological gender, and the members of each pair are basically identical to one another. Each gene has a fixed normal position, or locus, on a specific chromosome. The genes that occupy the corresponding loci on any given pair of chromosomes (and that transmit the same trait) are said to be homologous.

The autosomes are numbered from 1 to 22 in the order of decreasing length. Each is divided into a long arm (q) and a short arm (p), which are further divided into regions, bands, and subbands for the purpose of designating gene loci.

In the formation of human sex cells (female ovum, male sperm), but in no other cells, the chromosome pairs divide by a process called meiosis, which results in cells having only 23 chromosomes instead of 23 pairs of chromosomes. When sperm and egg unite, the full complement of 23 pairs of chromosomes is restored, one of each pair having come from each parent.

Body cells other than sex cells multiply by splitting into two identical daughter cells. Before this division takes place, the chromosomes replicate; each chromosome forms a copy of itself in a process called mitosis. This process, which occurs in several stages, results in the formation of two nuclei having identical sets of chromosomes, one for each daughter cell.

When homologous genes are identical (for example, when both genes for eye color are coded for blue eyes), the individual is said to be homozygous for the trait coded by that gene. When homologous genes are not identical (for example, one coding for blue eyes and the other for brown eyes), the individual is said to be heterozygous for eye color.

Some genes exert their effects only in homozygous individuals. That is, both genes at a given locus must be identical. Such a gene is said to be recessive, because if it appears on only one chromosome of a pair, the trait for which it codes is not expressed. An individual having only one recessive gene is called a carrier of that gene, because it can be transmitted to some or all offspring. A gene that has its effect even in a heterozygous individual, that is, when paired with a gene that is not identical to it, is said to be dominant. The basic pattern of normal inheritance is called mendelian, after Gregor Mendel (see box).

The fundamental concepts of the genetic transmission of traits from parents to offspring were evolved by a Bohemian amateur scientist, Johann Gregor Mendel (1822-1884). Mendel came of peasant stock and was unable to finish his college education for lack of funds. After becoming an Augustinian monk, he studied to be a teacher, but failed twice to obtain certification because his mind always went blank at examination time.

His leisure studies of the transmission of characteristics from one generation of peas to later generations provided the basis for his theories of the statistical distribution of parental characteristics among offspring and the notions of dominant and recessive genes and hybridization. He published his theories in 1865, but was rebuffed or ignored by professional biologists. Three years later he became the abbot of his monastery, and abandoned further research.

His work was rediscovered after his death and brilliantly vindicated by the studies of later scientists.

Geneticists distinguish between an individual's phenotype, which is the complex of traits as observed by inspection, measurement, biochemical testing, or other means; and the genotype, which is the actual genetic composition of the individual's chromosomes, as determined by chromosomal analysis.

GENETIC ABNORMALITIES

Many things can go wrong in the process whereby a new individual is formed through the transmission of more than 50,000 genes. A mutation is a permanent, transmissible change affecting (usually) a single gene. Through mutation, an individual with normal parents can acquire an abnormal trait at conception and pass it on to some offspring, not necessarily in the first generation. Genetic defects in autosomes are called autosomal (dominant or recessive). Defects in sex chromosomes are called sex-linked or (since they all affect the X chromosome) X-linked. Not all genetic mutations cause evident abnormality. Fetuses with severe disorders are usually lost through spontaneous abortion.

Some mutations occur with sufficient frequency that their presence in a subject's genotype (chromosomal makeup) can be inferred from the resulting abnormal phenotype (physical appearance and biochemical composition and function). It is estimated that human beings are subject to at least 4,000 inheritable diseases.

Chromosomal aberrations are variations from the expected number and composition of chromosomes. These occur sporadically and result in a wide variety of abnormalities.

Nondisjunction means failure of chromosomes to divide and then pair up correctly during mitosis or meiosis. It results in an abnormal number of chromosomes (either more or less than the expected 46), a condition called aneuploidy.

When the number is 47 (meaning that, for one of the chromosomes, three copies occur rather than two) the condition is termed trisomy. A common example is Down syndrome, also called trisomy 21 because individuals so affected have three copies of chromosome 21. Down syndrome is discussed later in this chapter.

When the number of chromosomes is 45, the condition is called monosomy. A common example is Turner syndrome (monosomy X), in which the individual has only one X chromosome and no Y chromosome. This disorder is also discussed later in the chapter.

Mosaicism denotes a form of nondisjunction in which some of the cells of an individual have one genetic constitution (karyotype) while other cells have a different genetic constitution.

Breaks along the course of one or more chromosomes result in aberrations in their structure. Deletion is the complete loss of part of a chromosome that has broken away. In inversion, a separated fragment rotates end-for-end before reattaching. Translocation is an exchange of fragments between two chromosomes.

A few inherited disorders are called multifactorial, nonmendelian, or both, because they apparently result from abnormalities in more than one gene, involve an interaction between genetic material and environmental factors, and are transmitted in patterns other than the classical mendelian one. Examples include cleft lip and palate (discussed later in this chapter) and spina bifida (discussed in Chapter 19).

DIAGNOSTIC PROCEDURES IN HEREDITARY AND CHROMOSOMAL DISORDERS

A number of diagnostic methods are available to establish or confirm a diagnosis of inherited disease or chromosomal aberration. Physical examination, measurements, or simple chemical tests may be sufficient to determine the presence of a specific genetic defect with reasonable certainty. The family history or pedigree of an individual, even an unborn one, can supply valuable clues about heritable disorders and patterns of transmission.

Cytogenetics (also called chromosomal analysis and karyotyping) is the examination of chromosomes by light microscopy. Cells can be obtained for chromosomal analysis in various ways: blood specimen, skin biopsy, and (from the fetus) amniotic fluid

by amniocentesis and placental tissue by chorionic villus sampling.

Cells are first cultured (made to grow and divide in an artificial laboratory medium). Mitosis is induced by application of one chemical agent and then abruptly arrested by another. Cells are transferred to a microscope slide and stained by various methods that allow bands of genes on chromosomes to be distinguished. The slide is examined microscopically, and if chromosomes are clearly visible in several cells undergoing mitosis, these are photographed. Individual chromosomes appearing in the photograph are cut out and pasted on a form in standard order, autosomes 1 to 22 followed by sex chromosomes (X and, if one is present, Y). See Figure 1.

The resulting **karyotype** shows the number of chromosomes and readily identifies gross structural aberrations such as deletion and inversion.

Figure 1. Karyotype

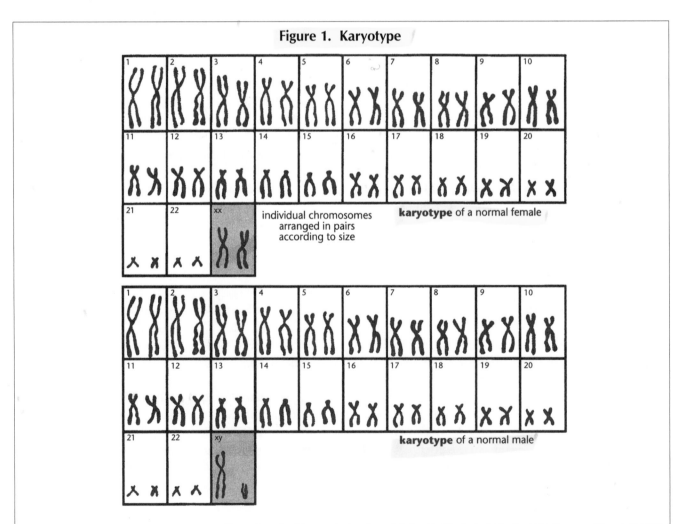

individual chromosomes arranged in pairs according to size

karyotype of a normal female

karyotype of a normal male

Reproduced with permission from *Melloni's Illustrated Medical Dictionary*, 4th ed. (2002)

Another diagnostic modality is biochemical genetics. Most if not all single-gene heritable disorders involve the absence or insufficiency (occasionally, overabundance or overactivity) of one single substance, usually an enzyme or other protein, in body cells or tissues. Early in the twentieth century, the term *inborn errors of metabolism* was applied to genetic diseases that were known to involve such biochemical flaws. The term is now falling into disuse as it becomes increasingly apparent that a majority of genetic disorders can be so characterized.

Biochemical genetics refers to the detection of abnormally high or low levels (or none at all) of certain proteins and other substances in body fluids or tissues. Seeking and finding these biochemical markers is a more precise measure than karyotyping. For example, the discovery that the subject's plasma contains a very low level of coagulation factor VIII solidly confirms the presence of hemophilia A (discussed in Chapter 16).

A still more sophisticated diagnostic method is **DNA analysis of chromosomes**, sometimes called *molecular genetics*. In this procedure, abnormal DNA sequences are identified in individual genes by chemical analysis. This is the most specific and also the most expensive method of genetic diagnosis now in use. Very small quantities of specimen material can be amplified through polymerase chain reaction (PCR) technology, and specific sequences of DNA identified by DNA probe, an artificially fabricated strand of DNA that finds and fuses with the sequence being sought.

Some or all of these diagnostic methods may be used to reveal a suspected hereditary disorder in children with evident congenital deformity, mental or physical retardation, or delayed puberty. Indications for prenatal genetic studies include advanced maternal age (which increases the risk of Down syndrome), genetic disease in either parent or in other offspring, and abnormal findings on prenatal ultrasound examination.

INHERITED DISEASES   *Hereditary*

In this section a few of the more common inherited disorders are discussed. This is not an exhaustive catalog of such disorders. Several diseases described in other chapters (diabetes mellitus, muscular dystrophy, sickle cell anemia) are also hereditary. The reason for surveying some genetic diseases here is to provide a notion of the broad variety of their signs, symptoms, and severity.

This section will also serve as an introduction to the format used for discussing individual diseases throughout the book. When you encounter a term with which you are unfamiliar, look it up in the Glossary at the end of the book. If you can't find it there, check the Index to find a definition or explanation of the term in the text.

Cystic Fibrosis

A disorder in which exocrine glands (bronchial mucous glands, pancreas, others) secrete abnormally thick mucus, which results in duct obstruction, damage to glandular tissue, and other adverse consequences. The most common lethal genetic disease in the United States, with an average incidence of one case for every 2000 Caucasian births.

Cause: Absence of a substance called cystic fibrosis transmembrane conductance regulator from mucous gland cells throughout the body. Autosomal recessive inheritance. Most patients have a family history of the disease.

History: In infancy, meconium ileus (bowel obstruction due to abnormally thick meconium, the stool formed in the fetal intestine before birth). In childhood, failure to thrive, cough, dyspnea on exertion, recurrent respiratory infections (bronchitis, pneumonia), bronchiectasis (abnormal, irreversible dilatation of bronchi, related to chronic infection), atelectasis (collapse of part or all of a lung), pneumothorax (air between a lung and the wall of the chest cavity), cor pulmonale (dilatation or failure of the right ventricle due to acute or chronic pulmonary disease). Malabsorptive nutritional deficiency, flatulence, steatorrhea (passage of excessive fat in stools, because the necessary enzymes are prevented from reaching the intestine by biliary and pancreatic obstruction). Infertility in males (due to spermatic duct malfunction and obstruction).

Physical Examination: Pallor, nutritional deficiencies, abdominal distention, basilar rales (crackling or bubbling sounds heard on auscultation of the lung bases, due to the presence of fluid in air passages), hyperexpansion and hyperresonance of the thorax, digital clubbing (club-shaped deformity of the fingertips; see box), nasal polyps.

Diagnostic Tests: Anemia, hypoalbuminemia (deficiency of the protein albumin in the blood), low

Clubbing of the digits refers to a deformity of the tips of all ten fingers in which the distal phalanges are swollen, spongy, and warm to the touch, and the angles between the distal phalanges and the nails are flattened out.

Clubbing is a hereditary trait in certain families, but it usually points to some systemic disease, particularly in the pulmonary or cardiovascular system, such as congenital heart disease with inadequate oxygenation of the blood, infection of heart valves (bacterial endocarditis), chronic hepatic or intestinal disease, and malignancy or infection (particularly bronchiectasis or lung abscess) within the thorax.

When clubbing results from pulmonary disease it is sometimes called hypertrophic pulmonary osteoarthropathy.

An alternative term is hippocratic clubbing, referring to the Greek physician and medical writer Hippocrates (460-377 BC). The oldest known description of digital clubbing, in a case of empyema (local pus-forming infection in the pleural cavity), appears in Hippocrates's work *Prognostic*.

"Patients with empyema invariably present with the following symptoms and signs: unremitting fever, which is worse at night; drenching sweats; racking nonproductive cough; sunken eyes; flushed cheeks; abnormal curvature of the nails and warmth of the fingers, especially at the tips…"

levels of fat-soluble vitamins (A, D, E, K) in serum. Arterial oxygen tension is reduced, and pulmonary function tests show reduction in forced vital capacity and in flow rate. Plasma levels of immunoreactive trypsinogen may be elevated. Chest x-ray may show peribronchial cuffing (thickening of bronchial walls), emphysema (trapping of air within cavities formed in lung tissue by breakdown of the walls of air sacs), bronchiectasis, atelectasis, or pulmonary infiltrates (spread of inflammatory fluid or exudate into air cavities of the lung, producing cloudiness of lung tissue on chest x-ray). The sweat chloride level is elevated.

Course: Recurrent respiratory infections, nutritional deficiencies. Only one-half of patients survive beyond the age of 20. Complications and sequelae: cor pulmonale, hepatic cirrhosis, asthma, nutritional deficiency.

Treatment: Vigorous attention to general health and avoidance of respiratory irritants and infections. Physical therapy, postural drainage, aerosols, bronchodilators, prophylactic use of influenza and pneumococcal vaccines; corticosteroids for exacerbations of pulmonary symptoms. Nutritional supplements, pancreatic enzyme supplements.

Phenylketonuria (PKU)

An inborn error of metabolism causing mental retardation unless diagnosed and treated in early life.

Cause: Decreased activity of phenylalanine hydroxylase, an enzyme that normally converts phenylalanine to tyrosine. Phenylalanine is an essential amino acid whose principal dietary source is milk. In phenylketonuria, abnormally high levels of phenylalanine accumulate and cause irreversible damage to the central nervous system. Transmitted as an autosomal recessive trait, it occurs in one of 10,000 Caucasian births. Several clinical patterns are recognized.

History: The child appears normal at birth, but within a few months may display psychomotor retardation (delayed development in muscle strength and coordination and impairment in the ability to understand and learn), hyperactivity (increased mobility, restlessness, inability to sit or lie still), seizures, movement disorders, paralysis, and abnormally fair skin with a tendency to eczema.

Physical Examination: Fair skin, mental retardation, muscle weakness or paralysis, myoclonus (involuntary jerking or twitching of certain muscles or muscle groups), eczema (an acute or chronic inflammation of the skin with itching, redness, blistering, weeping, crusting, and scaling). The urine has a mousy odor.

Diagnostic Tests: The serum level of phenylalanine is abnormally elevated, the level of tyrosine reduced. The urine contains phenylketones (phenylpyruvic acid and 2-hydroxyphenylacetic acid), hence the mousy odor and the name of the disease. Early detection of phenylketonuria is mandatory if treatment is to be successful (see box).

Course: With dietary restriction of phenylalanine begun early, most patients lead normal lives. Sensitivity to phenylalanine may be outgrown in some cases.

Treatment: Restriction of dietary phenylalanine by feeding low-phenylalanine substitutes for milk. Avoidance of the artificial sweetener aspartame. Treatment should be begun before one month of

Testing of newborn blood for **phenylalanine** is standard pediatric practice. Testing is required by law in many states before hospital discharge of the newborn. With hospital stays for uncomplicated delivery restricted to 24 hours, many infants are tested before phenylalanine levels have begun to rise. Repeat testing must therefore be done a few days later in an outpatient setting.

age and continued as long as blood tests show a rise in phenylalanine after consumption of milk.

Acute Intermittent Porphyria

An inborn error of metabolism causing crises of abdominal pain after ingestion of certain drugs.

Cause: Deficiency of the enzyme porphobilinogen deaminase, which normally breaks down porphyrins (products of red blood cell metabolism), leads to a rise of porphyrins in blood (see box), with resulting neurologic symptoms, most often attacks of severe abdominal pain. Such attacks can be triggered by ingestion of alcohol, various medicines (barbiturates, sulfonamides, and many others), or a low-carbohydrate diet. Autosomal dominant inheritance. Many if not most persons carrying the gene for acute intermittent porphyria have no symptoms. Most patients with symptoms are women, and symptoms often begin before age 25.

History: Attacks of severe abdominal cramps, often with vomiting and constipation; the pain arises in the middle of the abdomen but may radiate widely; less commonly, paralysis, seizures, or psychosis. Occasionally seizures or hallucinations. Urine turns deep pink, brick red, or brown on standing. Between attacks, no symptoms.

Physical Examination: During abdominal crises, evidence of severe distress, usually without abdominal tenderness, spasm, distention, or fever. Rarely,

The term **porphyria** (from Greek *porphyra* 'purple') refers to the color of the urine after standing. Several other diseases, not all hereditary, are also called porphyrias because they cause a rise in the level of porphyrins in the blood and of their products in the urine. The symptoms of the porphyrias vary widely.

jaundice. Weakness or paralysis of muscles, including respiratory muscles. Between attacks there are no abnormal signs.

Diagnostic Tests: The white blood cell count and differential count are normal. Porphyrin levels are elevated in blood, urine, and stool. Urinary excretion of porphobilinogen and delta-aminolevulinic acid is increased. The blood level of sodium may be far below normal.

Course: With avoidance of low carbohydrate intake (starvation diets), alcohol, and drugs known to precipitate crises, patients should be able to lead normal lives.

Treatment: Strict avoidance of alcohol and precipitating medicines, and maintenance of normal carbohydrate intake. For crises, supportive treatment as needed; intravenous glucose (to raise blood sugar) and hematin (to inhibit the synthesis of porphyrins).

Marfan Syndrome

An inherited disorder of connective tissue affecting primarily bones, the cardiovascular system, and the eye.

Cause: Abnormal synthesis of the protein fibrillin (a major component of connective tissue) due to an abnormal gene on chromosome 15. Autosomal dominant inheritance.

History: Lax joints, subject to dislocation; unusually tall stature. Dislocation of ocular lens, severe myopia, (nearsightedness), retinal detachment. Symptoms of cardiac failure.

Physical Examination: Characteristic habitus (body build, physique, overall appearance): long, spindly extremities and digits, often with pectus excavatum (funnel chest, hollow chest) and scoliosis (lateral curvature of the spine). Lax joints. Evidence of ectopia (abnormal location or position) or dislocation of ocular lens(es); there may be mitral regurgitation (leakage of blood from the left ventricle back into the left atrium during contraction of the ventricle because of an incompetent mitral valve, discussed in Chapter 8) or evidence of aortic dilatation or aortic regurgitation (backward leakage of blood into the left ventricle between contractions of the ventricle because of an incompetent aortic valve).

Diagnostic Tests: There are no known biochemical markers. In most patients echocardiography reveals mitral valve prolapse (abnormal mobility or floppiness of the valve), with or without regurgitation of blood during left ventricular contraction. Chest x-ray may show dilatation of the aorta.

Course: Progressive dilatation of the aorta often leads to aortic rupture in middle life. Recurrent dislocations may damage joints. Scoliosis may become severe and is irreversible after adolescence. Ocular abnormalities often lead to severe visual impairment. An abnormal valve may become the site of endocarditis (bacterial infection of valve leaflets, discussed in Chapter 8).

Treatment: Avoidance of strenuous physical exertion and prophylactic use of beta-blockers to delay aortic dilatation. Close observation of vision and correction of myopia with glasses. Monitoring of aortic diameter and cardiac valvular function. Prophylactic grafting of the aorta when dilatation is severe. Endocarditis prophylaxis before surgery or dental work.

Cleft Lip and Palate

A group of congenital deformities of the face and the roof of the mouth.

Cleft lip is a gap in the upper lip near the midline, and cleft palate is a similarly located fissure dividing part or all of the roof of the mouth. Either may occur without the other. Deformity is evident at birth and may cause severe feeding difficulties. Some cases are due to chromosomal abnormalities, and may occur in conjunction with other heredofamilial disorders of the lower jaw, eyes, or ears. Other cases may be related to maternal ingestion of alcohol or certain drugs (for example, phenytoin). Treatment is surgical repair of cleft lip before the age of 3 months and of cleft palate by the age of one year. Patients with cleft palate usually require speech therapy and orthodontic treatment.

CHROMOSOMAL ABERRATIONS

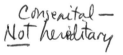 Congenital — Not hereditary

Down Syndrome (Trisomy 21, Mongolism)

A genetic aberration producing characteristic physical stigmata and mental retardation.

Cause: The presence of an extra chromosome 21. In most instances the mother is over 40.

Physical Examination: Small head, characteristic facial features (slanted eyes, flattened bridge of nose, small ears, large tongue with gaping mouth), short flat hands with single transverse "simian" crease, hypotonia (diminished muscle tone), retarded physical and mental development (IQ around 50). Brushfield spots (small white spots in the irises of the eyes) during first year of life.

Course: Life expectancy is reduced (under 50). Heart disease, acute leukemia, and an Alzheimer-like dementia often develop before age 30.

Turner Syndrome

A chromosomal aberration consisting of loss of an X chromosome (XO pattern). All patients are female. Several variants occur, some due to mosaicism. Signs and symptoms include short stature, facial abnormalities, webbed neck, failure of ovarian development with amenorrhea (absence of menstruation) and sterility (inability to conceive), and structural abnormalities of the skeleton, the cardiovascular system, and the kidneys. Treatment with growth hormone and estrogen leads to correction of some deformities but does not restore fertility.

Klinefelter Syndrome

A chromosomal aberration consisting of an extra X chromosome (XXY pattern). All patients are males. At puberty, the arms and legs grow disproportionally long, the testicles fail to develop, and gynecomastia (abnormal development of the male breast) occurs. All patients are sterile; many have subnormal intelligence or learning disorders. There is a higher risk of breast cancer and diabetes mellitus than in the general population. Diagnosis is confirmed by karyotyping. Treatment with testosterone may correct abnormalities of habitus but will not reverse sterility.

Oncogenes and Tumor Suppressor Genes

Some individuals inherit a predisposition to certain malignancies. Oncogenes are abnormal autosomal genes that arise by mutation from pre-existing normal genes (proto-oncogenes) and, under certain conditions, can induce neoplastic transformation of cells. Oncogenes cause certain body cells to secrete abnormal proteins (or normal proteins, such as cellular growth factors and regulators, in abnormal amounts), with resultant uncontrolled growth and development. The most important oncogene thus far identified is p53, which is believed to be involved in more than 50% of human cancers.

Various factors can lead to the formation of an oncogene. Some viruses (such as the human papillomavirus) contain oncogenic strands of DNA in their chromosomal makeup. Infection with one of these viruses can cause incorporation of such abnormal genetic material into body cells. Some oncogenic mutations are triggered by exposure to ionizing radiation or to toxic chemicals (carcinogens), such as benzo[a]pyrene in cigarette smoke, benzene, and asbestos. Genetic instability (a heightened risk of chromosomal aberrations) occurs in some inherited diseases, such as Down syndrome, in which the risk of leukemia is 20 times that in the general population.

Tumor suppressor genes (anti-oncogenes) are normal genes whose function is to suppress transformations in cells that could lead to malignancy. Their inactivation through deletion or mutation results in increased risk of such malignant transformation.

Most familial cancers are due to an inherited mutation in one allele of a tumor suppressor gene. If the second allele is inactivated by mutation or deletion, malignant proliferation of cells can take place. BRCA1 and BRCA2, which predispose to early-onset breast cancer and ovarian cancer, are tumor suppressor genes.

It is now possible to identify a number of oncogenes, and to detect inactivation of anti-oncogenes, by DNA analysis.

QUESTIONS FOR STUDY AND REVIEW

1. Distinguish *congenital* (but not inherited) *disorders* from *hereditary disorders*, and give examples of each type.
   a. congenital disorders *Beginning, occurring, or first being evident at birth. Not necessarily transmitted genetically. Herpes simplex, cerebral palsy, mental retardation due to mother on drugs, physical disabilities due to medication taken by mother, Down syndrome*
   b. hereditary disorders *genetically acquired - Transmitted by genes of one or both parents. Cystic Fibrosis, diabetis, muscular dystrophy, PKu, Marfan, Down syndrome.*

2. Define or explain these terms:
   a. karyotype _____
   b. gene _____
   c. autosomal dominant_____
   d. nondisjunction _____
   e. trisomy_____

3. What are the three basic laboratory methods of genetic diagnosis?
   a. _____
   b. _____
   c. _____

4. Give two examples of genetic diseases that cause obvious physical deformity:

5. Give two examples of genetic diseases that cause problems only intermittently:

6. What are some advantages and disadvantages of the medical progress that has enabled many persons with cystic fibrosis to survive past puberty?

_____

_____

_____

_____

_____

_____

CASE STUDY: YOU'RE THE DOCTOR *Read*

Ron and Linda Woehler, the parents of a child with cystic fibrosis, visit you, a pediatrician with a subspecialty in medical genetics, to discuss the advisability of having further children. According to them, their 3-year-old has already had many bouts of respiratory infection and is underweight and undersized for her age.

1. Why is it important for you to have precise medical documentation of their child's diagnosis and current condition before proceeding?

_____

_____

_____

2. What are the characteristics of *cystic fibrosis?*

_____

_____

_____

The Woehlers would like to have at least one more child, but are concerned that future offspring will be similarly afflicted.

3. What questions might you ask them about their personal health and family histories?

_____

_____

_____

_____

Linda, who appears to be more knowledgeable about the genetics of the disease, is mainly interested in knowing the statistical risk that a second child will also have cystic fibrosis. Ron feels that the first step should be for you to do genetic testing on both of them so that you will have objective data on which to base predictions and recommendations. Linda resists the idea of testing, stating repeatedly, "I'm not sure I want to know."

4. Cystic fibrosis is transmitted by an *autosomal recessive gene.* Explain this term.

5. What might be the implications for this couple's future if it were to turn out that Ron does not carry the gene?

SUGGESTIONS FOR ADDITIONAL LEARNING ACTIVITIES

1. Find a picture of a normal karyotype or photocopy the illustration on page 18. Use scissors to cut out the chromosome pairs and then separate them into individual chromosomes. Leave enough margin so you can clearly identify each chromosome. As you separate each one, pencil in the name of the pair on the back of each so you can check your work later. Then shuffle the chromosomes and lay them out face up. You are now a geneticist and must assemble the karyotype into its original form. For an extra challenge, perform this activity using an abnormal karyotype, one with additional or missing chromosomes. Exchange abnormal karyotypes with another student or family member and see if you can arrive at a diagnosis after assembling the karyotype.

2. Many genetic disorders have one or more advocacy groups formed by patients and their families. Locate an advocacy group for a disorder that interests you by searching on the Internet or checking the resources of your public library. What services and information does this group provide?

3. Examine your own family history for any indication of inherited disorders by interviewing relatives. Draw a pedigree chart (you can find an example in an encyclopedia or on the Internet), indicating which relatives are affected in each generation.

Infectious Diseases

LEARNING OBJECTIVES

Upon completion of this chapter, you should be able to

- explain the general concepts of infection, transmission of infectious diseases, and immunity;

- identify types of infecting organisms and the ways in which they cause disease;

- describe patterns of transmission;

- discuss the diagnosis of infectious diseases;

- summarize general principles of treatment of infectious diseases.

INFECTIOUS DISEASES

AN OVERVIEW OF INFECTIOUS DISEASE

An infection is a disease or process resulting from the growth of certain microorganisms (sometimes, larger organisms) in the living body. Infections may be local (an abscess of the elbow), generalized (septicemia, defined later in this chapter), or local with systemic effects (pulmonary tuberculosis). They may be trivial and self-limiting (the common cold), life-threatening (acute bacterial meningitis), or uniformly lethal (AIDS). They may be readily responsive to treatment (strep throat) or essentially untreatable (rabies).

The subject of infectious disease is far too broad to be fully explored within the scope of a single chapter. The following pages provide a survey of basic concepts. The chapter concludes with discussions of selected infectious diseases, to provide some notion of their variety. Most of the remaining chapters in this book also contain discussions of infectious diseases. If you encounter an unfamiliar term that is not immediately defined in the text, look in the Glossary at the end of the book. Terms not found in the Glossary should be looked up in the Index.

The term *pathogen* denotes any organism that is capable of inducing disease through infection. The following types of pathogens cause infections in human beings:

Bacteria (singular, bacterium): One-celled organisms on the borderline between animals and plants, varying enormously in structure, physical and chemical properties, and disease-causing capabilities. Examples: staphylococci (staph), streptococci (strep), chlamydia.

Fungi (singular, fungus): Simple microscopic mold- or yeast-like organisms. Examples: ringworm fungus, yeast causing thrush and vaginitis.

Parasites: Members of the animal kingdom, including one-celled organisms, worms, and arthropods (insects and related animals), that live on or in the human body, deriving their nourishment from it and often causing severe or chronic disease in the process; the term infestation is usually preferred to infection with respect to parasites. Examples: *Trichomonas*, pinworm, pubic lice.

Viruses: Fragments of genetic material incapable of independent existence; they cause disease by entering living cells, taking over their operation at the molecular level, and using them as breeding grounds for hundreds of thousands of new viral particles, ultimately destroying them. Examples: herpes simplex virus, chickenpox virus.

Pathogenic microorganisms induce disease by a wide variety of mechanisms. They may cause local erosion or destruction of tissue; interfere with the functions of cells, tissues, or organs; or elicit an inflammatory reaction in the host that becomes the dominant clinical problem.

Inflammation is a complex but stereotyped pattern of reaction whereby living tissue responds to injury in the broad sense (direct physical injury, burning or freezing, chemical or biological irritants, or poisons). In local inflammation there is generally an increase in blood flow through the affected part, causing redness, warmth, and (because fluid is released from the circulation into tissue spaces) swelling.

The nature of the tissue in which an inflammatory reaction occurs determines in some measure the resulting symptoms: in the respiratory tract, congestion and increased secretions; in the digestive system, abdominal pain, vomiting, and diarrhea; in the skin, itching, blistering, and crusting. An inflammatory reaction also includes production by the patient's tissues of chemical substances that attract white blood cells to the area to repel, engulf, or destroy invading or proliferating microorganisms.

Suppuration refers to the process of pus formation. Pus is a mixture of white blood cells, dead tissue, and killed or inactivated pathogens. A local accumulation of pus, surrounded by a wall of inflamed tissue, is called an abscess.

Many pathogens have "inborn errors of metabolism"—that is, they are biologically defective in some way, so that they depend on their host for sustenance, or produce waste products that are harmful to the host, or both. Such waste products, considered from the point of view of the host, are called toxins. A toxin (as the term is used here) is a chemical substance produced by pathogenic organisms and causing harmful effects to the host. These effects vary widely from one pathogen to another, and include local inflammation, rash, and muscular paralysis. Some microorganisms (for example, some streptococci) produce toxins that break down body proteins and permit spread of the pathogens through tissue spaces. An infection characterized by such wide infiltration of tissues by pathogens is called cellulitis. Toxin formation is an important mechanism of disease production by many pathogens.

Any severe or systemic infection may produce nonspecific symptoms such as fever, chills, headache and muscle aches, loss of appetite, nausea, vomiting, and general malaise.

TRANSMISSION OF INFECTION

Some infections (chickenpox, genital warts) can be spread from one person to another by various routes; others (sinusitis; pyelonephritis, an infection of the kidney and ureter) cannot. The following terms relate to the transmission of infectious diseases.

Airborne: Referring to infections that can be spread through the air, usually by droplets of respiratory secretions but sometimes on particles of moisture or dust, or free-floating.

Bloodborne: Referring to infections transmitted by blood transfusion, surgical or dental instruments contaminated with the blood of an infected person, needles shared by intravenous drug abusers, and occasionally through sexual or other intimate contact, with transfer of blood from one person to another.

Carrier: A person who has recovered from a communicable disease (hepatitis B, typhoid fever) but still harbors living and virulent organisms and can transmit them to others.

Communicable disease: An infection that is capable of being transmitted in any way from one person to another.

Congenital: Referring to infections acquired before or at birth.

Contagious: Transmitted by close exposure (direct touch, sexual contact, exposure to respiratory, digestive tract, or other secretions).

Droplet spread: Transmission of respiratory and other infections by fine mists of respiratory secretions expelled into the air by coughing or sneezing.

Epidemiology: The branch of medicine and public health that deals with patterns of disease causation and spread (not necessarily infectious diseases).

Fecal-oral route: The route by which some intestinal and other pathogens are transferred from person to person; contamination of food or water, or direct physical contact, with the infected person's feces leads to ingestion of the pathogen by the second host.

Fomite: Any inanimate object, such as a washcloth, drinking glass, or doorknob, that can be the means whereby pathogenic microorganisms are transmitted from an infected person to others.

Host: A living organism on or in which another organism, usually a parasite, lives.

Infectious disease: Any disease caused by infection; sometimes used in the narrower sense of transmissible disease.

Period of communicability: The length of time, often beginning before the appearance of symptoms, during which a person with an infectious disease can spread it to others in some way.

Sexually transmitted disease (STD): Any infection that is transmitted from person to person through sexual activity.

Transmissible: Able to be spread from person to person.

Tropical disease: An infection or infestation that occurs predominantly or exclusively in tropical latitudes.

Vector: A living organism that transmits pathogens from an infected person to a healthy person (such as mosquitoes that transmit the causative organisms of yellow fever or malaria).

CLINICAL FEATURES OF INFECTIOUS DISEASES

Numerous factors influence the signs and symptoms of infectious diseases, their course and severity, the diagnostic procedures whereby they can be identified, and their response to treatment. By and large, the most important of these factors is the identity of the infecting organism. That is, any given pathogen (chlamydia, hepatitis A virus, ringworm fungus) tends to produce the same basic disease or group of diseases in all infected persons.

But the extent and severity of the basic disease process can be modified by a number of variables. The virulence of a pathogen is its innate capacity to do harm. Some strains of an infecting organism may be more virulent than others, and may thus be better able to overcome the resistance of the host and to escape destruction by medicines. The mode of exposure (inhalation, ingestion, introduction into the bloodstream) and the dose (100 organisms or 100 billion) have a bearing on the extent and severity of illness produced, if any.

Host resistance refers to the whole gamut of defenses by which a living body is able to repel, inactivate, or destroy pathogens that threaten to invade it. General state of health, nutritional status, the integrity of skin and mucous membranes, and most importantly the effectiveness of the immune system, all influence host resistance.

Immunity (discussed more fully below and in the next chapter) is a biological response of the living body to invading microorganisms or other noxious materials. Some types of immunity protect the body by repelling or excluding potential invaders. Others neutralize or destroy organisms that have invaded, and still others confer a lasting, perhaps lifelong, ability to resist future infections by an organism that has once gained entry. When the immune system is impaired by congenital or acquired disease, infections may prove much more severe, even lethal. In addition, organisms that are ordinarily unable to infect human beings may produce opportunistic infections in persons with deficient immunity.

The interval between invasion by microorganisms and the first appearance of symptoms is called the incubation period of an infection. For some infections (the common cold, viral gastroenteritis) this may be less than one day; for others (malaria, leprosy) it may be more than six months.

Once a pathogenic organism has gained entrance to the body, it can spread by various routes, depending chiefly on the nature and virulence of the organism but also on host defenses. Some pathogens are spread by the hematogenous route (through the bloodstream). Others move through lymphatic channels. Bacteremia denotes the presence of bacteria in the blood, as detected by laboratory tests. Toxemia means the presence of toxic products of an infecting organism in the blood. When large numbers of virulent organisms and their toxic products are circulating in the blood, the condition is called septicemia. Microorganisms can also spread along the surface of skin or mucous membranes.

IMMUNITY TO INFECTION

The topic of immunity will be more fully discussed in the next chapter. Here it will suffice to state a few general principles.

Immunity is the capacity of a living body to repel or destroy invading microorganisms or other nox-

ious substances, and in particular to resist a second attack by a pathogen that has already invaded and caused disease. Immunity involves a large number of processes depending primarily on white blood cells (cellular immunity) and antibodies (humoral immunity). An antibody is a complex protein, formed by cells of the immune system, that can recognize a specific target organism, combine with it, and bring about its inactivation or destruction.

Immunity plays three important roles with respect to infectious disease:

1. It can strongly influence and alter the course and prognosis of an infectious disease.
2. An antibody produced by the immune system in response to a specific pathogenic organism, and circulating in the patient's blood, can be used diagnostically to identify the organism.
3. Vaccines consisting of killed or inactivated pathogens can cause the immune system to produce antibody conferring resistance to those pathogens, just as if the subject had already had the disease and developed natural antibody.

THE DIAGNOSIS OF INFECTIOUS DISEASE

Besides the basic diagnostic procedures described in Chapter 1, the physician uses numerous other measures to diagnose infections. These can only be sketched here; specific examples and elaborations will be given throughout the remaining chapters of the book.

The findings of the basic physical examination can be supplemented by various diagnostic tests. X-rays, scans, and endoscopy can provide more specific information about the location and character of an infection. Blood tests such as the white blood cell count, the differential white blood cell count, and the erythrocyte sedimentation rate can provide nonspecific clues to the presence of infection.

But generally the principal goal of diagnostic maneuvers in infectious disease is to identify the pathogen. For many if not most infections, knowing the exact identity of the causative organism leads to the most accurate prediction of the course of the disease and the most precise selection of effective therapy. The causative organism can be identified in one of two ways: by removing a specimen from the body and visually observing the pathogen in the specimen, or by detecting antibody to the pathogen in the patient's blood.

Methods leading to direct visual identification of pathogens pertain to the field of microbiology. Technologists in this field process and examine specimens of blood, urine, stool, or tissue obtained at surgery or by biopsy; and secretions, pus, or any other material that is likely to contain visible organisms. A smear may be made from the specimen on a microscope slide and inspected by light microscopy. Ordinarily a microbiologic smear is prepared for examination by the application of one or more stains. These are variously colored dyes that render microorganisms more readily visible or that bring out distinctive structural or biochemical features.

The Gram stain is a standard bacteriologic procedure that highlights structural features of bacteria and permits them to be separated into two large categories. Gram-positive organisms take up crystal violet stain in the presence of iodide, and hence appear blue or purple in a smear. Gram-negative organisms do not take up crystal violet in the presence of iodide, and so would be invisible in a smear if a second stain (counterstain) in a contrasting color (red or pink) were not applied after the first.

The acid-fast stain is used to identify mycobacteria, which cause tuberculosis and leprosy. These organisms take up fuchsin and certain other organic dyes so avidly that they cannot be washed away with acid-alcohol. (Mycobacteria, and often the infections they cause, are thus loosely termed "acid-fast.") Many other specialized staining procedures are available for the identification of certain organisms, including fungi and parasites.

Viruses cannot be seen by light microscopy. Some viruses, however, induce changes in cells (inclusion bodies, vacuolization) that can be seen in preparations of tissue or certain fluids, and can strongly support the diagnosis of a specific viral infection. Viruses can be seen by electron microscopy, but the principal method used to identify viral infection is testing for antibody in the patient's blood.

When a specimen is thought to contain too few pathogenic microorganisms for them to be observed in a smear, their number can be amplified by allowing them to multiply under controlled laboratory conditions. A culture is a colony of microorganisms grown in a laboratory. A culture grows on or in a medium (plural, media): a mixture of nutrients and other substances (minerals, antibiotics, agents to modify the texture of the medium) that is designed to favor the growth of certain organisms of interest and often to inhibit the growth of others.

Cultures are grown in specially designed dishes, bottles, or tubes. Media may be solid, semisolid, or liquid. Media for growing viruses and chlamydias contain living cells. A culture medium into which microorganisms are introduced is said to be inoculated with them. Growth of organisms in a culture medium is called incubation, especially when the culture is placed in an incubator that maintains a specific temperature (usually around human body temperature, 37°C).

Examining blood serum or other specimens for evidence of antibody to specific infectious organisms pertains to the field of immunology or serology. A number of highly precise techniques are currently available to find and measure antibodies to a large number of pathogenic organisms. Space does not permit elaborate discussion of this complex subject.

TREATMENT OF INFECTIOUS DISEASE

Physicians use numerous medicines to control or mitigate symptoms of infectious disease such as fever, pain, inflammation, cough, respiratory congestion, intestinal spasm or irritability, itching, and so forth. But for many infectious diseases, modern medicine has antimicrobial agents: specific drugs intended to destroy or inactivate pathogenic microorganisms in or on the body.

All antimicrobial agents are poisons. The basic principle underlying their use is selective toxicity: the drug must be able to combat the infecting organism without harming the host. Some antimicrobial agents, such as alcohol, hexachlorophene, and povidone-iodine, are effective against a wide variety of pathogens but are used only on skin or mucous membranes (for example, as a preoperative scrub) because they are too toxic to the host for systemic use. These are called disinfectants.

Most of the antimicrobial drugs in current use are effective against a narrower range of organisms but have low enough toxicity for the host that they can be administered systemically (by mouth or by injection). These are the antibiotics, the sulfonamides, and certain chemotherapeutic agents.

All natural antibiotics are produced by molds and are toxic to certain classes of microorganisms, sometimes including other molds. Modern technology can greatly amplify the yield of antibiotic from a culture of mold, and chemical alteration of the antibiotic molecule can produce a drug that is less toxic to the host than the parent molecule, more potent and specific in attacking pathogens, or both.

Sulfonamides (see box) are chemicals produced in the laboratory that work much like certain antibiotics. Some drugs used to treat malaria and other parasitic diseases are also laboratory products. Along

During the years immediately following the discovery of penicillin by Alexander Fleming in 1928, researchers around the world were testing thousands of substances, natural and synthetic, for activity against pathogenic microorganisms.

In 1932 Gerhard Domagk (1895-1964), a physician and biochemist at one of Bayer's chemical plants in Germany, found that a red dye for leather, marketed as Prontosil, had such activity.

Domagk conducted exacting experiments in mice and showed that Prontosil and its derivatives were both effective and safe in controlling infections, including those due to streptococci (discussed elsewhere in this chapter).

The usefulness of the new drug in human patients was put to a dramatic test when Domagk's own daughter Hildegarde injured her finger on a knitting needle and developed severe septicemia. She was dying when Domagk injected her with Prontosil. The experiment was brilliantly successful. The child recovered rapidly and completely.

Further research on Prontosil showed that in the body it split into two compounds, and that one of these, sulfanilamide, was responsible for its antimicrobial activity. This was the beginning of the sulfonamide era, which continues to this day.

Numerous other sulfa compounds with greater effectiveness and fewer side-effects have been synthesized. Drugs in this class are widely used nowadays in the treatment of respiratory and urinary tract infections and other conditions. However, the sulfonamides are no longer considered appropriate treatment for streptococcal infections.

Gerhard Domagk received the Nobel Prize for Medicine or Physiology in 1939, but was forbidden by Adolf Hitler to accept it.

with the sulfonamides, these are sometimes called chemotherapeutic agents in contradistinction to antibiotics, all of which originally came from molds. (Some antibiotics, such as chloramphenicol, were originally natural mold products but are now synthesized "from scratch" in the laboratory.)

Antibiotics and chemotherapeutic agents destroy pathogens or inhibit their growth by various mechanisms: by preventing them from forming cell walls (penicillins, cephalosporins), by affecting cell wall permeability (amphotericin B, polymyxin B), by inhibiting protein synthesis (erythromycin, tetracycline), or by inhibiting nucleic acid synthesis (sulfonamides, nalidixic acid). No antibiotic is effective against all pathogens. Virtually no antibiotic or sulfonamide is effective against any virus.

The range of organisms against which an antibiotic can be used is called its spectrum. The sensitivity of infecting organisms to antibiotics can be tested in the laboratory by applying small paper disks impregnated with various antibiotics to the surface of a culture medium inoculated with the organism in question, and observing which ones inhibit bacterial growth.

The dose, route of administration, and duration of treatment with an antibiotic depend on many considerations: the identity of the pathogen, the severity of the infection, the patient's general condition, other drugs the patient is already receiving, the antimicrobial spectrum of the drug, its physical and biochemical properties, its expected side effects, and even its cost. Some antibiotics are not adequately absorbed from the digestive system and so must be given by injection.

Prophylactic administration of antibiotics refers to their use in preventing rather than in treating infection. Antibiotic prophylaxis is generally considered inappropriate except in a limited number of circumstances: before or after certain types of surgery (particularly if the patient has a chronic condition such as valvular heart disease) and in certain disorders in which recurring infection is likely (emphysema, chronic bronchitis, certain urinary tract problems).

Two factors limit the usefulness of antibiotics in combating human infections: drug resistance and side effects. Many pathogens resist the toxic effects of some or all antimicrobial agents simply because of their innate biochemical makeup. But most cases of drug resistance in pathogens are due to genetic mutation. That is, one or more organisms undergo a change in their genetic composition that confers on them and their offspring the ability to escape the toxic effects of certain antimicrobials.

If microorganisms that are resistant to a certain antibiotic emerge in a patient who is taking that antibiotic, then the organisms that have not undergone mutation will die, while those that have developed resistance will quickly multiply and form a whole colony of resistant organisms. From then on, the antibiotic in question will be of no use in treating that patient's infection. Drugs chemically related to the first antibiotic may also prove ineffective, by a phenomenon called cross-resistance. Moreover, if resistant organisms are transmitted to other persons and cause infection, antibiotics to which they are resistant will be ineffective in treating those persons.

Adverse effects of antimicrobial drugs on the host are of various types. They may cause chemical toxicity, as when streptomycin and related drugs damage the eighth pair of cranial nerves, with resulting impairment of hearing or loss of balance sense. Peak and trough (maximum and minimum) blood levels of certain antibiotics may be monitored by laboratory testing to ensure that the dose is adequate (high enough to control the infection) but not excessive (that is, not likely to cause serious adverse effects).

Many adverse effects of antibiotics and sulfonamides are due to allergy, an acquired hypersensitivity to a drug, leading to rash, respiratory distress, or other problems, some of which can be fatal, when that drug is administered. Finally, an antimicrobial agent may so alter the patient's normal microbial flora (population of nonpathogenic microorganisms) that organisms not affected by the drug overgrow and produce symptoms. For example, antibiotic treatment often suppresses normal intestinal or vaginal germ populations so that virulent and toxigenic strains of resistant bacteria, or *Candida* and other yeasts, can become the predominant organisms present and produce disease.

As mentioned earlier, antibiotics and sulfonamides are ineffective against viruses. Physicians have a limited but growing arsenal of antiviral agents, most of them chemical substances synthesized in the laboratory:

acyclovir, used in chickenpox and herpes simplex
amantadine, rimantadine, and zanamivir, in influenza
famciclovir and valacyclovir, in zoster

foscarnet and ganciclovir, in cytomegalovirus retinitis
idoxuridine, in herpetic infections of the cornea
didanosine, indinavir, zalcitobine, and zidovudine, in AIDS

Interferons are natural substances, induced in human beings by viral and other types of infection, that boost and regulate host defense. Synthetic interferons are now used in various viral infections, including hepatitis B and C and genital warts.

Antibodies, usually in the form of immune globulin (the globulin fraction derived from the pooled serum of many persons who have already had the infection and have formed antibody against it), may be administered to some persons after exposure to certain diseases (hepatitis A, hepatitis B, rabies) to prevent or modify infection. Antitoxins are antibodies directed against toxins rather than against the organisms that produce them. They are useful in modifying certain uncommon diseases, such as botulism and diphtheria.

EXAMPLES OF SOME INFECTIOUS DISEASES

The chapter concludes with discussions of selected examples of infectious diseases. Many infectious diseases are discussed in following chapters.

Infectious Mononucleosis (IM)
A contagious viral infection involving primarily the lymphatic system (spleen, lymph nodes, and liver).

Cause: The Epstein-Barr virus (EBV), a member of the herpesvirus family. The virus is transmitted from person to person chiefly in saliva, hence most often through kissing or sharing of food, or of eating or drinking utensils.

History: After an incubation period of about 6 weeks, fever, headache, sore throat (often severe), glandular swelling, malaise, and a sense of fatigue. Less often, rash, jaundice, palpitation, chest or abdominal pain.

Physical Examination: Fever; inflammation of the pharynx with redness, swelling, and exudate; swelling of lymph glands, particularly on the back of the neck, but sometimes also in the groins and axillae (armpits); enlargement and tenderness of the spleen and, less often, the liver; occasionally jaundice (due to liver involvement), rash, or both; sometimes rapid or irregular pulse (due to cardiac involvement).

Diagnostic Tests: The lymphocyte count is elevated, with many atypical lymphocytes (also called reactive lymphocytes or virocytes). A few patients develop transitory hemolytic anemia. Liver function tests show slight or marked elevation of bilirubin and of hepatic enzymes, particularly alkaline phosphatase. Heterophile antibodies (nonspecific and nonprotective against further attacks of illness) appear in the blood by the second week of illness. More specific antibodies directed against components of EBV (viral capsid antigen, viral nuclear antigen) appear eventually, some persisting throughout life and conferring immunity to further attack. Chest x-ray may show enlargement of hilar lymph nodes. The electrocardiogram may demonstrate abnormalities if there is involvement of heart muscle (myocarditis) or of the conduction system of the heart.

Course: Despite the severity of symptoms in the acute phase, most cases resolve completely in 2-3 weeks. Complications such as severe hemolytic anemia, airway obstruction, rupture of the spleen, and severe liver involvement occur rarely.

Treatment: Largely supportive: symptomatic medicines for relief of pain and fever; rest, fluids, and diet as tolerated during the acute phase (7-10 days). With severe swelling of the neck and throat and high fever, nonsteroidal anti-inflammatory drugs are often supplemented with corticosteroids.

Lyme Disease (Lyme Borreliosis)

An acute and chronic infectious disease affecting successively the skin, the nervous system, and the joints.

Cause: *Borrelia burgdorferi*, a spirochete, which is transmitted by ticks of the genus *Ixodes*. Nymphs and larvae of the tick vector feed on the white-footed mouse, adults on the white-tailed deer. Infected ticks in any of these stages of development can transmit spirochetes to human beings, but usually only after feeding on the human host for at least 24 hours.

History: During the initial stage (starting about one week after infection), most patients develop either a characteristic expanding rash called erythema chronicum migrans, or a flu-like illness with fever and muscle aches, or both. In some infected persons, this stage passes without any symptoms. In the second stage, days or weeks after infection, spread of spirochetes to certain organs and tissues causes a highly variable clinical picture. Fever,

headache, muscle and joint pains, secondary skin lesions not related to tick bites, irregular heartbeat, and involvement of the central and peripheral nervous systems (encephalitis, Bell palsy) all may occur during this stage. The third stage, which occurs months or years after infection, causes painful chronic inflammation in joints, tendons, and muscles.

Physical Examination: Expanding red or purple rash at site of tick bite, often with a bull's-eye appearance. Fever, other nonspecific rashes, evidence of muscle weakness or abnormal reflexes, cardiac irregularities. Signs of local inflammation in joints.

Diagnostic Tests: Blood cell studies are nonspecific. The electrocardiogram or electromyogram may detect abnormalities in conduction. Antibody to the causative spirochete appears early in the disease, but currently available methods of detecting it often fail to meet acceptable standards of sensitivity, specificity, or reproducibility. Hence the diagnosis should be based on clinical findings, not laboratory studies.

Course: This has already been described under History. Some patients, particularly those in whom diagnosis and appropriate treatment are delayed, have residual musculoskeletal, neurologic, or mental impairment.

Treatment: Tetracyclines, azithromycin, ampicillin, and other antibiotics generally produce a cure within 2-3 weeks if administered during the first stage. Chronic symptoms may be less amenable to antibiotic therapy. A variety of treatments may be prescribed for symptoms, including physical therapy.

Streptococcal Disease

A group of infections caused by bacteria of the genus *Streptococcus*.

Streptococci are gram-positive bacteria with a broad range of potential effects on human hosts. Many species are highly virulent and aggressive. Streptococci are involved in infections of the skin (impetigo, cellulitis, erysipelas), the respiratory tract (streptococcal pharyngitis or "strep" throat, pneumococcal pneumonia), the ears and sinuses, heart valves (endocarditis), joints (infectious arthritis), and many other tissues. Particularly invasive strains of streptococci can spread from skin to underlying fascia and muscle, causing rapid destruction of tissue (necrotizing fasciitis) with systemic effects (toxic shock).

Group A beta-hemolytic streptococci (GABHS) are both widespread and highly virulent. One strain produces a toxin that induces a generalized red rash (scarlet fever). Pharyngeal or other infections with

GABHS, unless adequately treated, can stimulate the host's immune system to produce antibodies that attack the heart and the joints (acute rheumatic fever, discussed in Chapter 4) or the kidney (acute glomerulonephritis, discussed in Chapter 12).

The diagnosis of streptococcal infection is based on clinical findings and laboratory studies, particularly identification of the organism by smear, culture, or antibody tests. The strep screen, a rapid slide test for streptococci in pharyngeal secretions, permits prompt and reliable identification of streptococcal pharyngitis, a highly prevalent disease, particularly in children.

Several antibiotics are effective in controlling streptococcal infections, but not all of these are approved for prevention of rheumatic fever. Penicillin (intramuscularly in long-acting form, or orally), erythromycin, and some cephalosporins reliably prevent rheumatic fever. When given orally these drugs must be administered for ten days.

Varicella-Zoster

Two infections caused by the same virus, but with different manifestations: varicella and zoster.

Varicella (Chickenpox)

A febrile exanthem (that is, a skin eruption accompanied by fever) usually contracted in childhood.

Cause: The varicella-zoster virus, which can be spread from persons with chickenpox by direct contact or by respiratory droplets. It can also be acquired by direct contact with the lesions of zoster.

History: After an incubation period of about two weeks, fever for a day or two before and after the appearance of a rash consisting of small vesicles that rapidly evolve into pustules and then slough to form crusted ulcers. Three or four crops of lesions may appear over the next 3-5 days. The face, scalp, and trunk are most prominently involved; lesions may also appear in the mouth and throat. Itching can be severe, and scratching can result in secondary bacterial infection. Fever, headache, malaise, and cough are variable.

Physical Examination: Characteristic lesions involving the face and trunk more than the extremities. An early (vesicular) lesion resembles "a drop of honey on a rose petal." Crops appear on 3-5 successive days.

Diagnostic Tests: The white blood cell count may be low. A Tzanck smear of material from skin lesions shows multinucleated giant cells. Virus can be cultured from vesicle fluid, but identification of viral antigen by immunofluorescence is simpler.

Course: Fever generally disappears within one week of onset, and the skin lesions heal completely in 2-3 weeks. Secondary bacterial infection of lesions can lead to scarring or septicemia. Other possible complications are pneumonia, meningitis, and (after treatment with aspirin) Reye syndrome (a severe metabolic disorder resulting in vomiting, brain swelling, seizures, and often death). Maternal varicella during pregnancy can lead to death or deformity of the fetus.

Treatment: Largely symptomatic and supportive. Aspirin is withheld because of the risk of Reye syndrome. The antiviral drug acyclovir mitigates symptoms and shortens the period of illness. Patients are isolated from susceptible persons. Varicella is reliably prevented by a live vaccine recommended for all children at age one year and for susceptible household contacts of patients. Varicella-zoster immune globulin (VZIG) is given to exposed persons with immune deficiency.

Zoster (Herpes Zoster, Shingles)

A reactivation of varicella-zoster infection, with local involvement of nerves and skin.

Cause: After recovery from chickenpox, the varicella-zoster virus remains in the body for life, lying dormant in cells of the dorsal spinal nerve roots or in ganglia of cranial nerves. Reactivation of the virus leads to the clinical syndrome known as zoster.

History: Stinging or burning pain, almost always in the distribution of a single dorsal nerve root; usually on the trunk but occasionally on the face or in the ear. Before or after the onset of pain, a rash appears within the dermatome (skin distribution) of a single nerve root. On the trunk, this is a band 6-8 cm in width, running around half of the body from back to front (see box). Pain and rash are both in the same dermatome, but not necessarily in exactly the same places within that dermatome.

Physical Examination: Fever is generally absent. Skin lesions are highly typical, consisting of one or more clusters of vesicles, each cluster surrounded by a zone of erythema. Involvement of the geniculate ganglion of the facial (seventh cranial) nerve can lead to facial paralysis and lesions of the outer ear.

Diagnostic Tests: Diagnosis is clinically evident. Fluid from vesicles gives a positive Tzanck test (see under *Varicella*).

When the rash of **zoster** appears on the trunk of the body, it is so distinctive that the diagnosis can hardly be missed. Even many laypersons can accurately recognize it. When fully developed, the cutaneous eruption looks like a belt or sash running around half of the body.

Zoster is a Greek word for 'belt'. Another is *zone*, which in its latinized form *zona* was formerly used as a name for this condition. The lay English term *shingles* is a corruption of Latin *cingulum*, which also means 'belt, girdle'.

Course: Symptoms are more severe in persons over 40. Pain and skin lesions usually resolve within 2-6 weeks. However, one-half of patients over 60 develop postherpetic neuralgia, with chronic pain that can persist for months or years.

Treatment: Mild cases in younger persons are treated symptomatically. In severe disease, in older or immunodeficient persons, or when there is involvement of the eye or ear, antiviral agents (famciclovir, valacyclovir) shorten the duration of symptoms and reduce the risk of postherpetic neuralgia.

QUESTIONS FOR STUDY AND REVIEW

1. Name four general classes of pathogen:

   a. _____

   b. _____

   c. _____

   d. _____

2. Name four routes by which infecting organisms can be transmitted from person to person:

   a. _____

   b. _____

   c. _____

   d. _____

3. Name four classes of drugs used in infectious disease:

   a. _____

   b. _____

   c. _____

   d. _____

4. What are some nonspecific symptoms or signs that occur in many different infections? Do these always indicate the presence of infection?

   _____

   _____

   _____

   _____

   _____

   _____

5. What is the most important single piece of information that the physician needs in order to make a rational forecast of the course of most infectious diseases, and an informed choice of therapeutic agents? How can this information be obtained?

   _____

   _____

   _____

   _____

   _____

   _____

6. Name several infectious diseases that readily respond to treatment with antimicrobial agents:

_____

_____

_____

_____

7. Name several infectious diseases that do not respond at all to treatment with antimicrobial agents:

_____

_____

_____

_____

8. What factors have been responsible for the emergence of many drug-resistant strains of pathogenic micro-organisms? What can be done to combat this problem or prevent it from getting worse?

_____

_____

_____

_____

_____

_____

_____

CASE STUDY: YOU'RE THE DOCTOR

Kevin Graffner, a 22-year-old single graduate student, visits a public health clinic where you are on duty. He complains of mild urinary burning and a thin, watery urethral discharge, both of 5 days' duration. He has had no fever, chills, urinary frequency, hematuria, or abdominal or pelvic pain.

1. What type of disorder does this history most strongly suggest? (Hint: Refer to Chapter 12.)

_____

_____

_____

_____

_____

_____

Past history is significant in that Mr. Graffner has been treated twice in the past year for chlamydial urethritis, confirmed on both occasions by DNA probe examination of material obtained by urethral swab. He states that he has been in a stable, monogamous relationship with his girlfriend, to whom he refers as his fiancée, for the past 2¹/₂ years. He vigorously denies other sexual contacts and rejects the suggestion that his girlfriend may have had other contacts. On both of the prior occasions when he was treated for chlamydia, his girlfriend saw her private physician, had laboratory studies, and was told that she was free of disease and required no treatment.

2. Does this set of historical facts render the diagnosis of an STD more probable or less so? Why or why not?

_____

_____

_____

_____

_____

3. What does the abbreviation *STD* stand for?

_____

_____

Physical examination reveals no lesions of the external genitalia, inguinal lymphadenitis, or abnormalities of scrotal structures. Abdominal and rectal examinations are unremarkable. You obtain material for laboratory study and before Mr. Graffner leaves the clinic you administer azithromycin in a single oral dose of 1 g for presumed chlamydia urethritis. You give him an appointment to return to the clinic in 72 hours for laboratory results and followup.

4. What are some reasons that might justify giving medicine before laboratory test results are available?

_____

_____

_____

_____

_____

_____

_____

_____

_____

_____

_____

5. What are some objections to doing this?

_____

_____

_____

_____

_____

_____

When Mr. Graffner returns, he tells you that his symptoms have largely disappeared. His urethral swab was positive for chlamydia and negative for gonorrhea. He is virtually certain that he has been infected by his girlfriend on three occasions in the past year. Since an STD can't arise de novo between two entirely monogamous sexual partners, either Mr. Graffner or his fiancée must have had sexual contact with a third person.

6. Choose one of the following courses of action and justify your choice:

   a. Tell Mr. Graffner that either he is lying to you or his girlfriend is lying to him.

   b. Tell him that, even though his girlfriend's laboratory tests have been negative, she is apparently serving as an asymptomatic reservoir of infection, and must also be treated in order to eliminate his recurrent infections.

_____

_____

_____

_____

_____

_____

_____

_____

_____

_____

SUGGESTIONS FOR ADDITIONAL LEARNING ACTIVITIES

1. The Centers for Disease Control and Prevention (CDC) is the federal agency responsible for collecting data on infectious diseases. Visit their Web site (**http://www.cdc.gov**) or write to this agency with the assistance of your local librarian and obtain a Fact Sheet on an infectious disease that is not discussed in this chapter. Use this information to write an entry for this disease following the format used throughout this book. Include sections for Cause, History, Physical Examination, Diagnostic Tests, Course, and Treatment. As a group project, collect entries made by individual students and assemble an infectious disease reference notebook for your classroom.

2. This grade-school science experiment provides an opportunity for you to see how organisms grow. Start by washing your hands. Collect dust from your desk or any household surface on a cotton swab. Rub the dust on a lemon rid and place it in a Ziploc sandwich bag. Use an eye dropper to add 5 or 6 drops of water. Seal the bag and place it in a paper milk carton. Seal the carton with masking tape. Leave the carton at room temperature for a few days. Be sure to cover your mouth and nose so you don't inhale any mold spores when you examine your results.

3. Review the section on Transmission of Infection in this chapter. For each method of transmission listed, determine the best method of control. Give at least one example of an infectious disease that is transmitted by each of these methods.

The Immune System

LEARNING OBJECTIVES

Upon completion of this chapter, you should be able to

- describe the basic structure and function of the immune system;

- define immunodeficiency;

- discuss the nature and various manifestations of allergy;

- describe the features of autoimmune diseases.

THE IMMUNE SYSTEM

After a brief survey of normal immunity, this chapter discusses immunodeficiency (especially AIDS), allergy, and autoimmune disorders. If you encounter unfamiliar terms, look them up in the Glossary or the Index.

DESCRIPTION OF THE IMMUNE SYSTEM

Immunity was briefly described in the previous chapter. Here a more elaborate discussion is in order.

Immunity refers to a set of protective responses in the living body by which infections and other threats from outside can be repelled or inactivated. Human immunity has three cardinal features: it is stimulus-activated, directed against a specific target, and persisting. Immunity is a response: it does not come into play until some assault has been launched on the integrity of the body from without. Moreover, the response is specific: the immune system not only recognizes invading microorganisms as being foreign to self, but reacts to them in ways that are closely linked to their biochemical structure. Finally, the immune system has a memory: it retains the ability to recognize and repel previous invaders long after the first assault is over.

The immune system consists of the spleen, lymph nodes, and smaller aggregations of lymphoid tissue throughout the body; lymphocytes, which are white blood cells formed in lymphoid tissue; and other white blood cells formed in bone marrow. Lymphocytes are of two basic types: B lymphocytes, which (after being converted into plasma cells) produce antibodies; and T lymphocytes, which have a variety of subtypes with various functions.

The most important protective responses of the immune system are classified as either humoral or cell-mediated. Humoral immunity depends on the formation of antibodies by B lymphocytes. (Subtypes of T lymphocytes, called helper T cells and suppressor T cells, help to regulate antibody formation.) An antibody is a complex protein that reacts with a specific foreign material or organism by meshing chemically with it. Any substance that elicits the formation of an antibody is called an antigen.

Antibodies are part of the globulin fraction of plasma. The immune globulins are subdivided on the basis of chemical structure and immune function

into five classes. IgG, the largest group, includes antibodies and antitoxins that are important in providing lasting protection against infection. IgA antibodies protect surfaces and membranes. IgM antibodies are formed early in the immune response and often fade soon after recovery from infection. IgD is chemically bound to lymphocytes and serves as their link or attachment to antigens. IgE is concerned in allergic and hypersensitivity reactions and in protection against parasites.

The chemical structures of various immunoglobulins are shown in Figure 2. Each IgG molecule consists of two identical heavy chains (long strings of amino acids) and two identical light chains (shorter strings of amino acids). The N terminus of each chain (the end of the chain with a free amino group) is called the antigen-binding fragment (Fab) because it is responsible for recognizing and locking onto the target. The C terminus, at the other end of the chain, contains the constant fragment (Fc), which carries out the chemical mission of neutralization or destruction.

Cell-mediated immunity depends on a direct attack by cytotoxic or killer T lymphocytes on foreign cells. Killer T lymphocytes recognize these cells as foreign and react specifically to them, but without the involvement of antibodies. Other white blood cells (neutrophils, eosinophils, basophils, monocytes) and certain tissue cells (macrophages, mast cells) serve specialized functions. These cells function either by phagocytizing (engulfing and destroying) foreign cells and materials or by releasing into the blood or the tissues chemical mediators (histamine, prostaglandins, leukotrienes, cytokines) that trigger or modulate various features of the immune response.

Not all infections lead to the formation of protective antibodies. A mild infection may elicit only feeble or transitory immune response, so that some time after recovery the subject becomes vulnerable to the same pathogens. Other infections (the common cold, staphylococcal infections) generate no protective immunity at all.

A vaccine is a material administered to stimulate immunity (see box on p. 46). A live vaccine contains living pathogenic organisms that have been attenuated (weakened, chemically or otherwise, so as to be unable to cause disease). A killed vaccine contains only nonliving pathogens, and sometimes only part of their protein structure. Some vaccines currently in

Figure 2 Structures of Immunoglobulins

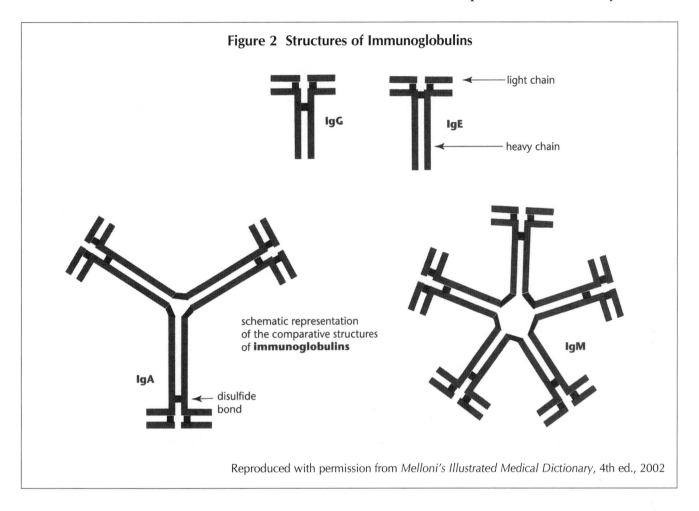

light chain

heavy chain

schematic representation
of the comparative structures
of **immunoglobulins**

IgG

IgE

IgA

disulfide
bond

IgM

use are chemical fabrications, made by recombinant DNA technology. They duplicate part of the protein structure of a pathogen, but are not derived from pathogens and are therefore incapable of inducing infection. A toxoid is a preparation of a weakened toxin (for example, the paralytic toxin produced by tetanus organisms) that causes the immune system to form antibody to the toxin (antitoxin) rather than to the pathogen. Use of these materials is called active immunization, since they all elicit an active response from the host's immune system.

In contrast, passive immunization is the administration of antibodies, including antitoxins, that have been formed by an immune system other than that of the recipient—that is, by human subjects or animals (rabbits, horses, sheep). Passive immunization is used when the patient's immune system is impaired, when protection against a specific infection is needed immediately and cannot wait for the formation of antibody after active immunization, or when no active vaccine is available.

It is currently recommended that all children receive active immunization against 10 diseases (diphtheria, hepatitis B, measles, mumps, poliomyelitis, *Haemophilus influenzae* type b infection, pertussis (whooping cough), rubella, tetanus, and varicella-zoster) by the age of 15 months, with booster doses for some of these at prescribed intervals throughout life.

IMMUNODEFICIENCY

Immunodeficiency is a general term for impairment of any part or function of the immune system that leaves the body vulnerable to infectious diseases. Persons with immunodeficiency are more susceptible than normal persons to certain bacterial, viral, and fungal infections. In addition, they may be subject to opportunistic infections (infections due to pathogens to which persons with intact immune systems are virtually invulnerable).

The term **vaccine** comes to us from *vaccinia*, the Latin name for cowpox. Late in the 18th century, the English physician Edward Jenner (1749-1823) made experiments to test the folk belief that infection with cowpox (a skin eruption of cattle sometimes contracted by herdsmen and milkmaids) could confer protection against smallpox.

At that time smallpox was one of the most dreaded diseases in the world. Caused (as we now know) by a virus, it had a mortality rate as high as 30% and usually left survivors marked with pits or scars for life. Down through history, epidemics of smallpox wiped out entire royal families, entire armies, and entire nations.

Inoculation of healthy persons with material from smallpox lesions had been imported into England from Turkey several decades before Jenner made his experiments. Although inoculation did elicit immunity, it might also bring on a disfiguring or fatal case of the disease.

Jenner's experiments were brilliantly successful. In 1806, the American President Thomas Jefferson wrote to Jenner, "You have erased from the calendar of human afflictions one of its greatest . . . Future nations will know by history only that the loathsome smallpox existed."

But resistance to "vaccination" (for which no scientific rationale then existed) was violent among both the medical profession and the lay public. Not until 1979 did an official declaration that smallpox is extinct fulfill Jefferson's prophecy of 173 years earlier.

Immune deficiencies are divided into two large classes: congenital and acquired. Congenital disorders of immunity are due to inherited defects in some component of the immune system. The following are some of the more common congenital immunodeficiency syndromes.

Agammaglobulinemia: Inability to form antibodies, due to inherited B lymphocyte dysfunction. Serum levels of immunoglobulin are low, and patients are subject to recurrent bacterial infections, including abscesses and purulent infections of the ears, sinuses, and lower respiratory tract.

Chédiak-Higashi disease: Reduction in the number of circulating neutrophils, with impairment of their ability to destroy bacteria due to enzyme deficiencies and failure to respond to chemical signals. Children with this disorder also have congenital abnormalities of the skin and central nervous system.

DiGeorge syndrome (thymic hypoplasia): Inherited T lymphocyte dysfunction, leading to susceptibility to local or systemic infection with fungi, viruses, mycobacteria, and protozoan parasites.

Job syndrome: A disorder of neutrophil function, with eosinophilia and increased IgE antibodies. Children with this disorder are vulnerable to recurrent staphylococcal infections of the skin and respiratory tract.

Severe combined immunodeficiency disease (SCID): Failure of both B and T lymphocyte function, with heightened risk of certain infections (bacterial diarrhea, *Pneumocystis carinii* pneumonia). Even a seemingly trivial infection can prove lethal, and few patients survive beyond childhood.

Wiskott-Aldrich syndrome: Combined B and T lymphocyte dysfunction complicated by thrombocytopenia and eczema.

Treatment of these disorders is limited to supportive care, avoidance of exposure to infectious organisms (sometimes by lifelong isolation), and vigorous treatment of infections when they occur.

Acquired immunodeficiency can result from malignancies affecting the immune system, radiation therapy, prolonged administration of corticosteroids, and deliberate suppression of immune function with cytotoxic drugs and antimetabolites in the treatment of autoimmune disorders and malignant tumors. The best-known and most significant form of acquired immunodeficiency is that caused by the human immunodeficiency virus (HIV) and known as AIDS (acquired immunodeficiency syndrome).

The following discussion begins with general remarks on history, physical findings, results of diagnostic tests, and treatment, and concludes with more detailed information about several of the more common opportunistic infections that occur in AIDS.

Acquired Immunodeficiency Syndrome (AIDS)

A lethal impairment of T lymphocyte function caused by a virus.

Cause: The human immunodeficiency virus (HIV), which is transmitted almost exclusively by sexual contact or by sharing of needles among intravenous drug abusers. After a latent period of 10-12 years, the virus causes wholesale destruction of helper T cells, with resultant loss of immunity to many opportunistic pathogens.

History: Primary HIV infection sometimes causes a self-limited flu-like illness and later, dementia. Any of a number of opportunistic infections may induce symptoms of weakness, weight loss, diarrhea, pneumonia, or cutaneous lesions.

Physical Examination: Fever, weight loss, and muscle wasting may occur in primary disease. Other findings depend on the presence of opportunistic infections.

Diagnostic Tests: The serum contains antibody to HIV. The absolute lymphocyte count is low, and in particular the CD4+ (T4, helper T) lymphocyte count is below 800/µL. Measurement of viral load by plasma HIV RNA assay provides quantitative information on viral replication. Other findings (anemia, abnormal chest x-ray, organisms in sputum or stool) depend on specific infections contracted.

Course: Without treatment, recurrent and increasingly severe infections lead to death within three years after diagnosis in most patients. With highly active antiretroviral therapy (HAART), lethal complications can be postponed indefinitely. However, such treatment is expensive, requires close adherence to complicated drug regiments, and has objectionable side-effects including elevation of serum cholesterol. In addition, viral resistance even to combinations of three or more drugs is an increasing problem.

Treatment: Combination regimens including nucleoside analogues (didanosine, lamivudine, ribavirin, stavudine, zidovudine), non-nucleoside reverse transcriptase inhibitors, (delavirine, efavirenz, nevirapine) and protease inhibitors (crixivan, indinavir, ritonavir, saquinavir). Prophylaxis against opportunistic infection (pentamidine, atovaquone, trimethoprim-sulfamethoxazole against *Pneumocystis carinii* pneumonia).

Opportunistic Infections in AIDS

Bacillary angiomatosis: Formation of vascular tumors in the skin, bone, liver, and other tissues, due to infection with species of *Rochalimaea*, which are rickettsias. Erythromycin, doxycycline, and other antibiotics provide a measure of control.

Candidosis: A superficial fungal infection due to *Candida albicans* and related species. This is a common pathogen in the general population, where it causes oropharyngeal lesions (thrush) and cutaneous and vaginal candidosis. In persons with AIDS, Candida often extends into the esophagus and the intestine. Superficial infections are treated with clotrimazole, miconazole, nystatin, and other topical antifungals. Amphotericin B and ketoconazole are used in systemic infection.

Cytomegalovirus (CMV) infection (cytomegalic inclusion disease): A common mild or subclinical infection in the general population. In AIDS, the virus causes disease of the respiratory system (pneumonia), gastrointestinal tract (ulcerative enterocolitis with bloody diarrhea), the eye (retinitis leading to blindness), and the nervous system (ascending polyradiculopathy). Treatment with ganciclovir or foscarnet slows progression of disease, particularly retinitis.

Herpes simplex: The familiar cold-sore and genital herpes are both caused by herpes simplex viruses. In AIDS, herpes simplex can present as an extensive and chronic ulceration of skin or mucous membrane (mouth or esophagus), bronchitis or pneumonia, or as systemic infection. Acyclovir and foscarnet provide some antiviral effect.

Histoplasmosis: Infection with *Histoplasma capsulatum*, a fungus that causes mild or subclinical respiratory infection in persons with intact immunity. In AIDS it is sometimes associated with severe pulmonary disease and respiratory failure. It may also become disseminated throughout the body. Treatment is with amphotericin B and itraconazole.

Kaposi sarcoma (KS): A malignant tumor caused by infection with human herpesvirus-8. Tumors appear as pink or purple plaques or nodules and consist of tangles of cutaneous or mucosal blood vessels. Kaposi sarcoma occurs in about one-third of all AIDS patients. The tumors may spread to the respiratory and digestive system and the abdominal viscera. Some control may be provided by treatment with interferon alfa.

Oral hairy leukoplakia: A shaggy whitish plaque of abnormal oral mucosa, induced by infection with the Epstein-Barr virus (also the cause of infectious mononucleosis) in AIDS. Antiviral drugs may suppress the lesion satisfactorily, but in about 5% of cases it progresses to oral cancer.

***Pneumocystis carinii* pneumonia (plasma cell pneumonia, PCP)**: An infection of the lungs due to a protozoan parasite, which eventually affects about three-fourths of all AIDS patients and is the cause of death in many. Symptoms include fever, cough, and progressive respiratory failure. There may be no specific findings on physical examination or x-ray. Silver stains demonstrate the causative organism in smears of respiratory secretions or bronchoalveolar washings. Treatment is with adrenocortical steroids, atovaquone, pentamidine, primaquine, and trimethoprim-sulfamethoxazole.

Toxoplasmosis: Infection with the intracellular parasite *Toxoplasma gondii*, which causes encephalitis (manifested as headaches, seizures, and personality change), pneumonitis, myocarditis, and disseminated infection. Treatment is with clindamycin, pyrimethamine, sulfadiazine, and other agents.

Tuberculosis: Pulmonary infection due to *Mycobacterium tuberculosis* and, more commonly, intestinal or disseminated infection due to *M. avium*, *M. intracellulare*, or other members of the *M. avium* complex (MAC). Multidrug regimens including isoniazid, rifampin, ethambutol, and other antibiotics or chemotherapeutic agents are commonly required to control tuberculosis in AIDS.

Varicella-zoster infection: The virus that causes chickenpox (varicella) and herpes zoster can produce a severe and protracted form of zoster in persons with AIDS. Treatment is with acyclovir, famciclovir, foscarnet, or valacyclovir.

ALLERGY AND DELAYED HYPERSENSITIVITY

An immunologically mediated sensitivity to a foreign antigen (allergen), with resultant tissue inflammation and organ dysfunction.

Allergy includes a broad variety of local and systemic reactions to foreign materials, which may be inhaled (dusts, pollens, molds), ingested (foods, medicines), injected (medicines, insect venoms), or brought into contact with skin (household or industrial chemicals, plant toxins). In all true allergy, prior exposure and sensitization must have occurred before the allergen can elicit a reaction. Two basic types are distinguished.

In IgE-mediated (immediate) hypersensitivity reactions, release of histamine and other substances from mast cells leads to local or systemic symptoms within minutes after exposure. Examples are allergic rhinitis (hay fever, nasal allergies to cats), atopic dermatitis (intensely itchy rashes), urticaria (hives), anaphylaxis (a life-threatening syndrome of urticaria, swelling of respiratory mucosa, and shock), and serum sickness (fever, urticaria, joint pains, swollen lymph nodes).

In T-cell-mediated (delayed) hypersensitivity, a latent period of 48-72 hours elapses between exposure and onset of symptoms. Examples are allergic contact dermatitis (poison ivy rash) and hypersensitivity pneumonitis.

History: Depending on the inciting cause and target organ, the range of symptoms includes watery rhinorrhea, sneezing, wheezing and cough, itching and rash, intestinal cramping and diarrhea, joint pain and swelling, dyspnea, hypotension and collapse.

Physical Examination: May show tachycardia, hypotension, edema, erythema, wheals, copious nasal secretion, nasal polyps, bronchial wheezing, fever, or other local or systemic signs of allergy.

Diagnostic Tests: The eosinophil count may be elevated, and eosinophils may be seen in smears of nasal scrapings or nasal or bronchial secretions. Provocative skin testing or challenge with certain foods may confirm specific causal agents. Radioallergosorbent testing (RAST) can identify specific antibody in serum.

Treatment: Avoidance of known causes is paramount in preventing allergic disorders. Antihistaminic drugs are used to control local and generalized symptoms due to histamine release. Cromolyn and related drugs stabilize mast cells and exert a protective effect if administered before exposure. Sympathomimetic drugs (epinephrine, albuterol) can block some of the local or general effects of histamine and other mediators of allergic symptoms. Adrenocortical steroids are used topically (as nasal spray) in allergic rhinitis and systemically in severe allergy. Immunotherapy consisting of periodic injection of known allergens in increasing doses provides an apparent desensitization in some patients.

AUTOIMMUNITY

Autoimmunity results when the body's immune system forms antibodies against some component of itself. Autoimmune disorders are common and exceedingly diverse. The formation of antibodies against self can come about through various mechanisms: failure of suppressor T cells to regulate the immune process; failure of the immune system to recognize some component of the body as self; formation of antibody to an infecting organism that happens to have a similar protein composition to some body tissue, which is then attacked by the antibody; and disorders of lymphocytes causing them to form abnormal antibodies that happen to attack body tissues.

Susceptibility to autoimmune disease runs in families, and persons who have one autoimmune disorder tend to have others. The so-called collagen or connective-tissue diseases (rheumatoid arthritis, lupus erythematosus, and others) are all caused by autoimmune phenomena.

The following survey of autoimmune diseases is by no means exhaustive. Discussions of several autoimmune disorders (insulin-dependent diabetes mellitus, Graves disease, Hashimoto disease, pernicious anemia, chronic hepatitis B) appear in other chapters of this book.

Rheumatoid Arthritis

A chronic systemic disease causing inflammatory changes in many tissues, particularly joint membranes.

Cause: Formation of antibody to one's own tissues, particularly synovial membranes. About 1-2% of the population are affected, and the disease is three times more common in women. It tends to run in families. Onset is typically between 20 and 40, and may be triggered by emotional or physical stress, surgery, or childbirth.

History: Gradual onset of pain, stiffness, and warmth in joints, particularly smaller joints (proximal interphalangeal and metacarpophalangeal joints, wrists, knees, ankles, and toes). Stiffness is worse in the morning ("gelling"). Malaise, fever, and weight loss may accompany the onset of the disease.

Physical Examination: Tenderness, warmth, stiffness of affected joints. Enlargement and deformity of joints, including ulnar deviation of finger joints, may occur late. About 20% of patients have subcutaneous nodules over bony prominences on extremities.

Diagnostic Tests: The erythrocyte sedimentation rate is elevated. A mild anemia is common, and platelets may be increased. Testing for rheumatoid arthritis (RA) factor is positive in about 75% of patients, and for antinuclear antibody in about 20%. Serum protein studies may detect an increase in immune globulin. X-rays are normal early in the disease but eventually show osteoporosis of bone near affected joints, erosion of joint surfaces, and narrowing of joint spaces.

Course: In as many as one-half of all patients, symptoms remit largely or completely within two years. Patients in whom symptoms continue may have intermittent or persistent pain and stiffness,

with increasing deformity and fusion of affected joints. Extra-articular manifestations include pericarditis, pleurisy with effusion, lymphadenopathy, splenomegaly, vasculitis, dry mouth and eyes (Sjögren syndrome, discussed below) and peripheral nerve entrapment problems such as carpal tunnel syndrome (see Chapter 19).

Treatment: The standard treatment is aspirin (ASA), but other nonsteroidal anti-inflammatory drugs (NSAIDs) may also be used, including COX-2 inhibitors (celecoxib, rofecoxib). In refractory cases other drugs may prove useful, including immunosuppressants (azathioprine, cyclosporine, methotrexate), antimalarials, gold salts, and adrenal corticosteroids. All of these drugs have problematic side effects or toxicities. Physical therapy is important in maintaining mobility. Surgery may be needed to correct severe deformity.

Polymyalgia Rheumatica

A syndrome of chronic muscle pain and stiffness, fatigue, weight loss, and fever.

Cause: An autoimmune cause is presumed. The disease occurs primarily in persons of white race over 50, and women are affected twice as often as men.

History: Pain and stiffness in the neck, shoulders, and hips, worse in the morning or after prolonged sitting. Headache, fatigue, weakness, anorexia, weight loss, mild fever.

Physical Examination: Fever, tenderness of affected muscles.

Diagnostic Tests: The erythrocyte sedimentation rate is usually elevated. Anemia is usually present. Liver function tests, particularly alkaline phosphatase, may be abnormal.

Course: The disease tends to burn itself out after 3-5 years. A serious complication is temporal arteritis, a related autoimmune disorder affecting the temporal artery and adjacent cranial vasculature. Temporal arteritis causes headache with scalp tenderness, jaw pain, and visual symptoms, and can lead to blindness.

Treatment: Adrenocortical steroid corrects symptoms of polymyalgia rheumatica and temporal arteritis promptly, but treatment must be continued for a long period. Alendronate may also be prescribed to protect the patient from osteoporosis induced by long-term corticoid use.

Lupus Erythematosus (LE)

A chronic inflammatory disorder of connective tissue due to formation of antibody to nucleoprotein.

Cause: Unknown. Ninety percent of patients are young women. Antinuclear antibody and anti-DNA antibody are found in the serum.

History: Gradual or abrupt onset of widely varying symptoms: joint pain, butterfly rash over the cheeks, discoid lesions and other skin changes (purpura, alopecia), fever, chest pain, mood changes and other psychiatric symptoms.

Physical Examination: Fever, signs of swelling and inflammation in joints, malar "butterfly" eruption, lymphadenopathy, splenomegaly, pericardial or pleural friction rub heard on auscultation.

Diagnostic Tests: The erythrocyte sedimentation rate is elevated, white blood cells (particularly lymphocytes) and platelets are decreased. Tests based on detection of abnormal antibodies (LE-cell preparation, antinuclear antibody, anti-DNA antibody) are often positive. Serologic test for syphilis may be falsely positive. Urinalysis may show proteinuria, red blood cells, and casts.

Course: The disease is chronic and relapsing, with spontaneous remissions and exacerbations. With treatment the 10-year survival rate is about 95%. Most patients eventually develop kidney disease (lupus nephritis), and death is usually due to renal failure.

Treatment: Nonsteroidal anti-inflammatory drugs (NSAIDs) and general supportive measures may suffice to control symptoms. Antimalarial drugs (hydroxychloroquine and others), adrenal corticosteroids, and immunosuppressive drugs (azathioprine, cyclophosphamide) are useful in more severe cases.

Discoid Lupus

A variant of systemic lupus erythematosus in which abnormalities are confined to the skin.

The disease occurs almost exclusively in young women. Round erythematous papules with plugging of oil gland ducts occur on the cheeks, nose, ears, and other cutaneous surfaces, particularly those exposed to sunlight. Involvement of mucous membranes and of the scalp (sometimes leading to alopecia) may also occur. About 10% of patients with these symptoms are found on evaluation to have systemic lupus erythematosus; in the rest, disease is limited to the skin eruption. Treatment is avoidance of sunlight, use of sunscreens, and, when necessary, topical steroids and oral antimalarials.

Sjögren Syndrome (Keratoconjunctivitis Sicca)

An autoimmune disorder of certain exocrine glands, causing dryness of the mouth and eyes.

Nearly all patients are middle-aged women. Dysfunction of lacrimal glands causes dryness and burning of the eyes. Abnormality of salivary glands leads to swelling of the glands (particularly the parotids), dry mouth, dysphagia, and dental caries. Other gland tissue impairment may affect the skin, the pancreas, the lower respiratory tract, and the vagina. The disorder frequently occurs in association with other autoimmune diseases (rheumatoid arthritis, systemic lupus erythematosus, Hashimoto disease). Many patients eventually develop renal disease or lymphoma. Treatment is supportive, with artificial tears, strict oral hygiene, and attention to diagnosis and treatment of associated disorders.

Acute Rheumatic Fever

An autoimmune disorder affecting the heart, the joints, and the skin.

Cause: Antibody formed to group A beta-hemolytic streptococci (during streptococcal pharyngitis) attacks certain tissues of the patient's body. Rheumatic fever follows streptococcal infection after an interval of 2-4 weeks. It occurs almost exclusively in children and adolescents. The incidence is higher during cold, damp weather and in children from lower socioeconomic levels. Susceptibility to acute rheumatic fever seems to run in families.

History: Fever, joint pain, rash, nontender subcutaneous nodules, weakness, shortness of breath, chest pain, rapid pulse, cough, chorea (see box).

Physical Examination: Fever, tachycardia, a macular rash called erythema marginatum, swelling and tenderness in certain joints, irritability, muscle twitching, heart murmurs indicative of mitral or aortic valve disease or both, evidence of congestive heart failure. (Valvular disease and congestive failure are fully discussed in Chapter 8.)

Diagnostic Tests: Neutrophilia, mild anemia, elevated erythrocyte sedimentation rate. The serum contains C-reactive protein during the acute phase, and eventually the antistreptolysin O (ASO) titer rises. Chest x-ray may show cardiomegaly, pericardial effusion, or signs of cardiac failure. Electrocardiography, echocardiography, and cardiac catheterization provide more specific clues to the extent and severity of disease.

Chorea (from Greek *choreia* 'dancing') denotes a clinical disorder manifested by recurring sudden, intricate, well-coordinated but involuntary and purposeless muscle movements, which may affect gait, use of the arms and hands, and even speech. Several forms of chorea are recognized and distinguished.

Huntington chorea, named after the American physician George S. Huntington (1850-1916), is inherited as an autosomal dominant trait. Onset usually occurs in the 30s or 40s and death, due to progressive neuromuscular dysfunction and dementia, follows in about 15 years.

Sydenham chorea, named after the English physician Thomas Sydenham (1624-1689), is the type that occurs in acute rheumatic fever. (Another name for this disorder is St. Vitus dance, after the Christian martyr whose intercession was believed to be helpful in various forms of movement disorder and "dancing mania" during the Middle Ages.) Patients display abrupt, jerky, complex, involuntary movements of the trunk and extremities, and often mild personality changes. This type of chorea is invariably self-limited, resolving without neurologic, psychologic, or muscular sequelae.

Course: Most of the manifestations of acute rheumatic fever resolve spontaneously. However, various forms of carditis (inflammation of the heart), which occur in about one-half of all patients, can lead to severe heart damage, with chronic, progressive, or even rapidly fatal malfunction of heart valves. About 20% of persons recovering from acute rheumatic fever will have a recurrence within five years.

Treatment: Streptococcal infection must be eradicated with penicillin, erythromycin, or another antibiotic known to be effective in preventing rheumatic fever. Bed rest is enforced until resting pulse, temperature, sedimentation rate, and electrocardiogram have returned to normal (often longer than one month). Most symptoms can be controlled with aspirin; corticosteroids are used as needed. Valvular heart disease and congestive heart failure may require vigorous treatment during the acute phase. Severe chronic involvement of the mitral or aortic valve may require long-term treatment, including surgery. Monthly injections of repository penicillin are continued for five years or until age 25, whichever comes first, to prevent recurrences of acute rheumatic fever.

QUESTIONS FOR STUDY AND REVIEW

1. Give a brief definition of *immunity*, including its three cardinal features:

   _____

   _____

   _____

   _____

   _____

   _____

2. Name three kinds of congenital immunodeficiency:

   a. _____

   b. _____

   c. _____

3. Name three opportunistic infections typical of the acquired immunodeficiency syndrome (AIDS):

   a. _____

   b. _____

   c. _____

4. Define or explain these terms:

   a. allergy _____

   _____

   b. anaphylaxis _____

   _____

   c. antibody _____

   _____

   d. antigen _____

   _____

   e. autoimmunity _____

   _____

   f. opportunistic infection_____

   _____

5. Name and briefly describe three autoimmune disorders:

a. _____

_____

_____

b. _____

_____

_____

c. _____

_____

_____

6. Discuss the pros and cons of having an immune system:

a. pros_____

_____

_____

_____

b. cons_____

_____

_____

_____

_____

CASE STUDY: YOU'RE THE DOCTOR

Monica Bellamy calls your pediatrics office and asks to talk to you about her 13-year-old son Wade, who has been a patient of yours since infancy. Although your receptionist has instructions to deal with telephone calls whenever possible without interrupting your appointment schedule, Ms. Bellamy insists on an immediate phone conversation with you.

1. At what point does being inaccessible to patients by phone become a liability for a physician?

_____

_____

_____

2. Which do you think is the more important determinant of a parent's insistence on talking to the child's pediatrician on the phone—the severity of the health problem or the personality type and parenting style of the caller? Explain your choice.

_____

_____

_____

_____

_____

_____

Wade has a long history of respiratory allergy and recurrent respiratory infections, and at age 9 was diagnosed with selective IgA deficiency. This is a fairly common congenital disorder of the immune system, which predisposes to bacterial upper respiratory infections. Year in and year out, you see Wade every few weeks with sinus or ear infections, and because of his known immune disorder you nearly always prescribe antibiotic treatment. Ms. Bellamy tells you that she kept Wade home from high school this morning because he woke up with a fever (100.2° orally), headache, and muscle aching. He does not have a sore throat or cold symptoms but has a mild dry cough. He has no nausea, abdominal pain, rash, or stiff neck.

3. Which symptoms support a diagnosis of a sinus or an ear infection?

_____

_____

4. Which symptoms support a diagnosis of a viral infection?

_____

_____

Ms. Bellamy asks you to telephone a prescription for an antibiotic to her local pharmacy. Her husband is out of town; she has two younger children, one of whom is also home from school with a flu-like illness; and she seems to be coming down with it herself. You tell her that, like her daughter and herself, Wade probably has an acute viral syndrome, for which antibiotic treatment is not indicated, even in the presence of IgA deficiency. You advise her to give him acetaminophen for fever, a light diet, and plenty of fluids. You ask her to call back again between 4 and 5 p.m. to report progress, and offer to make a house call on your way home from the office if he isn't doing better. Ms. Bellamy says, "By four or five this afternoon he could have a 104° fever and be needing IV antibiotics," referring to an isolated incident that occurred when Wade was 7 years old and required inpatient treatment for severe tonsillitis and otitis media.

5. Explain the implications of each of the following courses of action:

   a. Give in and phone an antibiotic prescription so that you can get on with your office practice.

_____

_____

_____

_____

_____

   b. Spend more time on the phone with Ms. Bellamy in an effort to explain the difference between the acute viral syndrome that Wade almost certainly has and the wholly unrelated recurrent bacterial upper respiratory infections to which his immune deficiency makes him prone.

_____

_____

_____

_____

_____

6. Which of the above courses of action would you choose? Defend your choice.

_____

_____

_____

_____

_____

SUGGESTIONS FOR ADDITIONAL LEARNING ACTIVITIES

1. You have won a whirlwind tour of the inhabited continents in the world. Draft an itinerary by choosing one country on each continent. Determine what vaccines you must receive in order to make this trip. Consult a local travel agency, your country health department, or the Internet to gather information on vaccination requirements for each of your destinations.

2. In the section of this chapter that discusses the treatment for rheumatoid arthritis, it mentions the side effects and/or toxicities that go along with drug therapy. Research the drugs commonly prescribed for rheumatoid arthritis, beginning with those listed in this section as well as from information available in other textbooks, drug reference books, medical journals, and the Internet. For each drug you find, prepare a two-column chart on an $8^1/_2$" x 11" sheet of paper. On the left-hand side, list the benefits of treatment with that medication. On the right-hand side, list any adverse effects. When your charts are completed, place them in order beginning with the drug that offers the most benefits with the least overall negative impact. Use your own judgment to make this ranking.

3. Using only your local telephone book and a newspaper, determine what resources are available in your community for AIDS patients and for AIDS prevention and education. Assemble this information in outline form and provide a copy to your own physician's office or local community groups as a service project.

5

Neoplasia

LEARNING OBJECTIVES

Upon completion of this chapter, you should be able to

- give the meaning of neoplasia;

- distinguish benign from malignant neoplasms;

- explain the diagnosis, grading, staging, and treatment of malignant diseases;

- identify the features of common cancers.

NEOPLASIA

THE NATURE OF NEOPLASIA

Neoplasia refers to any growth of cells or tissues that is erratic, not in accord with normal bodily needs or patterns of growth and development, and not under the control of normal regulatory mechanisms. Neoplasia results in the formation of a neoplasm (growth, tumor).

The causes of neoplasia are not fully understood. The process begins with normal cells. Cellular mutation, induced by chemical toxins (carcinogens), radiation, chronic inflammation, or certain infections, can lead to formation of a clone or colony of cells whose internal structure and biochemical nature are aberrant or atypical and whose proliferation and behavior do not respond to normal controls. An inherited tendency to develop some kinds of neoplasm has been recognized for many years. Oncogenes were discussed at the end of Chapter 2. Many neoplasms result from cell stimulation by abnormal growth factors, or by normal hormones in abnormal amounts. A tumor is said to be hormone-dependent if it develops in a tissue that is stimulated by a hormone normally present, and can be suppressed by withdrawing that hormone (for example, prostate cancer, discussed later in this chapter, is androgen-dependent).

Neoplasms are divided into two large classes: benign and malignant. A malignant tumor is one that, if unchecked, tends to cause death; a benign tumor has no such inherent tendency.

A more precise delineation of malignancy can be seen in the following four distinctions:

1. A malignant tumor is found on histologic examination to contain cells that are more primitive, undifferentiated, or anaplastic than those composing a benign tumor, or a higher proportion of such cells than in a benign tumor.
2. A malignant tumor enlarges by infiltrating and invading adjacent tissues, whereas a benign tumor simply gets bigger, without sending out neoplastic extensions into adjacent normal tissue.
3. A malignant tumor characteristically grows much faster than a benign one arising from the same cell type.
4. A malignant tumor can spread by metastasis—transmission of malignant cells or groups of cells by the bloodstream, the lymphatic channels, or other routes to establish new foci of malignancy at remote sites in the body.

These distinctions are not absolute. Although most cancers arise as malignant tumors, some develop by malignant degeneration of benign tumors. Skin cancers other than melanomas, though they are histologically malignant, seldom metastasize or cause death. A benign tumor can prove lethal if it compresses a vital structure or causes severe hemorrhage.

Malignant tumors, commonly called cancers (see box), can arise in virtually any cell, tissue, or organ of the body. A malignant tumor can cause death in a broad variety of ways: by outgrowing its blood supply and undergoing necrosis and hemorrhage, by producing toxic substances, by eroding into a major blood vessel, by invading or metastasizing to a vital organ such as the brain, or by impairing nutrition, immunity, or some other life-sustaining biochemical function.

Because of their built-in lethal potential, the diagnosis and treatment of malignant tumors are

---

The term **cancer**, the Latin word for 'crab', was used for malignant ulcerations by the Roman medical writer Celsus (1st century AD). Much earlier, Greek writers including Hippocrates used the Greek word *karkinos*, also meaning 'crab', and its derivative *karkinoma*, for malignant disease.

The association between malignancy and crabs has been variously explained. One theory is that malignant tumors were thought to gnaw or erode tissue like the claws of a crab. According to another view, the dilated veins on the surface of a cancerous breast seemed to suggest the outline of a crab with outstretched claws.

Cancer nomenclature is highly complex and constantly changing. Two main types of malignant tumor are distinguished on the basis of their tissues of origin. Carcinoma (by far the more common) develops from epithelium, either glandular (adenocarcinoma) or squamous (squamous carcinoma). Sarcoma (from a Greek word meaning 'to become fleshy') denotes a tumor arising from connective tissue (muscle, bone).

more critical than those of benign tumors. The branch of medicine devoted to the prevention, diagnosis, and treatment of malignant disease is called oncology. The remainder of this chapter will be devoted to more information about malignant tumors and detailed discussions of the four most common cancers. Various benign and malignant tumors are discussed in other chapters.

DIAGNOSIS OF MALIGNANCY

The signs and symptoms of malignant disease are highly variable. Many kinds of cancer (lung, pancreas) cause no symptoms until they have invaded surrounding tissues or spread by metastasis and have become essentially untreatable. The seven warning signals publicized by the American Cancer Society (see box) are all potential indicators of malignancy.

Cancer's Seven Warning Signals (American Cancer Society)

C Change in bowel or bladder habits
A A sore that does not heal
U Unusual bleeding or discharge
T Thickening or lump in the breast or elsewhere
I Indigestion or difficulty in swallowing
O Obvious change in a wart or mole
N Nagging cough or hoarseness

They are, however, highly nonspecific, and in any given instance, a benign explanation for one of these signs or symptoms is far more probable than a malignant one.

Cancer screening is the testing of apparently healthy persons for subtle indications of malignant disease. The following screening procedures are currently advised for all persons, at specified ages or intervals:

Breast: Monthly breast self-examination, yearly examination of the breasts by a physician, and mammography.

Uterine cervix: Pap smear.

Prostate: Digital examination of the prostate, blood test of PSA (prostate specific antigen) level.

Colon and rectum: Digital examination, sigmoidoscopy or colonoscopy, and examination of stools for occult blood.

When cancer is suspected, prompt and vigorous diagnostic evaluation is in order, unless the age or general health of the patient makes this inappropriate. Imaging techniques (x-ray, MRI, CT, ultrasound, nuclear imaging) can provide highly specific information about the nature, location, and extent of malignant disease. Blood tests that detect or measure immunologic or biologic markers (abnormal tumor products, immunoglobulins) can provide valuable further information.

But the diagnostic procedure par excellence for malignant disease is **biopsy**: Removal of a specimen of tissue from the patient's body for microscopic examination. Punch or shave biopsies are used to obtain skin specimens. Specimens from the interior of the digestive tract and the urinary tract can be obtained through endoscopes. Needle biopsy, performed with a specially designed instrument that passes through the skin and removes a sliver of tissue from the area of interest, enables the diagnostician to assess internal structures without performing open surgery. Laparoscopy permits sampling of tissue in the abdominal or pelvic cavities. In many instances, however, an adequate biopsy can only be obtained at exploratory surgery. Sampling of tissue by biopsy may include removal of numerous or extensive specimens—for example, regional lymph nodes or areas of suspicious tissue change.

A biopsy specimen is examined by a pathologist, first grossly (with the naked eye) and then (after fixation, embedding in a medium such as paraffin, thin sectioning, and staining) microscopically to determine whether it contains malignant cells, from what type of normal cells they have arisen, how undifferentiated they are, what tissue abnormalities they show (cyst formation, abortive attempts at organization, tissue death), and how far they have extended or invaded. For certain types of cancer (breast cancer), pathologic examination of surgically removed material can be performed immediately (before the surgical wound is closed) by the frozen section technique, which substitutes freezing of tissue for the more time-consuming paraffin process.

Diagnostic information obtained about a cancer is generally formulated according to a rigorous and highly specific scheme. The type of a cancer is its histologic nature: what kind of cells (squamous epithelium, gland tissue, duct tissue) have undergone malignant change? The **grading** of a cancer is a measure of its degree of malignancy, based on histologic evaluation of its cells. Higher-grade malignancies contain more primitive cells, showing a higher amount of undifferentiation (anaplasia). The higher the grade, the greater the probability of invasion and metastasis. The Broders classification of squamous-cell carcinomas is an example of a simple grading system:

grade 1	25% of cells undifferentiated
grade 2	50% of cells undifferentiated
grade 3	75% of cells undifferentiated
grade 4	100% of cells undifferentiated

Grading a tumor often permits a fairly accurate estimate of its future behavior, the likelihood of spread by invasion or metastasis, and the probable response to radiation or chemotherapy.

Staging is a measure of the extent of a malignant disease at the time of evaluation, expressed in arabic numerals (1, 2, 3…) with or without qualifying letters. Staging takes into account the type, size, and extent of the primary tumor; the degree of lymph node involvement, if any; and the number and location of any distant metastases. The presence of associated symptoms, such as weight loss and fever, may be relevant to the staging of certain malignancies. A basic framework used in expressing the staging of a wide variety of malignancies is the T-N-M (tumor, nodes, metastases) classification, mentioned in Chapter 1. In this system, subscript numbers indicate the extent of involvement, according to criteria that are specific for each type of tumor. Thus, T2 might represent a primary tumor that is larger than 5 cm in diameter but has not invaded locally; N2, involvement of lymph nodes at two distinct sites; M0, no evidence of distant metastasis.

Arriving at an accurate prognosis for a malignant tumor depends on precise typing, grading, and staging; on other diagnostic information (imaging and laboratory studies); and on due consideration of the patient's age and general health. The compilation of cancer statistics by national and international tumor registries has made possible the publication of survival information for each type of tumor depending on grade and stage. The 5-year survival rate is a familiar index of prognosis. If a given type, grade, and stage of tumor has a 5-year survival rate of 56% with a given treatment, that means that 56% of persons with such a tumor who undergo such a treatment will still be living after 5 years.

TREATMENT OF MALIGNANCY

The goals of treatment in malignant disease are to effect a cure when possible and to conserve the patient's comfort in all cases, with due attention to nutrition, hydration, and control of symptoms such as pain, nausea, and dyspnea.

Surgery has always been the principal method of treating cancer. Complete resection of a primary tumor that has not spread or metastasized usually proves to be curative. But adequate resection may involve damage to or removal of much normal tissue, with resulting functional impairment or disfigurement; on the other hand, conservative surgery may fail to remove all cancer cells. Moreover, metastases may only be discovered months or years after surgery has been performed. When curative surgery is not feasible, a palliative procedure may be undertaken to reduce the volume of the tumor (debulking) or to remove devitalized, necrotic, bleeding, or infected tissue. In certain types of malignancy, a palliative effect may be achieved by surgical removal of certain endocrine glands: the testes in metastatic carcinoma of the prostate, the ovaries in breast cancer.

During the past generation, **chemotherapy** of cancer with a wide variety of agents has become firmly established as a valuable and often curative resource. Useful cancer drugs include alkylating agents (nitrogen mustard, chlorambucil, busulfan), antimetabolites (methotrexate, 5-fluorouracil, 6-mercaptopurine), antibiotics (doxorubicin, dactinomycin, mithramycin), plant alkaloids (vinblastine and vincristine from periwinkle), hormones (adrenal corticosteroids, estrogens, androgens), and others (enzymes, platinum complex).

Most of these agents are toxic to cancer cells, and most of them can also damage normal cells and tissues. Because cancer is a life-threatening disease, a higher risk of severe side effects is tolerable. Most cancer chemotherapy must be administered by injection and continued over a period of weeks. During and after treatment, red and white blood cell counts and other diagnostic tests are performed regularly to monitor drug effects and detect severe bone marrow depression or other toxic effects of the drugs on normal tissues.

A course of chemotherapy typically includes three or more drugs given according to a precise regimen or protocol. The drugs used in such combinations are represented by their first letters in initialisms such as MOPP (mechlorethamine, Oncovorin, procarbazine, and prednisone); note that Oncovorin is a brand name for vincristine.

Because rapidly proliferating tissue is particularly subject to damage by ionizing radiation, x-ray and other forms of radiation have long been used as an adjunct to surgery and chemotherapy in the treatment of many malignant tumors. The dose and delivery site of **radiation therapy** must be carefully adjusted to ensure maximal therapeutic response with minimal side effects and risk of delayed complications.

CANCER STATISTICS

Reporting of malignant disease by healthcare providers to local and regional tumor registries enables the American Cancer Society to publish highly accurate statistics on the incidence and mortality of various types of cancer. Such statistics do not include data on skin tumors other than melanomas, since these typically respond to local treatment and do not cause death.

In a given year in the United States, about 1,400,000 new cases of cancer are diagnosed, and about 560,000 persons die of cancer. The relative incidence of the four commonest cancers, by gender, is as follows:

Men	Women
Prostate, 31%	Breast, 31%
Lung, 14%	Lung, 13%
Colon & Rectum, 10%	Colon & Rectum, 11%

Of all cancers causing death, the relative frequency with which these four cancers prove lethal is as follows:

Men	Women
Lung, 31%	Lung, 25%
Prostate, 11%	Breast, 15%
Colon & Rectum, 10%	Colon & Rectum, 11%

COMMON CANCERS

Bronchogenic Carcinoma

A malignant tumor of the lung arising from bronchial epithelium. Bronchogenic carcinoma ranks first as a cause of cancer death in both men and women in the United States.

Causes: Cigarette smoking is by far the most common cause of bronchogenic carcinoma. About 10% of regular smokers will develop lung cancer. Prolonged inhalation of second-hand smoke causes about 3000 deaths a year in the United States. Inhalation of industrial carcinogens (particularly asbestos, silica, chromium, nickel, and polyvinyl chloride) and exposure to ionizing radiation or radon are other known causes.

History: Gradual onset of cough (or change in a chronic cough), dyspnea, wheezing, hemoptysis, anorexia, weight loss, chest pain.

Physical Examination: May indicate weight loss, muscle wasting, or signs of bronchial obstruction, pneumonia, atelectasis, cavitation, or pleural effusion.

Diagnostic Tests: Chest x-ray or CT scan demonstrates a solitary nodule, infiltrate, atelectasis, cavitation, or pleural effusion. Cytologic examination of bronchial washings or pleural fluid, or histologic examination of biopsy material obtained by bronchoscopy or needle aspiration through the chest wall, shows malignant tissue arising from bronchial epithelium. Screening of high-risk populations (for example, smokers over age 60) with low-radiation, high-resolution CT, sputum cytology, or both can often detect disease early enough for cure.

Course: Bronchogenic carcinoma is typically advanced and inoperable when first diagnosed. The 5-year survival rate is only 10-15%. Obstruction of airways commonly leads to atelectasis and pneumonia. Complications include obstruction of the vena cava (superior vena cava syndrome) or esophagus, cardiac tamponade or arrhythmia, neurologic disorders (phrenic nerve palsy, Pancoast syndrome due to involvement of the brachial plexus), and paraneoplastic syndromes (Cushing syndrome, hypercalcemia) due to production of hormone-like agents by tumor cells.

Treatment: Surgery, radiation, and chemotherapy.

Other diseases of the lung are discussed in Chapter 10.

Breast Cancer

A malignant tumor of the female breast, arising most frequently from ductal epithelium. The commonest cancer in women, and the second-commonest cause of cancer death (after lung cancer) in women. One in eight or nine women will develop breast cancer.

Cause: Women who have no children, or whose first pregnancy occurs late in the childbearing years, are at increased risk of breast cancer. So are women who have a family history of breast cancer, particularly cancer occurring at an early age in one or more female relatives, which may be associated with the BRCA1 or BRCA2 oncogene. According to most authorities, the risk of breast cancer is slightly increased by estrogen replacement therapy after menopause.

History: A solitary, firm, nontender mass in the breast, usually discovered by the patient accidentally or during breast self-examination. (All women over 20 should practice breast self-examination monthly.) Sixty percent occur in the upper outer quadrant of the breast. Occasionally nipple discharge is the presenting symptom. With advancing disease, swelling and local pain. Bone pain, weight loss, and jaundice are symptoms of systemic spread through metastasis.

Physical Examination: There may be enlargement or abnormal contour of one breast on inspection. The tumor is felt as a hard, ill-defined, nontender solitary mass. There may be skin or nipple retraction, fixation of the tumor to the underlying chest wall or the overlying skin, and signs of local inflammation (swelling, redness, ulceration). Axillary lymph nodes may be found enlarged if cancer cells have spread to them.

Diagnostic Tests: Mammography (a specialized x-ray procedure) can identify changes indicative of breast cancer (calcification, mass, or both) as long as 2 years before a tumor becomes palpable, and is therefore a valuable screening procedure for asymptomatic women over 50, and for younger women believed to be at increased risk because of a family history of early-onset breast cancer or presence of BRCA 1 or 2 as detected by genetic testing. Ultrasound examination can supply valuable additional information. Biopsy is required for confirmation of malignancy and precise identification of tumor type. A biopsy can be obtained through the skin by either a large-needle or fine-needle technique. Excisional biopsy (removal of the tumor followed by frozen-section examination before closure of the surgical site) is the method usually chosen when clinical and mammographic evidence supports a diagnosis of cancer.

Course: An untreated breast cancer typically enlarges, invades surrounding and underlying tissues, and causes extensive cutaneous ulceration. Breast cancers spread to axillary and mediastinal lymph nodes, liver, bone, and brain. For a solitary, localized tumor, the 5-year survival rate is 95% and the 10-year survival rate is 90%. The figures for disease that has become systemic before treatment is instituted are 5% and 2% respectively. Five-year and even 10-year rates do not adequately reflect the long-term mortality of breast cancer, which is eventually the cause of death in most patients, except when cancer is discovered very early by screening procedures.

Treatment: The basic treatment of breast cancer is surgical removal of the tumor. Various further procedures, including radical mastectomy (removal of the entire breast as well as surrounding and underlying tissues and axillary lymph nodes) may be appropriate with certain types and stages of cancer. Both radiation treatments and chemotherapy are usually administered after surgery. Radiation is not usually needed after radical mastectomy, but the procedure is mutilating and psychologically devastating. In metastatic disease, elimination of estrogen stimulation through either oophorectomy (removal of the ovaries) or administration of tamoxifen, a chemical anti-estrogen, delays progression of disease and mitigates symptoms.

Other diseases of the breast are discussed in Chapter 13.

Adenocarcinoma of the Prostate

A malignant tumor arising from glandular epithelium of the prostate gland.

Cause: Adenocarcinoma of the prostate is the most common cancer in men (31% of all cancers diagnosed). The incidence of prostatic cancer found at autopsy in men over 50 is about 40%. However, prostate cancer causes only 11% of all cancer deaths in men. The risk of developing prostatic carcinoma is higher in men with a family history of it and in those who have undergone vasectomy. The tumor is testosterone-dependent (that is, it does not occur in men who have undergone orchidectomy). Adenocarcinoma of the prostate does not arise from benign prostatic hyperplasia.

History: There may be no symptoms. Diminished urine flow, urinary frequency, nocturia, and dribbling of urine may occur as in benign prostatic hyperplasia. The first symptom may be bone pain due to metastasis.

Physical Examination: The prostate, as palpated on digital rectal examination, may be unusually firm, nodular, or asymmetric.

Diagnostic Tests. The level of prostate specific antigen (PSA) or acid phosphatase or both in the serum is elevated in many cases of prostate carcinoma, particularly when metastasis has occurred. Transrectal ultrasound may detect abnormally dense areas within the prostate gland, representing tumor. Transrectal biopsy discloses zones of malignant tissue. The Gleason grading system gives a histopathologic estimate of malignancy and likely future behavior. X-ray studies and radionuclide bone scans may show metastases to bones of the spine or pelvis.

Course. Progression of disease is typically slow, and most patients die of other causes before the prostatic cancer has reached a lethal stage. Metastasis to lymph nodes and to the spine or pelvis eventually occurs. Urinary obstruction may lead to urinary tract infection and even renal failure.

Treatment. Surgical excision (usually radical prostatectomy), radiation by external beam or implanted radioactive needles; in advanced (metastatic) disease, castration or administration of estrogen (or an anti-androgen such as flutamide) to suppress tumor growth.

Other diseases of the prostate are discussed in Chapter 12.

Adenocarcinoma of the Colon and Rectum

A malignant neoplasm arising from glandular epithelium in the large intestine. In both men and women, colon cancer ranks second as a cause of cancer deaths in the U.S. One-half of all colon cancers are situated in the sigmoid colon or rectum. These tumors tend to grow slowly, but may eventually become bulky; they may encircle and constrict the bowel.

Causes: Most colon cancers arise by malignant transformation of benign polyps (adenomas). Several oncogenes are associated with heightened risk of developing primary cancer in the colon; some of these predispose to formation of multiple malignant tumors, which may involve organs other than the bowel. Risk factors for developing colon cancer include age over 40, a history of adenomas (benign polyps) of the colon, a family history of colon cancer, and a history of ulcerative colitis.

History: Depending on the location of the tumor, crampy abdominal pain, change of bowel habits, bloody stools, weakness, fatigue.

Physical Examination: A mass may be felt on abdominal or digital rectal examination. The liver may be enlarged or irregular if hepatic metastases are present.

Diagnostic Tests: The red blood cell count may be low as a result of hemorrhage. Chemical examination of the stool may detect occult blood. The carcinoembryonic antigen (CEA) titer in the serum may be elevated. This is not a reliable diagnostic indicator of colon cancer, but is useful in watching for recurrence or metastatic disease after surgery. With extensive hepatic metastases, liver function tests become abnormal. Barium enema demonstrates mucosal defects, a space-occupying lesion, or an encircling obstruction. Abdominal CT scan may provide additional information. Endorectal ultrasound is valuable in distal lesions. Chest x-ray may show pulmonary metastases. Colonoscopy with biopsy provides definitive diagnosis.

Course: The overall survival rate in treated colon cancer is about 35%. If complete resection of primary tumor can be carried out, the survival rate is about 55%.

Treatment: The procedure of choice is surgical resection. Rectal carcinoma may require abdominoperineal resection (removal of the entire lower bowel, including the anus) with sigmoid colostomy. Tumors higher in the colon may be able to be resected with simple anastomosis of normal bowel above and below the surgical site. Chemotherapy and radiation therapy are valuable adjuncts to surgery in colon carcinoma.

Other diseases of the colon and rectum are discussed in Chapter 11.

END-OF-LIFE CARE

Although the principal goal of all health care is to preserve and prolong life, it is often appropriate, in the presence of terminal illness, to abandon futile attempts at cure and to direct medical and nursing efforts toward palliative treatment, with adequate control of pain and other distressing symptoms, emotional and spiritual support, and preservation of the patient's autonomy and dignity. End-of-life care is a multidisciplinary approach to meeting the needs of persons with terminal cancer, end-stage renal or pulmonary disease, and other conditions.

The hospice movement provides formal programs and facilities to meet the needs of dying persons for comfort and care and also to afford support and counsel for caregivers and family members during and after the patient's final illness. Features of formal end-of-life programs include patient-controlled analgesia and anesthesia systems and advance dialog about the patient's wishes with respect to life-extending care, including resuscitation in the event of respiratory or cardiac arrest and long-term preservation after brain death has occurred. State legislatures have established procedures whereby persons nearing the end of life can give advance directives regarding the provision or withholding of such care in the event that they become incompetent or comatose.

QUESTIONS FOR STUDY AND REVIEW

1. Give a general definition of *neoplasia*:

   _____

   _____

   _____

2. State three differences between *benign* and *malignant neoplasms*:

   a. _____

   _____

   _____

   b. _____

   _____

   _____

   c. _____

   _____

   _____

3. What kind of cancer causes the largest number of cancer deaths in men? In women?

   _____

   _____

   _____

   _____

   _____

4. Define or explain these terms:

   a. carcinogen _____

   _____

   b. debulking _____

   _____

   c. grading _____

   _____

   d. oncology _____

   _____

   e. chemotherapy protocol _____

   _____

   f. staging _____

   _____

5. What are the three principal types of treatment used in cancer?

a. _____

_____

b. _____

_____

c. _____

_____

6. Distinguish between *curative* and *palliative therapy*:

_____

_____

_____

_____

7. List some of the physical, social, occupational, financial, and psychologic implications of a diagnosis of cancer:

_____

_____

_____

_____

_____

_____

_____

_____

_____

_____

CASE STUDY: YOU'RE THE DOCTOR

Carl Ostmund is a 57-year-old clergyman who consults you, a general internist, about increasing tiredness and weakness during the past 3 months. He has also lost about 15 pounds, but feels that that is because he has been trying to reduce. He denies fever, headaches, nausea, abdominal pain, change of bowel habits, bleeding, muscle or joint pain, numbness, vision or balance problems, tremors, and syncope. He has had no chest pain or cardiac palpitation, but gets out of breath when he climbs stairs.

1. Check the areas below for which you would like to have additional information on Dr. Ostmund:

___ Family medical history   ___ Smoking history

___ Birth and development   ___ Drugs and/or alcohol history

___ Childhood illnesses   ___ Dietary habits

___ Immunizations   ___ Activity level

___ Marital status   ___ Occupations, past and present

___ Education   ___ Chemical exposure

___ Military history   ___ Past illnesses

___ Hobbies   ___ Past surgeries

___ Foreign travel   ___ Past injuries

___ Sexual orientation   ___ Allergies

___ Sleep history   ___ Current medications

He is an ordained minister, scripture scholar, teacher, and writer. He was born in China, the son of medical missionaries, but has lived in the United States since age 20. His parents are in poor general health and live in a church-affiliated nursing facility. He is married and the father of two sons. He has never smoked or used alcohol. He takes no medicines regularly. His past medical history is essentially negative except for pulmonary tuberculosis in his teens (treated and subsequently pronounced inactive) and mild psoriasis, waxing and waning for many years and primarily affecting the scalp. He maintains an active schedule combining pastoral work, lecturing at a seminary, and editing two journals. He has noted considerable reduction in exercise tolerance during the past 3 months and has had to curtail some activities. He occasionally takes naps in the early afternoon.

2. What conditions might you suspect as causes for Dr. Ostmund's symptoms?

_____

_____

_____

_____

Vital signs are normal except for a resting pulse of 104 and a weight about 25 pounds above ideal weight-for-height. The patient is normally developed, above average height, and solidly built. He is alert, articulate, cooperative, and slightly apprehensive but in no apparent distress. His skin is pale, warm, dry, and of normal turgor. The scalp shows purplish patches of dermatitis with silvery scale, typical of psoriasis. Pupils are equal and reactive to light; extraocular muscle function is intact; visual fields are grossly normal by confrontation. The neck is supple, without masses, thyromegaly, or bruits. The thorax is symmetrical and respiratory excursions are full and equal. Breath sounds are normal throughout all lung fields but a pronounced pleural friction rub is heard over the left upper chest. The heart is regular at 104. The PMI is at the left midclavicular line. A faint (2/6) holosystolic murmur is heard best at the aortic valve area. No clicks, rubs, or gallop rhythm noted. The abdomen is moderately protuberant. No scars, tenderness, masses, organomegaly, tympanites. Extremities show normal development and no lesions or edema; peripheral pulses are full and symmetrical. Neurologic examination discloses no weakness, sensory loss, tremor, or pathologic reflexes.

3. On a scale of 1 to 10, where 1 is the weakest and 10 is the strongest, rate these diagnostic possibilities as likely explanations for Dr. Ostmund's tiredness and weakness:

___ a. congestive heart failure

___ b. disseminated tuberculosis

___ c. chronic fatigue syndrome

___ d. major depression

___ e. malignancy

You order laboratory studies and ask the patient to return in one week. Complete blood count shows a significant normochromic, normocytic anemia: hemoglobin 9.2 g/dL, hematocrit 29%, erythrocytes 3.8 million/mm³. White blood cell count and differential count and platelets are normal. Blood chemistries are essentially normal except for a uric acid of 10.3 mg/dL (normal 2.5-8.0). A chest x-ray is read by a radiologist as showing evidence of inactive pulmonary tuberculosis with prominent hilar lymph nodes, calcified and fibrotic parenchymal lesions in the left upper lobe, and pleural calcifications, but no infiltrate or space-occupying lesions; the heart is normal in size and configuration and the osseous structures appear normal.

4. What diagnostic possibilities now occur to you?

_____

_____

_____

_____

5. What additional studies might you order to sharpen the focus?

_____

_____

_____

_____

_____

You explain to Dr. Ostmund that he has a significant anemia which, in the absence of other explanations, is presumed to be due to blood loss. He denies any recent bleeding, blood donation, unusual bruising, or personal or family history of anemia or bleeding disorder. You order stool examinations for occult blood, and these are positive. Upper gastrointestinal series with small-bowel follow-through shows a 4 cm mass of the jejunum, encroaching slightly on the lumen. You refer Dr. Ostmund to a surgeon, who performs a segmental resection of the affected part of the small intestine and excises regional lymph nodes. Before surgery the patient receives 2 units of packed red blood cells, and during surgery he receives 2 units of whole blood. Histologic study of the tumor and nodes shows a diffuse, poorly differentiated non-Hodgkin lymphoma. Radiation and a course of chemotherapy (CHOP protocol) are administered postoperatively.

6. The CHOP protocol consists of which group of chemotherapeutic agents?

___

When you see him 3 months later he is doing well. He is taking only vitamins and iron. He has regained most of his energy and has now gone back to his usual schedule. He lost much of his scalp hair as a result of chemotherapy, but in exchange his psoriasis has cleared up almost completely. His weight has continued to drop slightly, partly because both you and the surgeon advised him to lose weight. Repeat red blood cell count, hematocrit, and hemoglobin are now normal.

7. What is Dr. Ostmund's likely prognosis at this point?

___

Dr. Ostmund returns to see you $3^1/2$ years later because of abdominal pain, a sensation of fullness in the upper abdomen, and weight loss. He has also noted some loss of appetite and nausea and a recurrence of weakness such as he experienced before his first visit. He has now retired from pastoral work and is teaching on a reduced schedule. He is pale and appears chronically ill. Vital signs are normal but his weight has dropped 31 pounds since you last saw him.

8. What do you think is happening?
    ___ a. reactivation of tuberculosis
    ___ b. hepatitis C from blood transfusions
    ___ c. congestive heart failure
    ___ d. recurrence of lymphoma

Your examination confirms the presence of a firm, irregular, slightly tender abdominal mass measuring about 5 x 8 cm in the epigastrium and left upper quadrant. The liver is not enlarged or tender. You refer him for laboratory studies and a CT scan of the abdomen. His hemoglobin has fallen again, and his white blood cell count is 48,000/mm^3 with 84% lymphocytes and many lymphoblasts. Imaging studies show a large irregular upper abdominal mass. You refer him back to the surgeon and the oncologist who supervised his care earlier.

9. What studies or procedures might the surgeon and oncologist pursue?

_____

_____

_____

_____

_____

Further studies including laparoscopy show that he has a recurrence or extension of his jejunal lymphoma, probably from a metastatic site not excised at the time of his first surgery. Hepatic metastases are also noted. Further surgery is not deemed advisable. Whole-body irradiation is administered in an effort to induce tumor regression. A repeat course of chemotherapy is prescribed, but the patient discontinues it because of severe nausea. He is admitted briefly to a hospice facility for increasing pain and nausea, but once these are improved he elects to return home with a patient-controlled narcotic analgesia system. Six weeks later he dies in his sleep.

10. Of the seven warning signs of cancer listed in this chapter, which ones, if any, applied to Dr. Ostmund?

_____

_____

_____

_____

_____

_____

_____

_____

_____

11. What routine procedures described in this chapter might have provided an earlier diagnosis in this case?

_____

_____

_____

_____

_____

_____

_____

_____

_____

SUGGESTIONS FOR ADDITIONAL LEARNING ACTIVITIES

1. Locate the nearest hospice facility in your community. Find out what services it offers and what qualifications are required for participation of patients with a cancer diagnosis.

2. Contact the local unit of the American Cancer Society and obtain information on a form of cancer that is not discussed in this chapter. Using this information and relying on additional sources of information, such as textbooks, library, and the Internet, prepare a brief report that contains a description of the condition, statistics indicating its occurrence in men and women with age breakdowns, if available, its cause, presentation and diagnostic features, treatment, and course. Include in your report a discussion of risk factors, including genetic factors.

3. Prepare a learning game on cancer diagnosis and treatment using the information in this chapter. On one side of a 3" x 5" index card, write the form of cancer. On the other side of the card, write three facts consisting of one subjective symptom, one objective physical finding, and one diagnostic test result. You should be able to come up with a dozen or more cards for each of these four diagnoses, repeating some pieces of information as necessary so long as the same three facts (symptom, finding, and test result) aren't repeated. Shuffle the cards, fact side up. Play with another student, ask a family member to test you, or test yourself by reviewing each set of facts and then sorting the cards into piles based on the diagnosis you make.

6

Trauma and Poisoning

Chapter Outline

TRAUMA AND POISONING

TRAUMA

CLOSED (BLUNT, NONPENETRATING) INJURIES

OPEN (PENETRATING) WOUNDS

SPECIAL TYPES OF INJURY
Head Injuries
Spinal Injury
Thoracic Injury
Abdominal Injury
Child Abuse (Battered Child Syndrome)
Rape
Cumulative Trauma Disorder (CTD)

INJURIES NOT DUE TO DIRECT APPLICATION OF FORCE
Suffocation and Drowning
Thermal Burns
Cold Injury
Electric Shock
Injury due to Radiant Energy
Multiple Trauma

POISONING

QUESTIONS FOR STUDY AND REVIEW

LEARNING OBJECTIVES

Upon completion of this chapter, you should be able to

- describe the various kinds of trauma to which the human body is subject;

- explain how physicians examine, diagnose, and treat victims of trauma;

- discuss chemical poisoning and its treatment.

TRAUMA AND POISONING

This chapter surveys a broad variety of injuries to which the human body is subject. Most of these injuries are due to direct force or violence, but a few result from heat, cold, or radiant energy of various kinds. The chapter ends with a brief consideration of chemical poisoning.

TRAUMA

Trauma is a general term for an injury of any kind (see box). In this section, the subject of trauma will be discussed under three broad classifications: blunt, closed, or nonpenetrating injuries due to

---

The Greek noun **trauma** comes from the verb *titrosko*, which means 'to wound'. In classical Greek it generally refers to wounds sustained in hand-to-hand combat or in other contact sports.

In modern medicine the word has a wider application. When physicians speak of repetitive trauma syndrome, emotional trauma, microtrauma, and chemical trauma, they are obviously taking the word in the sense of any assault on the integrity of the human organism from outside.

The Latin word *injuria*, from which our *injury* derives, is a compound of *in* (with the sense of 'against' or 'not') and *jus* 'legal right, law'. The original sense was something like 'any violation of a right'; often the term meant simply 'insult' or 'infringement on personal freedom'.

As in the case of *trauma*, the English word *injury* has undergone a considerable shift of meaning. Nowadays it almost always refers to direct physical violence, while the legal sense of 'crime against the person' has largely died out; we speak of accidental injury and of injuring oneself.

Finally, we often hear the phrase *traumatic injury*, which may seem redundant, since both words mean roughly the same thing. But the sense of this expression is 'injury (gross damage to tissue) that is due to violent application of physical force (rather than to heat, radiant energy, or chemical agents)'.

---

force; penetrating injuries due to force; and injuries of special types, or affecting special body parts or regions.

CLOSED (BLUNT, NON-PENETRATING) INJURIES

Nonpenetrating injuries result from a wide range of deliberate or accidental applications of force to the body: falls, automobile accidents, mishaps with bulky loads or machinery, criminal assault with fist or blunt instrument, and athletic injuries.

The direct application of blunt force to the body surface usually leads to a contusion: bruising or crushing of cutaneous and subcutaneous tissues, muscles, and other structures, as manifested by local swelling, discoloration due to leakage of blood from the circulation, pain, tenderness, and reduced mobility. Ecchymosis is the bluish discoloration that appears under the skin at the site of extravasated blood—that is, blood that has leaked from damaged blood vessels. A large accumulation of extravasated blood in tissues (under a fingernail, within a muscle) is called a hematoma.

Contusions vary in extent from mild to life-threatening, depending on the amount of force applied, the way in which it was applied, and the structures or area injured. A severe contusion of muscle, particularly in the thigh, can result in myositis ossificans, the formation of one or more painful lumps in the area of injury due to calcification of damaged muscle tissue or of slowly resolving hematomas. Treatment includes local ice; compression and immobilization as needed with elastic bandaging, padding, or splinting; elevation; rest of the injured part; analgesics (perhaps including narcotics), anti-inflammatory agents, and other drugs as dictated by special circumstances. Surgical drainage of hematomas or repair of damaged tissue is sometimes necessary.

Injuries to bones usually result from blunt force or from some violent twisting or straining action. Any break in a bone is called a fracture. A fracture usually causes severe pain and local swelling. There may be obvious deformity of the involved part and marked impairment of function.

Hundreds of qualifying terms may be added to the noun "fracture"; the following are among those more frequently used:

Comminuted fracture: A fracture resulting in more than two fragments.

Compound fracture: A fracture accompanied by an open wound, from which a bone fragment may protrude.

Displaced fracture: A fracture in which the relative positions of the fragments are significantly different from what they were before the fracture.

Hairline fracture: A fine crack in a bone, barely visible on x-ray examination.

Impacted fracture: A fracture in which the end of a long bone is driven into the body of the bone rather than being broken away from it.

Stress fracture: A crack in a bone induced by repetitive stress on the same bone (as in jogging or doing step aerobics) rather than by a single violent force.

The basis of all **fracture treatment** is immobilization during the period of healing. This may be a few days to a few months, depending on the site of the fracture, its size and shape, and the general health of the patient. If a fracture is not adequately immobilized, the result may be a nonunion—a failure of the fragments to join together in solid bony union. For many fractures, external fixation (plaster or fiberglass cast) suffices; for others, internal fixation (wires, screws, pins, or plates inserted through a surgical incision) must be used. Before immobilization is applied, the fracture may require reduction: manipulation of the bone fragments so as to bring them as nearly as possible into a normal anatomic relationship. Certain types of fracture (carpal navicular, femoral neck) may interrupt the blood supply to one of the bone fragments, with consequent delay or failure of healing. Ischemia (impairment of blood supply) may cause the affected fragment to undergo avascular necrosis (death of tissue due to lack of blood supply). Treatment may include a bone graft, in which the patient's own bone, taken from another site, is ground into small chips and packed into the bony defect. Bone grafting is also used in injury or disease of the spinal column.

Joint injuries commonly result from forces that tend to separate the bones making up the joint, or to drive them into a positional relationship that threatens to crush or tear supporting structures (ligaments, cartilages, joint membranes). Ligaments are nonyielding bands of connective tissue that limit the direction and range of movement of a joint. The articulating surfaces of bones are usually protected with pads or disks of cartilage, a tough, resilient tissue that serves to absorb shocks and protect bone ends. A joint is enclosed by synovial membrane, a delicate tissue that forms a sac-like envelope and contains a small amount of lubricating synovial fluid.

A **sprain** is a stretching or twisting injury to one or more of the ligaments supporting a joint, by some force that tends to deform the joint. The ligaments may be completely divided (particularly in knee injuries), but usually ligament tears are only partial. A sprain usually causes pain, swelling, and restriction of movement of the joint. A severe sprain may lead to chronic or permanent deformity or disability. Sprains are treated with rest and immobilization (usually by means of splinting or bandaging), compression and elevation of the injured part, ice, analgesics, and nonsteroidal anti-inflammatory agents. Severe ligament tears or damage to articular cartilage may require surgical repair.

When the relationship between two bones at a joint is radically altered by some violent force, the result may be a **dislocation**: a deformity of the joint persisting after the initial application of violence. Often the bones become locked in an abnormal relationship because of their shapes, the pull of ligaments, or muscle spasm. A dislocation is often associated with severe sprain or ligamentous tearing. A subluxation is a dislocation of minor degree, without severe deformity.

A dislocation or subluxation causes local pain and more or less evident joint deformity, often with marked restriction in the range of motion. Initial treatment is reduction of the dislocation—restoration of the normal anatomic relationship between the bones involved. Sometimes this requires an open surgical procedure. After reduction, the injured joint is immobilized with splinting or bandaging while the supporting structures about the joint heal. Severe damage to joint structures can culminate in ankylosis, a rigid fusion of the tissues causing complete loss of joint mobility.

Violent stretching of a muscle or tendon may partially or completely disrupt its fibers. A **strain** is a muscle or tendon pull causing pain, spasm, and perhaps local swelling and discoloration. The injury usually heals promptly with rest, ice, support, and analgesics as needed. Complete tear or rupture of a muscle (such as the rotator cuff of the shoulder) or tendon (such as the calcaneal tendon of the heel) is less common. Disability can be severe, and surgical repair is often needed.

OPEN (PENETRATING) WOUNDS

Wounds that break the body surface are usually due to a scraping type of injury or to forceful application of something sharp, such as a knife or broken glass. They may also result from blunt trauma (especially over a bony prominence), from a gunshot, or from a fracture in which a bony fragment tears its way out through the skin (compound fracture). With any penetrating injury there is a risk of infection due to pathogens introduced from outside, including staphylococci, streptococci, and a variety of other organisms including those that cause tetanus and gas gangrene. In addition, a foreign body (needle, bullet, wooden splinter) may be retained within the tissues.

Scraping away of the surface of skin or mucous membrane by violent contact with a rough surface (concrete, gravel) is called an **abrasion**. A severe abrasion can remove or destroy all levels of the skin, resulting in scarring. Often particles of foreign material are embedded in an abrasion and contribute to the amount of damage and the risk of infection and scarring. A deep abrasion may injure tissues far below the skin.

A cutting injury caused by a sharp object is properly called an **incised wound**. (Many health professionals incorrectly call such a wound a laceration. Lacerations are discussed below.) In a cut, or incised wound, some or all layers of the skin are separated, and injury may extend to underlying subcutaneous tissues, muscles, tendons, nerves, blood vessels, and internal organs. When a penetrating injury is caused by a needle, nail, or similar sharp object of small caliber, it is called a puncture.

A **gunshot wound** results from penetration of the skin surface by a missile (or missiles, in the form of shot) driven at high velocity by expanding gases generated by the rapid combustion of a charge of explosive. The extent of damage depends on the type of firearm and ammunition, the distance between the firearm and the victim, the site of penetration, and the direction in which the missile is traveling. Gunshot wounds can penetrate or shatter bones, violently damage soft tissues, destroy internal

organs, and tear open major blood vessels, with resulting hemorrhage that can be rapidly fatal.

A **laceration** is a tearing of tissue due to blunt violence (collision with wall, furniture, or floor; being struck with a hard ball, a bat, or someone's knee) rather than to something sharp. The skin bursts at the site of a laceration because it is crushed between the injuring object and an underlying bony prominence (chin, elbow, knuckle) or a broad flat bony surface without subcutaneous padding (scalp, shin). Generally there is contusion of the wound edges.

Open wounds are treated by cleansing with surgical soap, irrigation or scrubbing to remove foreign material, application of sterile dressings, and administration of tetanus toxoid or tetanus immune globulin, prophylactic antibiotics, and analgesics as needed. Cuts and lacerations that penetrate all levels of the skin or deeper usually require surgical repair. Closure of an open wound must be performed within a few hours after injury; otherwise infection nearly always results.

Before surgical repair begins, tissue that has been crushed, shredded, or devitalized is excised, a procedure called **débridement**. If there is a significant tissue defect, grafting may be required. Each layer or type of tissue (tendon, muscle, fascia, subcutaneous tissue, skin) is separately sutured (sewed) with absorbable suture material (gut), silk, wire, or synthetic material. Wound repair includes careful attention to hemostasis (control of bleeding), avoidance of undue tension on wound edges, and obliteration of any dead space (open pockets, which may fill with blood or serum or become a site of infection) below the surface. Wound repair cannot always be carried out in such a way as to yield a result that is anatomically, functionally, and cosmetically satisfactory. The location and nature of the wound and other factors (for example, the patient's gender, occupation, or general medical condition) play a part in the surgeon's decision as to which of these ideal goals should be sacrificed.

SPECIAL TYPES OF INJURY

Head Injuries

Blunt or penetrating wounds of the head can cause irreversible damage to the brain, and hemorrhage within the brain or between the brain and the skull. Such injuries are frequently lethal, or result in permanent impairment of mental function.

Cerebral concussion is defined as a violent blow to the skull that causes brief unconsciousness but does no permanent damage to the brain or its supporting structures. In cerebral contusion, there is local injury to brain tissue, but again without lasting consequences. Cerebral laceration is a still more violent injury in which part of the brain is torn. The outcome is often death or severe permanent impairment (paralysis, seizures, dementia).

Intracranial **hemorrhage** can be extradural or epidural (between the outermost covering of the brain, the dura mater, and the skull), subdural (beneath the dura mater), subarachnoid (under the arachnoid membrane covering the brain), or intracerebral (within the substance of the brain). Extradural hemorrhage usually results from arterial bleeding and often proves rapidly fatal. Subdural hemorrhage is often venous, with chronic signs and symptoms (gradually progressing headache, stupor, personality change, or neurologic impairment). Subarachnoid hemorrhage is less often due to trauma than to rupture of a congenital aneurysm (abnormal bulge or weakness in a cerebral artery, present from birth). Any intracranial hemorrhage is life-threatening because of the danger of irreversible damage from compression of brain tissue within the rigid, nonexpanding skull.

The treatment of head injury demands prompt and decisive action to conserve brain tissue and arrest hemorrhage.

Spinal Injury

Injuries to the spinal cord, particularly at the cervical level, usually result from automobile accidents, falls, or diving accidents. Fracture or dislocation of one or more vertebrae can compress or even sever the spinal cord, with permanent loss of sensation and motor power (including the ability to breathe) at levels below the site of injury. Treatment includes rigid immobilization of the spine until diagnostic evaluation is completed, surgical reduction of dislocation or freeing of compressed nerve tissue, supportive care (including maintenance of breathing function if necessary by various types of respirator), and physical therapy to preserve joint and muscle mobility and restore function when possible.

Thoracic Injury

Blunt injury to the chest can fracture ribs and produce severe contusion of heart or lungs. Rib fractures may be so painful that the patient is unable to breathe deeply enough to maintain normal oxygen levels in tissues. Extensive rib fractures can lead to **flail chest**, in which normal respiratory efforts fail because part of the chest wall has lost its normal stability.

Penetrating wounds of the chest, due to stabbing, gunshot wounds, or accidents, endanger the heart and great vessels, the lungs, the esophagus, and other structures within the thorax. Puncture of the heart or a main blood vessel can be almost instantly fatal. Hemorrhage into the pleural cavity is called **hemothorax**.

An open wound of the chest wall can result in **pneumothorax** (presence of air in the pleural cavity). Under normal circumstances, inspiration results when the chest wall moves outward and the diaphragm moves downward, making the lungs expand. When there is an abnormal opening in the chest wall, inspiratory efforts suck atmospheric air into the pleural space so that the lung collapses. If the edges of the chest wound act as a valve, allowing air to enter but not escape, the pressure of the air in the pleural cavity may rise high enough to displace the mediastinum (the structures between the two lungs) to the opposite side, compressing the normal lung and adding to respiratory compromise.

Management of chest wounds includes vigorous efforts to maintain circulatory and respiratory function and to identify the precise nature, location, and extent of internal injuries so that adequate procedures can be applied in timely fashion to restore structural integrity.

Abdominal Injury

Blunt injury to the abdomen can cause bruising, laceration, or severe hemorrhage of internal organs (liver, spleen, kidney, digestive tract, urinary bladder). In penetrating abdominal injuries, the risk of damage and particularly of hemorrhage is much increased. Puncture of the stomach or intestine releases digestive fluids into the peritoneal cavity and causes chemical peritonitis. Hemorrhage into the abdominal cavity is called hemoperitoneum.

The diagnosis of abdominal injury depends on careful physical examination, x-ray studies and scans, and peritoneal lavage (injection of physiologic saline solution through a needle passed through the abdominal wall, followed by its withdrawal and laboratory examination). This procedure can detect blood, digestive fluids, urine, or other substances not normally present.

Management includes supportive care and prompt surgical intervention to repair leaking blood vessels or punctured organs.

Child Abuse (Battered Child Syndrome)

Child abuse is any action by an adult (parent, relative, caregiver, teacher, or other person) that jeopardizes the safety, mental or physical health, or general well-being of a child. This may include physical battering, harshly punitive actions, failure to provide a nurturing home life, inadequate attention to hygiene and nutrition, and gross neglect. Much child abuse results from impulsive or vindictive behavior by a parent, but it often becomes habitual. Often child abuse is a symptom of personality or mental disorder or of family pathology; alcohol, drug abuse, and a history of having been abused oneself as a child increase the risk that one will abuse children.

Child abuse may appear in numerous forms: severe malnutrition; scars, infections, digestive disorders, and other evidences of neglect; bruises, burns, abrasions, dislocations and fractures, and other evidences of direct physical violence. Shaken baby syndrome, resulting from violent shaking of an infant under two, can result in spinal cord injury or intracranial bleeding, with irreversible brain damage, blindness, hearing loss, seizures, learning disabilities, paralysis, or death. A special type of child abuse is sexual abuse, which may take many forms. Sexual abuse generally leads to both physical and emotional trauma.

The treatment of child abuse depends on the nature of the injuries sustained. Recognition that abuse has taken place is crucial. Abusing parents often lie about the way in which injuries have occurred, and the physician must constantly be alert to the possibility of abuse. Child abuse is a serious crime. In virtually all jurisdictions, healthcare personnel and others who report suspected child abuse to law enforcement authorities are immune to legal reprisals by the persons accused.

Rape

Rape is sexual intercourse, with penetration, that is against the will of the passive participant. The victim may be forced into submission by violence or intimidation, or may be rendered submissive or unconscious by intoxication with alcohol or drugs. Intercourse with a minor (usually legally defined in this context as a woman under the age of 16) is rape even if the victim consents. Date rape is rape in the setting of a social engagement. Often the phrase is misapplied to seduction (inducement to sexual intercourse by persuasion and enticement, without the use of force or intimidation).

Rape is a felony in all jurisdictions. Many cases go unreported and untreated because the victim is ashamed, or unwilling to submit to questioning by law enforcement officers or to medical examination for diagnosis and collection of evidence. Management includes identification and treatment of all injuries sustained, prophylaxis against sexually transmitted infection and pregnancy, and emotional support and counseling as needed.

Cumulative Trauma Disorder (CTD)

This term refers to various painful or disabling injuries that result not from sudden violent application of force but from repeated stresses and strains on certain body parts, particularly ligaments, tendons, and joints. Currently about one-half of all reported occupational disease conditions are the consequences of repetitive trauma. Lateral epicondylitis (tennis elbow) is a good example. Repetitive activities (usually occupational) that strain the origins of the wrist extensors at the lateral epicondyle of the humerus can induce chronic and disabling pain about the epicondyle. Treatment is rest, immobilization, use of nonsteroidal anti-inflammatory drugs or adrenal steroids, and occasionally surgery. Recovery may be protracted.

INJURIES NOT DUE TO DIRECT APPLICATION OF FORCE

Suffocation and Drowning

Suffocation is any stoppage of respiratory effort or obstruction to respiratory air flow. This can come about through chemical or drug effect or injury to the respiratory centers of the brain or from blockage of the airway by swelling, hemorrhage, foreign body, or severe injury. Drowning is suffocation due to filling of the airway and lungs with water. Suffocation is rapidly fatal, causing failure of both oxygenation of the blood and removal of carbon dioxide from tissues.

The treatment of suffocation must be applied promptly. Clearing of the airway is of paramount importance; this may require tracheotomy (cutting into the trachea to bypass the mouth, oropharynx, and larynx). Artificial ventilation must be provided if the patient's breathing efforts are ineffectual or absent. Underlying causes of respiratory arrest must be sought and corrected.

Thermal Burns

Thermal burns are caused by contact of skin or mucous membrane with hot objects, liquids, or vapors. The amount of injury depends on the degree of heat and the extent and duration of contact. High heat induces an intense inflammatory reaction with leakage of fluid into tissues. It also coagulates protein and destroys tissues by vaporization or carbonization. Skin burns are classified as first-degree (redness of the surface without blistering), second-degree (redness and blistering), and third-degree (redness, blistering, and charring). First- and second-degree burns normally heal without scarring unless they become infected. In third-degree burns, the nature and depth of injury usually lead to scarring. Deep burns can destroy tissues below skin level: subcutaneous fat, muscles, nerves, tendons, and even bone. Extensive burns, even when only first-degree, typically cause severe biochemical imbalance, due to sequestration of fluid in the burned area with proportionate reduction of blood volume. Dehydration, shock, toxemia, and severe local or systemic infection may complicate any severe burn.

Treatment is aimed at correcting fluid and electrolyte imbalances, relieving pain, and preventing or treating infection. Third-degree burns often require grafting.

Cold Injury

The harmful local effects of intense cold (frostbite) are similar to those of heat: local inflammation, often with blistering and tissue destruction. Treatment is similar to that for burns.

Exposure to atmospheric cold, or prolonged immersion in cold water, can induce systemic hypo-thermia, a drop in the rectal (core) temperature below 35°C. The basic treatment is rewarming. Severe hypothermia can lead to profound derangement of physiologic functioning, including cardiac and respiratory arrest. Vigorous resuscitation efforts may be necessary.

Electric Shock

Passage of electrical energy through body tissues (exposure to a source of direct or indirect current, lightning stroke) causes varying degrees of structural damage and functional impairment. At any given voltage, indirect current is much more dangerous than direct current. Lightning stroke involves very high voltage exposure for a very brief period. Conduction of electrical energy by living tissue can result in surface or deep burns, extensive damage to skeletal and cardiac muscle with release of myoglobin into the serum and cardiac arrhythmias or arrest, or loss of consciousness. Treatment is dictated by the nature and extent of injury and is largely supportive. The patient must be observed for several days for delayed evidence of damage.

Injury due to Radiant Energy

Depending on the dose, ionizing radiation (x-rays, gamma rays) can cause mild or irreversible damage to skin and other tissues. It can alter the chemistry of cells and tissues and induce abnormal cell division and even malignant change. Rapidly proliferating cells, such as those of bone marrow, lymphoid tissue, and the lining of the digestive tract, are particularly vulnerable to damage by radiation. Damage to sex cells (gametes) can lead to abnormalities in future offspring. Anemia, gastrointestinal ulceration, and blood cell malignancies are common consequences of excessive radiation exposure. Total body exposure to high doses of ionizing radiation can lead to a systemic response (radiation sickness) with vomiting, dehydration, weakness, anemia, and heightened susceptibility to infection. Treatment is purely symptomatic and supportive.

Sunlight and ultraviolet radiation from sunlamps or other devices can cause acute cutaneous burns similar to thermal burns. Prolonged or repeated exposure leads to tanning (increased pigment in skin), accelerates aging and degenerative changes in skin, and often induces malignant change. Severe sunburn can cause systemic symptoms (fever, vomiting). Treatment is similar to that for thermal burns, but otherwise supportive.

Multiple Trauma

A person who has been injured in an automobile or other high-speed accident, a natural disaster (flood, tornado), an explosion, a fire, the collapse of a building, or a fall from a considerable height, or who has been the victim of criminal assault or warfare, often has extensive trauma of various types and involving various body parts and systems. Patients with multiple trauma are generally treated in hospital emergency departments or trauma centers.

When many victims of multiple trauma must be treated at one facility within a brief period (for example, after a low altitude plane crash or a pileup of many cars on a highway), a procedure called triage (literally 'sorting') is used to ensure that available resources will be used for the greatest good of the largest number. Basically, triage means dealing first with those persons who are expected to survive but are most severely injured and in need of immediate treatment, and then with less severely injured persons. Triage also means not expending supplies or personnel time in futile efforts to save persons who are obviously injured beyond any hope of recovery.

The treatment of multiple trauma requires the coordinated efforts of many health professionals—physicians, nurses, technicians, and practitioners of surgical specialties such as orthopedic, thoracic, neurologic, and plastic surgery. Diagnostic procedures are carried out simultaneously with initial resuscitation efforts.

The physician's first concern is to ensure that the patient has a clear airway, since suffocation is rapidly fatal. Secondly, if the patient is not breathing, artificial ventilation must be started at once. The third priority is heart action and the adequacy of blood flow to tissues. (These can be remembered by the mnemonic ABC, for Airway, Breathing, Circulation.)

When respiration and circulation have been stabilized, a full assessment of the patient is undertaken to find and manage all injuries. Intracranial, thoracic, and abdominal injuries are carefully investigated and intensively treated. Bleeding sites are identified and surgically repaired. Fractures, dislocations, contusions, and lacerations are examined and treated with the same diligence and thoroughness as if each injury were the only one the patient had.

POISONING

A poison is any chemical substance that has a harmful effect on the body through contact with skin or mucous membranes, ingestion, injection, inhalation, or absorption by any other route. Poisoning can occur accidentally or with homicidal or suicidal intent. It may be due to inappropriate use of prescribed medicines; abuse of illicit drugs; exposure to insecticides, household chemicals, or industrial toxins or wastes; contamination of food or water; or inhalation of toxic gases, vapors, or dusts. A biologic poison is one that is produced by a living thing (plant or animal).

The effects of poisons on the body are extremely various. Strong mineral acids and alkalis have a rapid irritant or corrosive action on skin and mucous membranes. Benzene can impair the production of blood cells by bone marrow, but only after repeated or prolonged exposure. Inhalation of carbon monoxide interferes with the ability of red blood cells to carry oxygen. Some chemical poisons have broadly deleterious effects on many types of cells and tissues; others, particularly some drugs, cause highly specific injury or malfunction, such as paralysis, loss of vision, or abnormal heart rhythm.

The broad category of biologic poisoning includes envenomation by the sting or bite of an arthropod (bees, wasps, spiders, scorpions), snake, or other poisonous animal; symptoms due to cutaneous exposure to, or ingestion of, poisonous plants (mushrooms, poison ivy); and food poisoning due to the presence in food of contaminants produced by microbial growth (staphylococcal food poisoning, botulism). Allergy and anaphylaxis can contribute to the severity of biological poisoning, since most biological toxins are complex organic compounds capable to eliciting antibody reactions.

Snake venom typically causes erythema, ecchymosis, swelling, and severe pain at the site of the bite. Systemic effects include nausea, weakness, and other symptoms depending on the type of snake: hypotension and shock (circulatory toxins), paralysis and respiratory failure (neurotoxins), hemorrhage due to reduction in circulating fibrinogen and platelets. The bite of the brown recluse spider (*Loxosceles reclusa*) causes local inflammation with edema and often severe necrosis leading to scarring. The venom of the black widow spider (*Latrodectus mactans*) causes a milder local reaction but may have severe systemic effects, including headache and painful muscle spasms in the limbs and abdomen.

Many varieties of plants, including mushrooms (*Amanita, Psilocybe*), weeds (poison ivy, Jimson weed) and ornamental garden or house plants (philodendron, poinsettia, dieffenbachia, holly) can cause local irritation on contact with skin or oral mucous membranes, systemic toxicity if ingested, or both. Herbal teas and other botanical remedies are sometimes associated with severe or fatal toxic effects.

Food poisoning is usually due to toxins formed by microbial agents in foods that have been improperly prepared or preserved. Some *Salmonella* and *Staphylococcus* species produce toxins in food that can cause violent but usually short-lived gastroenteritis, with nausea, vomiting, abdominal cramping, and diarrhea. The toxin elaborated by *Clostridium botulinum* can also cause such digestive symptoms, but its effects on the neuromuscular system are more serious. Symptoms of botulism include dry mouth, blurring of vision and diplopia, and muscular weakness progressing to paralysis. Infantile botulism, which occurs typically in children under one year of age, is characterized by constipation and extreme loss of muscle tone, which can progress to respiratory paralysis. In this disorder, toxin is produced by *Clostridium* organisms residing in the intestine. A common source of such organisms is honey.

The treatment of poisoning begins with recognition that poisoning has occurred and identification of the poison and the amount taken or absorbed. Resuscitative efforts may take priority over other activities. Intensive evaluation and monitoring, with blood and other studies as needed, must be continued until the patient's condition is stable. General measures are emptying the stomach by lavage or by inducing vomiting, administration of drugs to stabilize heart action and blood pressure, and use of oxygen and artificial ventilation when indicated. More specific measures are available for a limited number of poisons in the form of antidotes. For example, acetaminophen poisoning is treated with acetylcysteine; cyanide poisoning with sodium thiosulfate and sodium nitrite intravenously; lead poisoning with edetate calcium disodium; rattlesnake envenomation with antivenin.

QUESTIONS FOR STUDY AND REVIEW

1. In a patient with multiple trauma, what is the treating physician's first concern?

   _____

   _____

   _____

   _____

   _____

   _____

   _____

   _____

2. Point out some major differences between *blunt* and *penetrating injuries* to the trunk of the body.

   _____

   _____

   _____

   _____

   _____

   _____

3. Define or explain these terms:

   a. concussion _____

   _____

   b. contusion_____

   _____

   c. laceration _____

   _____

   d. trauma _____

   _____

   e. triage _____

   _____

4. Which medical problems discussed in this chapter may have psychiatric or legal implications?

   _____

   _____

   _____

   _____

_____

_____

_____

5. Give examples of each of the following:

a. chemical and biological poisoning_____

_____

_____

_____

_____

b. local and systemic effects of poisons _____

_____

_____

_____

_____

c. specific and nonspecific treatment for poisoning _____

_____

_____

_____

_____

_____

_____

CASE STUDY: YOU'RE THE DOCTOR

Zora Gindra is a 6-month-old baby girl who is brought by her mother and her aunt to the neighborhood clinic where you are serving part of your pediatrics residency. They tell you that the baby has been irritable and lethargic for about 48 hours and has been nursing poorly. She has had no fever, cough, vomiting, or diarrhea during this time. In fact, she was constipated for about 3 days before the onset of the other symptoms.

1. What diagnostic considerations occur to you at this point?

_____

_____

_____

_____

The baby's parents belong to a migrant colony. She has had no well-baby care and no immunizations to date. She had been nursing normally and thriving until the past few days. Her mother thought she was teething and rubbed her gums with whiskey, but to no avail. The baby has had no seizures and no prior illnesses.

2. What further concerns might now be raised?

_____

_____

_____

_____

_____

The baby appears thin and chronically ill. She cries feebly when placed on the examining table. Her rectal temperature is 99.0°, pulse 108, respirations 15. She is at the 50th percentile for length but only the 12th percentile for weight. Head circumference is normal and the fontanels are flat. The skin is warm, dry, and of normal turgor. Some ecchymoses over the left cheek and the upper chest, several days old, are explained by the mother as the result of the child's rolling off a cushion to the floor about a week ago. No icterus is noted. The startle reflex is sluggish and muscle tone is poor. Head control is substandard for age.

3. Which of the following possibilities are you now considering?

___ a. cerebral palsy

___ b. encephalitis

___ c. meningitis

___ d. poliomyelitis

___ e. shaken baby syndrome

Examination of eyes, ears, throat, and lungs is unremarkable. The abdomen is slightly distended and tympanitic, and slightly tender all over. No masses or organomegaly is noted. Bowel sounds are hypoactive. Firm stool is palpable in the left colon through the abdominal wall. Neurologic exam shows general hyporeflexia and hypotonia without focal signs.

4. Which of the following steps would you now take first?

___ a. lumbar puncture

___ b. CT scan of the head and neck

___ c. barium enema examination

___ d. get more history

___ e. call the police

You discuss the baby's history further with the mother. She tells you that she has been nursing since birth with no problems until recently. Breast feedings are supplemented by baby food (cereals, vegetable and fruit purees) and by bottle feedings with 2% milk sweetened with honey. The baby also takes honey water by bottle.

5. Does this new information suggest a course of action?

_____

_____

_____

You arrange for admission to the children's hospital where your residency is based and order a complete blood count, a chemistry profile, and a stool examination (specimen obtained by saline irrigation of the colon) for botulinum toxin. The latter test is positive, and the child receives botulinum immune globulin in addition to supportive care. She is closely observed for respiratory paralysis, but respirator therapy is not needed. She is discharged well 16 days after admission.

6. If you could go back in time and change your initial diagnosis and treatment plan, what would you change and why?

_____

_____

_____

_____

SUGGESTIONS FOR ADDITIONAL LEARNING ACTIVITIES

1. Shock is a frequent and sometimes life-threatening complication of serious trauma. Find out as much as you can about shock, starting with information appearing in this and other chapters of this textbook and extending your research to the library, medical journals, and the Internet. Summarize your findings in a one-page report.

2. Contact the poison control center for your region. (Don't use the emergency telephone number; call their administrative offices.) Find out where the facility is located and how it is staffed. Ask for statistics about the population they treat, e.g., the age and sex of patients, geographic location, and the types of poisonings they encounter. Obtain literature on preventive measures to avoid accidental poisoning.

3. Set up a triage unit and assess patients by the type and severity of their injuries. You or your classmates can use dolls or any household objects to stand in for the real thing. If you are working with classmates, have them choose their own injury and describe to you their history and symptoms. Ask questions as necessary to determine the diagnosis. To work with objects, write historical notes and individual symptoms on slips of paper, putting all the slips for one "patient" in an envelope. Pull out and read as many slips as necessary to make a diagnosis. As you diagnose your patients, rank them in order of priority for life-saving treatment.

7

Diseases of the Skin

Chapter Outline

DISEASES OF THE SKIN

ANATOMY AND PHYSIOLOGY OF THE SKIN

CUTANEOUS SIGNS AND SYMPTOMS
Primary Skin Lesions
Secondary Skin Lesions

DIAGNOSTIC PROCEDURES IN DISORDERS OF THE SKIN

DERMATITIS
Atopic Dermatitis (Eczema)
Seborrheic Dermatitis
Contact Dermatitis

BACTERIAL INFECTIONS OF THE SKIN
Impetigo
Folliculitis
Other Bacterial Infections of the Skin

FUNGAL INFECTIONS OF THE SKIN
Tinea Corporis (Tinea Circinata,
    Ringworm of the Body)
Other Superficial Fungal Infections of the Skin

VIRAL INFECTIONS OF THE SKIN
Herpes Simplex
Warts (Verrucae)

(Outline continued on next page)

LEARNING OBJECTIVES

Upon completion of this chapter, you should be able to

- describe the basic anatomy and physiology of the skin;

- identify symptoms of diseases of the skin and the diagnostic procedures used to assess the skin;

- classify common diseases affecting the skin by their signs, symptoms, and treatment.

DISEASES OF THE SKIN *(continued)*

PARASITIC INFESTATIONS
Scabies
Pediculosis (Phthiriasis)

**BIRTHMARKS AND DISORDERS
OF PIGMENTATION**

SOME COMMON SKIN DISORDERS
Acne Vulgaris
Rosacea (Acne Rosacea)
Urticaria (Hives)
Psoriasis
Pityriasis Rosea

NEOPLASMS OF THE SKIN
Benign Neoplasms
Basal Cell Carcinoma
Squamous Cell Carcinoma
Malignant Melanoma

DISORDERS OF HAIR
Alopecia (Baldness)
Hirsutism

QUESTIONS FOR STUDY AND REVIEW

DISEASES OF THE SKIN

ANATOMY AND PHYSIOLOGY OF THE SKIN

The skin is the largest "organ" in the body, and the most accessible for diagnosis and treatment. It covers the entire body and consists of two layers, the outer epidermis and the inner dermis or true skin. (See Figure 3.)

The **epidermis** is a thin sheet of squamous (flat) epithelial cells, several layers thick, which are constantly renewed from the deepest layer, growing steadily outward to replace cells worn away. Most of the cells of the epidermis are keratinocytes, containing a horny material, keratin, that provides mechanical toughness to the outer skin surface. A few cells in the epidermis are pigment cells, containing melanin, which imparts to the skin its characteristic color, varying according to race, familial characteris-tics, age, sun exposure, and other factors. Pigment distribution is more intense in certain areas, such as around the nipples and in the anogenital region. At bodily orifices, the epidermis undergoes a transition to mucous membrane.

The **dermis** is a tough layer of connective tissue containing blood vessels, sensory nerves, hair follicles, and sebaceous and sweat glands. Hair protects the body surface and also provides some thermal insulation. Each hair follicle is accompanied by a sebaceous gland, which produces oil (sebum) that is discharged on the skin surface and exerts protective and moisture-retaining effects. Sweat glands secrete sweat, which helps in temperature regulation.

CUTANEOUS SIGNS AND SYMPTOMS

The skin is subject to numerous disorders, some of which are local while others are manifestations of

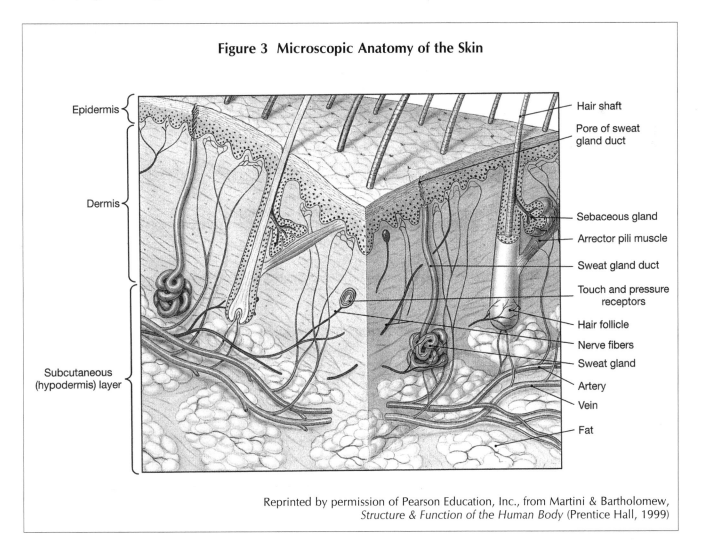

Figure 3 Microscopic Anatomy of the Skin

Epidermis

Dermis

Subcutaneous (hypodermis) layer

Hair shaft

Pore of sweat gland duct

Sebaceous gland

Arrector pili muscle

Sweat gland duct

Touch and pressure receptors

Hair follicle

Nerve fibers

Sweat gland

Artery

Vein

Fat

Reprinted by permission of Pearson Education, Inc., from Martini & Bartholomew, *Structure & Function of the Human Body* (Prentice Hall, 1999)

systemic disease. Despite the wide variety of these disorders and their causes, the signs of skin disease can be reduced to a relatively small number of distinctive lesions. Skin lesions are divided into primary (resulting from disease or injury of the skin) and secondary (resulting from complications of the basic disorder, including the effects of scratching and infection).

Primary Skin Lesions

Bulla (also, bleb): A blister; a thin-walled sac exceeding 1 cm in diameter and containing clear fluid.

Callus (not callous): A zone of thickened epidermis caused by repeated friction or pressure.

Comedo (plural, comedones): A papule consisting of a dilated sebaceous duct or gland plugged with keratin debris.

Cyst: An abnormal thick-walled structure containing fluid or semisolid material.

Ecchymosis: A broad zone of red or purple discoloration (more than 1 cm in diameter) due to hemorrhage under the epidermis.

Macule: A clearly defined zone of skin, less than 1 cm in diameter, differing from surrounding skin in color but not in texture or elevation.

Nodule: A firm elevation of the skin surface more than 1 cm in diameter.

Papule: A clearly defined zone of skin, less than 1 cm in diameter, that is raised above surrounding skin, and may differ from it in color or texture.

Petechia: A pinhead-sized, round, red or purple macule due to extravasation of blood under the epidermis.

Plaque: A clearly defined zone of skin, more than 1 cm in diameter, that is raised above surrounding skin, and may differ from it in color or texture; a plaque may consist of many confluent papules.

Purpura: A purple zone of hemorrhage in the skin, larger than a petechia but less than 1 cm in diameter; may be macular (flat) or papular (raised).

Pustule: A thin-walled sac containing pus.

Telangiectasis: Dilatation of one or more small blood vessels visible through the skin.

Vesicle: A small thin-walled sac containing clear fluid.

Wheal (weal, welt): A hive; a small zone of edema in skin, which may be red or white; wheals are typically multiple and appear and disappear abruptly.

Secondary Skin Lesions

Cicatrix (scar): A zone of fibrous tissue occurring at the site of a healed injury or inflammatory or destructive lesion extending into the dermis.

Crust: A hard, friable, irregular layer of dried blood, serum, pus, tissue debris, or any combination of these adherent to the surface of injured or inflamed skin.

Erosion: A surface defect in the epidermis produced by rubbing or scratching.

Eschar: The crust that forms on a burn.

Excoriation: Abrasion of the epidermal surface by scratching.

Fissure: A linear defect or crack in the continuity of the epidermis.

Keloid: A firm, nodular, irregular, often pigmented mass of fibrous tissue, the result of exaggerated or abnormal scarring at a site of injury.

Lichenification: Thickening, coarsening, and pigment change of skin due to chronic irritation, usually scratching.

Pit: A small depression in the skin resulting from local atrophy or scarring after trauma or inflammation.

Scab: See *crust*.

Scale: A flake of epidermis shed from the skin surface.

Scar: See *cicatrix*.

Ulcer: A cutaneous defect extending into the dermis.

DIAGNOSTIC PROCEDURES IN DISORDERS OF THE SKIN

Inspection with good lighting, natural if possible, and magnification as needed.

Diascopy: Inspection of red or purplish lesions through a transparent plastic or glass plate, which compresses the skin. If the color is due to dilated blood vessels, it blanches (fades) with compression; color due to deposition of pigment, including blood pigment, is not altered by surface pressure.

Wood light: An ultraviolet lamp with a filter that selects wavelengths under which certain funguses infecting skin or hair fluoresce brightly.

Microscopic examination of scrapings from the skin to identify fungal material, the mites of scabies, and distinctive kinds of scales; skin scrapings are usually treated with hot potassium hydroxide (KOH) solution, which partially or completely dissolves human tissue but leaves fungal elements unchanged.

Culture of exudate, pus, crusts, or scrapings for bacteria, fungi, or viruses.

Tzanck smear: A stained smear of material from an ulcer or vesicle. Changes in cells indicate viral infection but cannot distinguish varicella (discussed in Chapter 3) from herpes simplex (discussed below).

Blood studies may identify underlying, perhaps systemic, conditions, or provide additional information about the skin disorder.

Skin tests with various allergens (molds, pollens, medicines) administered by patch, scratch, or intradermal injection can identify and roughly measure skin sensitivity to these substances.

Biopsy: Removal of a specimen of abnormal skin by shaving away the surface with a fine blade or removing a plug of skin with a round punch. Sometimes the lesion is completely excised and submitted for pathologic examination.

DERMATITIS

Inflammation of the skin, a broad general term encompassing a variety of disorders. Three of the most common are discussed below.

Atopic Dermatitis (Eczema)
A chronic pruritic condition of the skin.

Cause: Unknown. Most patients have a personal or family history of allergy. May be exacerbated by irritants, emotional stress.

History: Recurrent itching, particularly affecting the back of the neck and the antecubital and popliteal areas, usually causing constant scratching.

Physical Examination: Patches of redness, sometimes with weeping, scaling, or vesiculation. Excoriations and lichenification from scratching. Sometimes evidence of secondary infection.

Diagnostic Tests: Scratch tests and RAST (radioallergosorbent test) may be positive for many allergens.

Course: Chronic, with remissions and exacerbations. Secondary infection may result from scratching, and very chronic lesions may progress to fibrosis or pigmentation.

Treatment: Avoidance of known allergens, irritants, strong soaps, excessive wetting of skin and excessive bathing. Moisturizers to restore texture of skin, and topical adrenocortical steroids to reduce itching and inflammation.

Seborrheic Dermatitis
A scaly dermatitis affecting parts of the skin richly supplied with oil glands.

Cause: Unknown. There is a genetic predisposition. The response to treatment with antifungal medicine suggests that the disease may be an inflammatory reaction to normal skin fungi such as *Pityrosporum ovale*.

History: Itching, oiliness, scaling of scalp, face, and other areas.

Physical Examination: Erythema, dryness or oiliness, scaling of the scalp, face, eyelids (marginal blepharitis), and body folds.

Course: Secondary infection, bacterial or fungal, may occur.

Treatment: Seborrheic dermatitis of the scalp is treated with selenium sulfide shampoos. On the skin, topical adrenocortical steroids and topical ketoconazole, an antifungal, are about equally effective in controlling symptoms.

Contact Dermatitis
Dermatitis resulting from contact with an irritant or allergen.

Cause: Numerous substances, including industrial chemicals, cosmetics, toiletries, and household products, can cause either an irritant or allergic type of contact dermatitis. Irritant contact dermatitis results from direct chemical attack on the skin and typically produces symptoms within minutes of exposure. Allergic contact dermatitis occurs only in sensitized persons, and there may be a latent period of 2-5 days between exposure and appearance of symptoms.

History: Itching, burning, stinging, with variable amounts of swelling, redness, and other physical signs, on parts of the skin that have been exposed to the causative agent.

Physical Examination: Redness, swelling, vesicles or bullae, weeping, crusting. Signs of damage from scratching or of secondary infection may be present.

Course: Secondary infection may occur.

Treatment: Avoidance of the cause, soothing applications, topical or even systemic adrenocortical steroids.

BACTERIAL INFECTIONS OF THE SKIN

The skin, being the first line of defense against bodily invasion, is exposed to numerous physical, chemical, and biological assaults. Many types of skin infection (bacterial, viral, and fungal) occur, some of them largely limited to the skin. In addition, the skin and hair are subject to parasitic infestation. Only the more common cutaneous infections and infestations are discussed here.

Impetigo

A spreading bacterial infection of the skin causing itching and crusted sores.

Cause: Staphylococci, sometimes streptococci. Infection may begin in a trivial cut or abrasion. Impetiginization refers to the development of impetigo in an area of skin already damaged by a noninfectious dermatitis. Scratching and poor personal hygiene, particularly among children, lead to rapid spread of lesions and often transmission to household contacts, schoolmates, or playmates.

History: Itching and crusted sores, especially on the face.

Physical Examination: Macules, vesicles, bullae, pustules, and copious gummy purulent exudate forming honey-colored crusts on an erythematous base. In severe infection there may be fever.

Diagnostic Tests: Smear and culture can identify the causative bacteria.

Course: Without treatment, increasing spread often occurs. Systemic effects (toxemia, dehydration) may occur in children, particularly those already debilitated by disease or malnutrition. A severe form of impetigo known as ecthyma may leave scars.

Treatment: Strict attention to personal hygiene and use of antibacterial soap; isolation may be appropriate. For most cases of impetigo, the antibiotic mupirocin applied as an ointment is curative. In the presence of extensive disease, fever, or toxemia, antibiotics are administered systemically.

Folliculitis

Bacterial infection in hair follicles.

Cause: Invasion of hair follicles (the weak point in the body's armor) by bacteria, usually staphylococci. Factors that tend to reduce the resistance of the skin to infection (prolonged pressure, friction, excessive perspiration, chemical irritation, diabetes mellitus) predispose to folliculitis. Any severe bacterial infection of the skin may spread to surrounding hair follicles (satellite folliculitis). Infection beginning in just one follicle can be widely propagated by shaving (face in men, legs in women). Hot tub folliculitis is often due to *Pseudomonas aeruginosa*. Folliculitis without demonstrable infection occurs in persons exposed to oil (industrial lubricants, cosmetics) and in those treated with adrenocortical steroids.

History: Itching and burning of hairy skin, with tiny painful red lumps at the bases of hairs.

Physical Examination: Pustules in hair follicles. Occasionally generalized erythema and crusting. Distribution of lesions provides clues as to underlying cause.

Course: May become chronic. Abscess formation may occur, and even bacteremia and septicemia.

Treatment: Topical mupirocin is generally effective. Shaving of affected areas should be discontinued until infection resolves. Systemic antibiotics may be needed for severe infections or those contracted from hot tubs. Hot tub water should be chlorinated.

Other Bacterial Infections of the Skin

Bacterial infections of the skin can take a number of other forms. Pyoderma is a general term for any purulent (pus-forming) infection of the skin. An abscess is a sharply localized bacterial infection, usually due to staphylococci, in which pus forms in a tissue space walled off from surrounding tissues by fibrin, coagulated tissue fluids, and eventually fibrous tissue. A furuncle is a deep, solitary abscess; a carbuncle is a spreading lesion made up of furuncles communicating by subcutaneous passages.

Cellulitis refers to a type of infection occurring in soft tissues, including the skin, whose cardinal features are diffuse and spreading tissue swelling, redness, pain, and fever. Cellulitis is usually due to streptococci; a particularly severe form, with a sharply circumscribed border, bulla formation, and often septicemia, is called erysipelas. Necrotizing fasciitis is a severe toxic complication of streptococcal infection in which superficial fascia and underlying muscle are rapidly destroyed. Local spread of infection is accompanied by high fever, shock, and evidence of systemic toxicity. Abscesses, furuncles, and carbuncles are treated by surgical incision and drainage. Cellulitis and erysipelas respond to antibiotics given orally or by injection. Antibiotic treatment is guided by results of cultures of pus, tissue fluid, or blood. In necrotizing fasciitis, débridement or amputation may be life-saving.

FUNGAL INFECTIONS OF THE SKIN

Tinea Corporis (Tinea Circinata, Ringworm of the Body)

Superficial fungal infection of the skin (see box).

The long-established lay term **ringworm** causes much misunderstanding and consternation. Skin diseases known by this name are not due to worms, and physicians never thought they were. The word *ring* in *ringworm* refers to the circular shape of the lesions, with central clearing. *Worm* is just a metaphorical allusion to the "moth-eaten" appearance of skin infected by various superficial fungi, clothes-eating moth larvae being incorrectly called worms. *Tinea*, the Latin term for ringworm, also means 'moth'.

Cause: Fungi of the genera *Epidermophyton*, *Microsporum*, and *Trichophyton*. Transmission from infected persons or animals sometimes occurs. Moisture and friction reduce resistance of the skin and favor invasion.

History: One or more slowly expanding round or oval patches of red, scaly skin, usually on exposed surfaces, with a variable amount of itching. There may be a history of recent new exposure to domestic animals or to persons with similar lesions.

Physical Examination: Lesions are pink, red, or tan, round or oval and sharply circumscribed, and covered with fine scales. The outer border of a lesion is raised slightly, and with continuing expansion of the margin, the skin near the center of the lesion gradually clears and assumes a normal appearance.

Diagnostic Tests: Scrapings of scales heated with hot potassium hydroxide (KOH) solution often show fungal material on microscopic examination. Culture on Sabouraud medium may be required to confirm the presence of fungi. Examination with Wood light shows characteristic fluorescence only when infection is due to species of *Microsporum*.

Course: Tinea may become chronic and widespread, with extension to scalp, hair, and nails. Secondary bacterial infection may complicate diagnosis and treatment. In some persons an autoimmune phenomenon called a dermatophytid or id reaction may cause eruption of vesicular lesions on areas not infected with fungus, particularly on the hands.

Treatment: Numerous antifungal medicines are effective in topical form. Topical adrenocortical steroids may also be used if inflammation and itching are severe. Systemic antifungal treatment may be needed when infection is severe or resistant to topical treatment.

Other Superficial Fungal Infections of the Skin

The fungal organisms responsible for tinea corporis can also cause more localized infections. In tinea capitis (ringworm of the scalp), infected hairs break off at the scalp surface, leaving patchy areas that appear bald, often with black dots representing the roots of broken-off hairs. Mild itching and scaling may occur. Treatment is with oral antifungals such as griseofulvin and selenium sulfide shampoo. Kerion is a possible complication, with boggy edema and exudation of pus though hair follicle openings. Tinea pedis (athlete's foot) causes erythema, itching, scaling, fissuring, maceration, and vesicle formation of varying degree, particularly between the toes. Tinea cruris (jock itch) is a similar infection of the groin. Tinea versicolor, caused by *Malassezia furfur*, consists of variable numbers of white to tan macules with very fine scales. Patches are lighter than surrounding tanned skin, but darker than surrounding untanned skin, hence the name versicolor 'changing colors'. Tinea pedis, tinea cruris, and tinea versicolor usually respond to topical antifungals.

Tinea unguium (onychomycosis) is probably the most important chronic nail disease. Fungal infection of fingernails and toenails causes discoloration, deformity, splitting, crumbling of nails, and separation from nailbeds, generally without other symptoms. Oral antifungal treatment, usually for several months, is standard. Topical methods and even avulsion of infected nails are sometimes used.

Candidiasis (or candidosis; infection of skin and mucous membranes with the yeastlike fungus *Candida albicans*) causes shiny, sharply delimited patches of intense erythema with itching or burning. Infection is more common in diabetics, and typically occurs on areas where two skin surfaces are in apposition, with trapping of moisture: under the breasts, in the anogenital area, and in skin folds of obese persons. Diagnosis is confirmed by microscopic examination for hyphae or culture. Treatment is with topical or systemic antifungal agents. Candidal infections in the mouth (called thrush) and in the vagina may be treated with antifungal formulations intended specifically for those areas.

VIRAL INFECTIONS OF THE SKIN

Herpes Simplex

Local viral infection of skin or mucous membranes, causing vesicular lesions, typically recurrent.

Cause: Herpesvirus type 1 (oral, labial, facial herpes) and type 2 (genital herpes). Transmission is by direct contact with an infected person, not necessarily with a person having visible lesions. Genital herpes is a sexually transmitted disease. The virus may lie dormant for months or years before causing symptoms. Viral activation, with ensuing skin eruption, may be triggered by physical or emotional stress, fever or respiratory infection (hence the lay terms "cold sore" and "fever blister"), sun exposure, and menstruation.

History: Clusters of small, painful vesicles about the nose or lips or on the genitals. These often recur in the same place, at greater or lesser intervals, in response to triggering factors mentioned above, or for no apparent reason. Vesicles may ulcerate. Women with genital herpes may have severe pain on urination. The first episode of infection is typically the most severe, and may be accompanied by fever.

Physical Examination: A cluster of 4-6 small vesicles or ulcers on an erythematous, edematous base. With a first infection there are often fever and regional lymphadenitis. Secondary infection may cause pustule formation, crusting, and even impetigo (discussed above).

Diagnostic Tests: Tzanck smear of material from lesions shows multinucleated giant cells with cytoplasmic inclusions, confirming viral infection but not specific for herpes. Viral culture yields more specific proof of herpes infection.

Course: An episode of infection typically runs its course in about a week, somewhat longer when it is the patient's first infection. Secondary bacterial infection may lead to exacerbation of symptoms. Intrauterine infection is associated with abortion or fetal damage. A child delivered through an infected birth canal may acquire localized or widespread neonatal infection, typically severe. Ocular infection with herpes simplex virus causes herpetic (dendritic) keratitis, a severe ulcerative disorder of the cornea that can lead to visual impairment.

Treatment: Analgesics and topical applications to control pain. Antiviral drugs topically (penciclovir) or systemically (acyclovir, valacyclovir).

Warts (Verrucae)

Virally induced coarse papules of the skin and mucous membranes.

Cause: Human papillomavirus (HPV), of which about 80 types can be distinguished immunologically. Most types preferentially affect particular areas (plantar warts on soles of the feet, genital warts on the external genitalia or uterine cervix). Transmission is by direct contact. Genital warts are transmitted sexually. Scratching and picking at lesions cause autoinoculation (implantation of infective viral material at new sites, with spread of lesions).

History: One or more papules on skin surface, or on anogenital mucosa. Mild itching may occur, and occasionally bleeding.

Physical Examination: One or more coarsely textured papules, varying from flat (on the sole of the foot or the face) to elevated (on the hands or the genitals). Typical genital warts are narrow-based, raised, and tend to come to a point; lesions of this type are called condylomata acuminata (singular, condyloma acuminatum). There may be evidence of excoriation or damage from scratching, picking, or crude attempts at removal. Secondary infection may occur.

Diagnostic Tests: Diagnosis is usually clinically evident, but biopsy can provide histologic confirmation. Wart virus cannot be cultured. Cervical infection produces characteristic changes on Pap smear, but the Pap smear is not an adequate screening test for HPV infection. Suspicious lesions treated with dilute acetic acid become chalky gray or white (aceto-whitening) if they are warts. These areas are examined with a colposcope (a low-power microscope with light source, adapted for viewing the cervix through a vaginal speculum) and biopsies are taken.

Course: HPV infection is chronic and difficult to eradicate. Infection may resolve spontaneously after a time, but meanwhile other lesions may have developed, or the condition may have been transmitted to others. Genital infection with certain types of HPV is now recognized as a leading cause of cervical carcinoma, and is also associated with genital cancers in men.

Treatment: Numerous treatments are available, none of them perfectly satisfactory. Choice of treatment depends partly on the site of infection. Surgical excision, electrocautery, laser ablation, and cryotherapy (freezing with liquid nitrogen or a cryoprobe) are currently the most popular methods. Others include destruction with caustic chemicals such as salicylic acid, bichloracetic acid, and podophyllin, and injection of interferon directly into lesions.

PARASITIC INFESTATIONS

Scabies

A chronic, pruritic eruption due to burrowing of mites in the skin.

Cause: The itch mite, *Sarcoptes scabiei*, a microscopic parasite that burrows under the skin surface and lays eggs. Transmission is from person to person by direct contact, probably also by indirect contact (sharing of toilets, showers, towels, clothing, bedding). Itching is due not to the mere presence of mites but to a sensitivity reaction to foreign mite protein; hence symptoms may not appear for about a month after infection.

History: Chronic itching, more intense at night, associated with formation of reddish papules and linear raised lesions.

Physical Examination: Reddish papules and burrows, found most often on the hands (finger webs), wrists, elbows, nipples, buttocks, and genitalia, never on the face or scalp. There may be evidence of excoriation, lichenification, or secondary infection.

Diagnostic Tests: The diagnosis is usually clinically evident. Microscopic examination of scrapings from lesions may show mites.

Course: Relentlessly chronic without treatment: an older name for scabies is "seven-year itch." In debilitated persons, especially children, secondary infection may cause extensive weeping and crusting.

Treatment: Topical treatment with permethrin, lindane, or crotamiton is generally curative. Itching may be treated with oral or topical antipruritics.

Pediculosis (Phthiriasis)

Human cutaneous infestation with lice.

Cause: The body louse (*Pediculus corporis*), the head louse (*Pediculus capitis*), and the pubic louse (*Pthirus pubis*; see box). These six-legged arthropods, visible to the naked eye, live and reproduce on the body surface and derive their sustenance from the host's blood, which they obtain by puncturing the skin. They remain in position by grasping body or scalp hairs, and also attach their nits (egg cases) to hairs. Eggs hatch in about two weeks and females become sexually mature in another two weeks; hence a single louse (if a pregnant female) can give rise to a substantial colony in about a month. Transmission is from person to person; pubic louse infestation is a sexually transmitted disease. Indirect transmission (from sharing bathroom facilities, clothing, hats, bedding) also occurs.

> The genus name *Pthirus* was derived incorrectly from *phtheir*, the Greek word for 'louse'.
>
> Although writers and editors constantly "correct" the spelling to *Phthirus*, the "wrong" spelling *Pthirus* is officially "right."
>
> The next time you use the expression "lousy" or "nit-picking" in a metaphorical sense, stop and think what you are saying.

History: Itching in the infested area. Visible, mobile lice on body or scalp hairs, possibly along with nits. Minute dark spots may be noted on underwear; these are deposits of louse feces.

Physical Examination: With adequate illumination, lice and often nits are plainly visible on hairs. Fine blue patches may be noted on skin at sites where lice have fed. There may be indications of excoriations or secondary infection.

Course: Without treatment, colonies can become very large. Lice do not burrow under the skin or penetrate body orifices. *Pthirus* does not transmit diseases. *Pediculus* is a vector of typhus and plague in parts of the world where these diseases are endemic.

Treatment: Topical pyrethrin or lindane, left on the skin long enough to kill both adult lice and eggs, is curative.

BIRTHMARKS AND DISORDERS OF PIGMENTATION

The term *nevus* (originally denoting a birthmark) has two meanings in dermatology. A vascular nevus is a pink, red, or purple birthmark—histologically a benign tumor (hemangioma) consisting of dilated blood vessels. Vascular nevi, though often not apparent at birth, appear within the first few weeks of life. Two types are distinguished. The capillary hemangioma (nevus flammeus, portwine stain) is typically flat but often widespread and disfiguring, particularly when on the face or neck. Cosmetic treatment may include cryosurgery (freezing with liquid nitrogen) or laser ablation. A cavernous hemangioma (giant nevus, strawberry mark) is a raised and much more conspicuous lesion, which generally regresses during the second year of life. For that reason, a cavernous hemangioma is usually left untreated unless it obstructs a body orifice.

A pigmented nevus is any mark or lesion on the skin, not necessarily present at birth, consisting of deposits of intensely pigmented cells (nevus cells). Pigmented nevi are commonly called moles. Small flat pigmented lesions appearing early in life are usually junctional nevi, so called because histologic examination shows that the nevus cells lie at the junction of the dermis and epidermis. Some of these may evolve into compound nevi, with additional deposits of pigment cells within the dermis. In intradermal nevi, found more commonly in the elderly, groups of nevus cells are confined to the dermis. Pigmented nevi are variously perceived as attractive ("beauty spots") or cosmetically objectionable. Their greatest medical significance is that they must be carefully distinguished from malignant melanoma (discussed below).

Abnormalities in the intensity and distribution of pigment in the skin can be congenital or acquired and may be due either to local or to systemic causes. Patchy or diffuse areas of increased pigmentation can occur in pregnancy and Addison disease. Darkening of skin color is not always due to increase of melanin. Cutaneous deposition of heavy metals (mercury in occupational poisoning, iron in hemochromatosis) can also cause darkening.

Freckles (ephelides; singular, ephelis) are small pigmented macules, common in children, that become darker with sun exposure. Lentigines (singular, lentigo) are pigmented macules that occur on the face and hands with aging.

Vitiligo consists of widely distributed patches of depigmented skin, due to destruction of pigment cells. The condition is found in about 1% of the population, and occurs with increased frequency in persons with diabetes mellitus, hyperthyroidism, hypothyroidism, hypoadrenocorticism (Addison disease), and gastric carcinoma. PUVA (psoralen + ultraviolet A) treatment, using topical methoxsalen and ultraviolet light, may provide some improvement. The best method of management is often judicious use of cosmetics.

SOME COMMON SKIN DISORDERS

Acne Vulgaris

A chronic eruption of comedones, papules, pustules, and cysts occurring primarily in adolescence.

Causes: The ultimate cause is unknown. There may be a genetic predisposition (identical twins are equally affected). The disease tends to be worse in males, but does not occur in castrated males. It comes on about the time of puberty and typically resolves within 5-8 years, but may persist into the middle and late 20s or beyond. Acne or acneform lesions develop in Cushing syndrome, including the type induced by treatment with adrenocortical steroids; in women with hyperandrogenism of any cause; and in persons exposed to certain chemicals (chloracne, due to industrial exposure to chlorine; iodism, due to medicinal administration of iodide). Acne typically gets worse during times of emotional stress.

The lesions of acne develop in oil (sebaceous) glands, apparently as a result of heightened sebum production that leads to retention of sebum and plugging of gland ducts. Plugged, enlarged glands are called comedones (singular, comedo). These are colloquially called whiteheads when closed, and blackheads when the gland orifices are open, exposing sebum plugs, which darken as a result of chemical changes (not dirt). Very large comedones form cysts. Retained sebum is broken down by bacteria (*Propionibacterium acnes*) or spontaneous chemical changes to form fatty acids, which cause local inflammation and induce a foreign body reaction. Surface bacteria (staphylococci) invade inflamed tissue to produce pustules. Symptoms are aggravated by application of greasy or oily cosmetics and by repetitive picking or squeezing of lesions. Healing of pustules may be protracted, and may leave pits or scars.

History: Appearance of lesions varying in type (blackheads, whiteheads, papules, pustules, cysts), number, distribution, and severity on the face, upper back, and chest; rarely elsewhere.

Physical Examination: Essentially as above.

Diagnostic Tests: Culture may be useful to identify unusual organisms causing secondary infection. Other laboratory studies may disclose underlying or contributing causes.

Course: Eventually, spontaneous remission occurs. This can take years, however, and in the meantime the patient may suffer severe emotional distress. The course of cystic acne may be especially protracted, and any severe case of acne is likely to leave some scarring.

Treatment: Diet is no longer regarded as having an important influence on the severity of the disease. Numerous topical and systemic medicines are used in the treatment of acne. Vigorous skin hygiene with greaseless soaps and cleansers is the foundation of treatment. Topical drugs include benzoyl peroxide, azelaic acid, retinoids (adapalene, tazarotene, tretinoin), and antibiotics (clindamycin, erythromycin). Antibiotics such as tetracycline, minocycline, and erythromycin may also be administered orally for long periods. Expression of sebum from comedones with a comedo extractor by a physician may reduce symptoms. Injection of adrenocortical steroid into lesions may also help by lessening local inflammation. In women, cyclical hormone therapy with an oral contraceptive containing norgestimate and ethinyl estradiol often provides long-term control. Isotretinoin taken orally for 4-6 months induces lengthy, usually permanent resolution of acne, but it is reserved for severe cases because of side effects (peeling of lips in 90%; elevation of blood cholesterol in 15%; abnormal liver function tests; grave risk of fetal damage if taken by a pregnant patient).

Rosacea (Acne Rosacea)

A reddish facial eruption occurring in the middle-aged and elderly.

Cause: Unknown. Occurs more commonly in persons with migraine headaches. Responds to antibiotic treatment. A rash similar to rosacea sometimes results from prolonged application of potent topical adrenocorticosteroids to the face.

History: Burning and flushing of the face, with patchy or diffuse rosy tint, papules, and sometimes pustules or excessive sebum production.

Physical Examination: As noted above. The cheeks, nose, and chin show a faint to bright inflammatory blush. Papules, pustules, telangiectases (visible patches of dilated skin vessels), and oiliness are usually present to some degree. Inflammation of the eyelids and even the cornea may occur. In some patients marked hyperplasia of the tissues of the nose (rhinophyma) eventually develops.

Course: Rosacea is highly chronic, but treatment provides a fair degree of control.

Treatment: Topical metronidazole or other antibiotics provide improvement in symptoms. Oral antibiotics and topical corticosteroids may be required. Lasers can obliterate telangiectases. For severe rhinophyma, plastic surgery is required.

Urticaria (Hives)

An acute, often transitory eruption of intensely itchy papules or wheals.

Cause: Urticaria is caused by a release of histamine from mast cells in the dermis, with resultant local edema, capillary dilatation, and stimulation of nerve endings. Many factors can incite this reaction: allergies to food (shellfish, strawberries), medicines (aspirin, penicillin), insect bites or stings (beestings), nonallergic sensitivity to medicines (atropine, codeine), parasitic infestation, sunlight, cold, heat (cholinergic urticaria), and even, in susceptible individuals, simple stroking of the skin (dermographism).

History: Sudden onset of a localized or generalized eruption of intensely itchy wheals or papules, which may be transitory.

Physical Examination: Wheals (raised white or red papules) surrounded by erythema. Wheals may be round or scalloped and confluent. Signs of scratching may be evident.

Diagnostic Tests: Blood studies and allergic screening may indicate the underlying cause, but usually do not.

Course: Urticaria often occurs in attacks at intervals of a few hours, but typically resolves within one or two weeks unless continued exposure to the causative agent occurs. Urticaria persisting beyond one month may point to occult infection or malignancy.

Complications: Secondary infection due to scratching.

Treatment: Severe urticaria responds to intramuscular epinephrine. Antihistamines such as diphenhydramine or hydroxyzine may be given orally or by injection to control an acute attack. Regular use of antihistamines prevents or mitigates further attacks. The nonsedating antihistamines fexofenadine and loratadine may be useful prophylactically even though they are ineffective in other forms of pruritus. Doxepin, a tricyclic antidepressant, is also effective either orally or topically. In severe cases, topical and systemic corticosteroids may be used.

Psoriasis

A chronic skin disorder characterized by scaly plaques.

Cause: Increased proliferation of epidermal cells. Evidently an autoimmune disorder, to which some persons are genetically predisposed.

History: Plaques of scaly thickening of the skin, particularly the scalp, knees, and elbows, with moderate itching. Nails and joints may also be affected.

Physical Examination: Reddish-purple thickened plaques of skin covered with silvery, firmly adherent scales. Pitting or stippling of nails and inflammation of joints, particularly the distal interphalangeal joints, may also be noted. In guttate psoriasis the plaques are small and numerous. Koebner phenomenon (formation of lesions at sites of trauma) may be noted.

Diagnostic Tests: Skin biopsy (usually unnecessary) shows characteristic changes in the epidermis.

Treatment: Topical steroids, calcipotriene, tar ointments; tar shampoos to the scalp. UVB (ultraviolet B); PUVA (psoralen + ultraviolet A). Oral methotrexate, etretinate, cyclosporine.

Pityriasis Rosea

A mild, benign, self-limited scaly eruption.

Cause: Unknown. More common in spring and fall. The male: female attack rate is 2:3. Person-to-person transmission has not been demonstrated.

History: Appearance of a solitary scaly patch (herald patch) on the skin, followed in 1-2 weeks by a generalized eruption of similar but smaller lesions. Itching is mild or absent.

Physical Examination: A widespread eruption of oval fawn-colored macules with fine scales on the trunk and proximal extremities. The hands, face, and feet are typically spared. Trunk lesions follow a segmental distribution, especially on the back, giving a "Christmas tree" appearance.

Diagnostic Tests: Because pityriasis simulates secondary syphilis, a serologic test for syphilis is often done to rule out that possibility.

Course: Lesions disappear spontaneously in about 6 weeks.

Treatment: Ultraviolet treatments, oral erythromycin, and topical or oral steroids may hasten clearing, but treatment is seldom needed since itching is mild, affected body parts can easily be covered by clothing, and spontaneous resolution within weeks is virtually certain.

NEOPLASMS OF THE SKIN

Benign Neoplasms

The skin is subject to many varieties of benign growth, most of them of only cosmetic significance. However, all must be carefully assessed to rule out malignancy.

Seborrheic keratosis is a tan, brown, or black plaque, of knobby or gummy texture, that seems to be stuck on the skin. Such lesions, common in the elderly, are benign and warrant treatment (cryosurgery or excision) only for cosmetic reasons. Actinic keratosis (senile keratosis) is a scaly, pigmented lesion, occurring on exposed skin (face, hands) in older persons. These lesions grow very slowly, but are considered premalignant; some evolve into squamous cell carcinoma. Treatment is with cryotherapy or application of 5-fluorouracil. Keratoacanthoma is a benign epidermal neoplasm that appears as a reddish nodule, grows rapidly, often ulcerates, and then resolves spontaneously within a few weeks. Treatment is usually by wide excision because of its similarity to squamous cell carcinoma.

Basal Cell Carcinoma

A slowly growing, waxy or pearly papule with telangiectatic vessels, appearing usually on parts of the body exposed to sunlight, particularly the face. Most appear in the middle-aged or elderly. Ulceration and widespread erosion may occur if treatment is delayed, but metastasis is rare. Treatment is by surgical excision, including Mohs chemosurgery and cryotherapy.

Squamous Cell Carcinoma

A hard red nodule appearing on sun-exposed skin, usually in a middle-aged or elderly person. The lesion may develop in a pre-existing actinic keratosis and may rapidly ulcerate. Metastasis is uncommon. Treatment is by excision.

Malignant Melanoma

A pigmented malignancy of the skin that develops in persons of all ages, progresses rapidly, metastasizes widely, and is fatal without treatment. Among malignancies melanoma ranks ninth in incidence, and incidence is increasing. At least some cases are due to sun exposure. It is estimated that, for a person under age 30, visiting a tanning parlor 10 or more times a year increases the risk of melanoma sevenfold. The risk is also higher in persons of white race, persons with many pigmented nevi, and persons with a family history or prior personal history of melanoma. Melanoma can arise anew or develop from a previously benign pigmented nevus. Features of a pigmented lesion that suggest malignancy are irregularity of shape or border, uneven distribution of pigment, pink, blue, or black color, bleeding or ulceration, and rapid enlargement. Treatment is by excision. Prognosis depends on the thickness of the tumor (Breslow classification) or the depth of invasion (Clark classification). In metastatic disease, radiation and chemotherapy may prolong survival.

DISORDERS OF HAIR

Although the visible part of scalp and body hair is not living tissue, the follicles in which hair is formed are subject to a number of disorders.

Alopecia (Baldness)

Hair loss leading to temporary or permanent, patchy or diffuse zones of baldness can result from scarring after trauma or after severe bacterial or fungal infection. It can also be a symptom of systemic disease (systemic lupus erythematosus, iron deficiency, pituitary deficiency). Male pattern baldness (affecting brow and vertex) is genetically determined; it may also affect genetically predisposed women with elevated blood levels of androgens from any cause. The condition often responds to oral finasteride in men and to topical minoxidil in persons of both sexes. Each hair follicle normally passes through cycles between anagen (active hair production, with increase in hair length), and telogen (resting phase). Telogen effluvium is a transitory generalized thinning of scalp hair due to a systemic condition that puts the growth of a large number of hairs into the telogen phase at the same time, with resultant increased shedding of hairs. Causes include pregnancy, oral contraceptives, excessive dieting, high fever, and any severe physical or emotional stress. Hair thinning becomes noticeable after a latent period of two to four months, and typically resolves spontaneously within a few months.

Hirsutism

Excessive or cosmetically objectionable hairiness (an excessive amount of hair; unusual darkness or coarseness of hair; abnormal distribution of hair—for example, on the face in women) is called hirsutism. In some cases it is a familial trait. Hirsutism in women is often due to increased levels of androgenic substances in the blood, generally as a feature of polycystic ovary syndrome, congenital adrenal hyperplasia, or functioning (hormone-producing) tumors of ovarian or adrenal tissue. In these disorders hirsutism is generally just one symptom of virilization, others being deep voice, male-pattern baldness, and hypertrophy of the clitoris. Treatment is with estrogens, often given as oral contraceptives, or antiandrogens (spironolactone, finasteride, flutamide).

QUESTIONS FOR STUDY AND REVIEW

1. Sweat glands, oil glands, hair follicles, and nails are sometimes called dermal appendages. What beneficial functions, if any, does each of these serve? In what way can they be a liability?

   _____

   _____

   _____

   _____

   _____

   _____

2. Distinguish between a *dermatitis* and a *dermatosis* and give three examples of each.

   dermatitis _____

   _____

   _____

   a. _____

   b. _____

   c. _____

   dermatosis _____

   _____

   _____

   a. _____

   b. _____

   c. _____

3. Define or explain these terms:
   a. alopecia _____

   _____

   b. cicatrix_____

   _____

   c. comedo_____

   _____

   d. dermographism_____

   _____

e. macule _____

_____

f. papule _____

_____

g. telangiectasis _____

_____

h. tinea corporis _____

_____

i. urticaria _____

_____

j. verruca _____

_____

4. Most cutaneous malignancies and many other skin problems occur primarily on sun-exposed skin. It is estimated that just one or two severe cases of sunburn in a lifetime increase the risk of skin cancer. Is there any such thing as a "healthy tan"? Explain your answer.

_____

_____

_____

_____

_____

5. Offer some examples to illustrate the saying that "the skin is the mirror of the interior of the body." What skin disorders are or can be symptoms of systemic disease?

_____

_____

_____

_____

_____

_____

_____

_____

CASE STUDY: YOU'RE THE DOCTOR

Erskine Yeazell is a 37-year-old construction laborer who consults you, a dermatologist, about several cutaneous problems.

1. What kinds of skin disorders might you expect to occur more often in a person of this age, and in a person with this occupation?

_____

_____

_____

_____

Mr. Yeazell shows you several deeply pigmented moles over his chest and back, which he says have been there since he was small. None of them have changed recently in size or appearance, but two of them sometimes get irritated and bleed as a result of friction from the straps of equipment he wears at work. He has also had a gradually enlarging lump on the side of his neck for about one year. Finally, he gets a recurrent scaly irritation of the backs of both hands. This burns and stings when he puts his hands into water but doesn't really bother him much. However, it concerns his wife and is the main reason he came in.

2. What specific questions would you now ask Mr. Yeazell?

_____

_____

_____

_____

He denies any personal or family history of skin cancer. He smokes one package of cigarettes daily and drinks two to five beers daily, more on weekends. He takes no regular medicine and has not seen a doctor for the past 10 years except for treatment of job-related injuries. He works outdoors much of the time. He wears protective equipment such as ear plugs for hearing protection around noisy machinery, filter masks when cutting or boring bricks or cement, safety glasses, and a hardhat "if somebody's watching," but often dispenses with these when working alone. He never uses sunscreen. He wears gloves for some jobs, but not when they reduce dexterity. In his work he is regularly exposed to wet cement, adhesives, solvents, fiberglass insulation, and mineral dusts.

3. What impact might some of these historical features have on Mr. Yeazell's cutaneous health? On his general health?

_____

_____

_____

_____

Mr. Yeazell is alert, cheerful, and normally developed. He is afebrile and his blood pressure is 150/97. His skin is deeply tanned and he is about 50 pounds overweight.

4. Since you are a skin specialist, do you

   a. Routinely ignore health concerns that are outside your area of specialization, such as this patient's cigarette smoking, carelessness about hearing protection and other safety measures, overweight, hypertension, and excessive drinking?
   b. Advise Mr. Yeazell that these are all potentially harmful issues that need to be addressed, and offer to provide at least initial assistance or referral for their management?

_____

_____

_____

_____

Mr. Yeazell has a number of benign-appearing pigmented nevi of the trunk. All have sharp borders, with regular distribution of pigment that is of uniform chocolate brown color. None currently show signs of inflammation. There is a 2.5 cm subcutaneous nodule of the left posterior neck that is nontender, slightly fluctuant, and fixed to the skin but not to underlying muscle. Your clinical diagnosis is a benign cutaneous cyst. You advise Mr. Yeazell that this can be excised for cosmetic reasons or simply because it seems to be enlarging, but that malignant disease is not a serious consideration. The skin of his palms is thick and callused. The dorsa of both hands show erythema and scaling. You believe this is probably due to recurrent exposure to cement.

5. Which of these other pieces of advice will you give Mr. Yeazell?

   ___ a. Seek a job change.
   ___ b. Wear gloves when working in wet cement.
   ___ c. Have all his moles removed in case some of them should be malignant.
   ___ d. Wear sunscreen on exposed skin surfaces when working outside.
   ___ e. Sue his employer for causing him to develop contact dermatitis on his hands.

SUGGESTIONS FOR ADDITIONAL LEARNING ACTIVITIES

1. Using the illustration on page 89 as a guide, draw your own diagram of the skin. Use crayons or colored marking pens to create a bright and interesting design. Color-code your picture by using a single color for the structures that are the same. Label the structures in your drawing and post it on your refrigerator or in another prominent place in your home until your study of human diseases is complete.

2. Engage in a collaborative reading activity with a partner or group. Take turns reading a section of the chapter aloud. As that section is being read, other participants jot down what they feel are the key points from that section, using a separate piece of paper for each section. When the reading of the entire chapter is complete, assemble all the notes for each section and compare them. Did everyone select the same key points? How do they differ? Why?

3. Using a sheet of graph paper as a grid, create a word search puzzle that contains every term used to describe primary and secondary skin lesions as well as the names of common skin disorders and the diagnostic tests associated with them. Scatter the terms throughout the puzzle, entering them forward, backward, up, down, and diagonally. Fill in blank squares with random letters. Exchange puzzles with someone else and see who can complete their puzzle first.

Diseases of the Cardiovascular System

(Outline continued on next page)

LEARNING OBJECTIVES

Upon completion of this chapter, you should be able to

- describe the basic anatomy and physiology of the cardiovascular system;

- explain diagnostic procedures and treatments for cardiovascular diseases;

- classify common diseases of the cardiovascular system by their signs, symptoms, and treatment.

DISEASES OF THE CARDIOVASCULAR SYSTEM
(continued)

CORONARY ARTERY DISEASE (ARTERIOSCLEROTIC HEART DISEASE, ISCHEMIC HEART DISEASE)
Angina Pectoris
Myocardial Infarction (Heart Attack, Coronary Thrombosis)

DISORDERS OF CARDIAC (MYOCARDIAL) FUNCTION
Myocarditis
Congestive Heart Failure
Acute Pulmonary Edema

PERICARDITIS
Acute Pericarditis
Pericarditis with Effusion

DISORDERS OF BLOOD PRESSURE: SHOCK AND HYPERTENSION
Shock
Hypertension

PERIPHERAL ARTERIAL DISEASE
Atherosclerosis
Aneurysm
Dissecting Aneurysm
Raynaud Phenomenon

THROMBOSIS AND EMBOLISM

THROMBOPHLEBITIS
Superficial Thrombophlebitis
Deep Thrombophlebitis

QUESTIONS FOR STUDY AND REVIEW

DISEASES OF THE CARDIOVASCULAR SYSTEM

ANATOMY AND PHYSIOLOGY OF THE CARDIOVASCULAR SYSTEM

The cardiovascular or circulatory system consists of the heart and the blood vessels (arteries, capillaries, veins). (See Figure 4.) The purpose of the system is to provide rapid delivery to the tissues of oxygen from the lungs, nutrients, minerals, vitamins, and water from the digestive system, hormones from glands, and white blood cells from bone marrow and lymphoid tissue, while removing waste products and delivering them to the lungs (carbon dioxide), liver (broken-down red blood cells), and kidney (nitrogenous wastes) for excretion.

The heart is a pump—actually two synchronized pumps each handling a different segment of the circulating blood at any given moment. The right atrium (antechamber) and the right ventricle receive venous blood from the systemic circulation and pump it into the lungs for gas exchange. The left atrium and left ventricle receive freshly oxygenated blood from the lungs and pump it through the arteries into the systemic circulation. The contraction of a heart chamber is called systole; relaxation and refilling is called diastole. Valves in the heart (one for each of the four chambers) prevent backflow of blood into a chamber during diastole. The heart is made up largely of muscle (myocardium), which receives its blood supply by way of the coronary arteries. (See Figure 5.) The heart is encased in a protective sac called the pericardium.

The normal pacemaker of the heart is the sinoatrial (SA) node, a nodule of specialized tissue located near the right atrium that generates a constant, regular succession of electrical impulses throughout life. Each impulse passes across the right atrium, triggering contraction (systole) of both atria. The impulse then reaches a second nodule, the atrioventricular (AV) node, from which it spreads through nervelike tissue trunks to the ventricles, causing them to contract. The rate and force of cardiac contractions are subject to change by neural and hormonal factors.

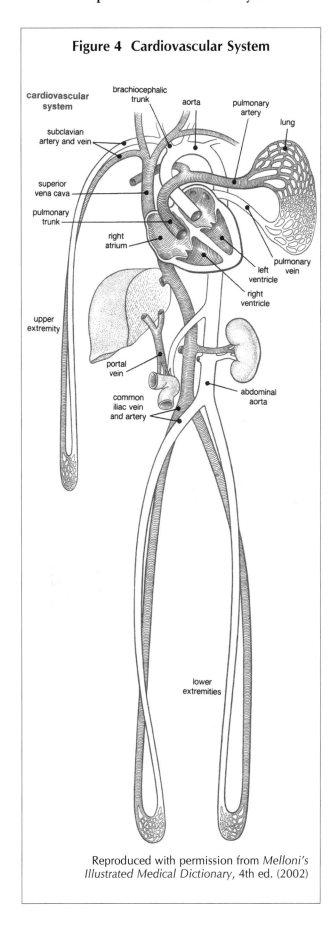

Figure 4 Cardiovascular System

Reproduced with permission from *Melloni's Illustrated Medical Dictionary*, 4th ed. (2002)

Figure 5 Coronary Circulation

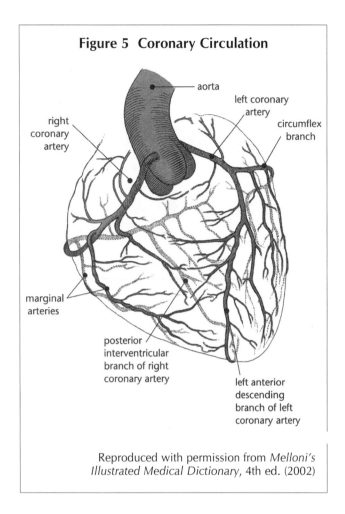

right coronary artery

aorta

left coronary artery

circumflex branch

marginal arteries

posterior interventricular branch of right coronary artery

left anterior descending branch of left coronary artery

Reproduced with permission from *Melloni's Illustrated Medical Dictionary*, 4th ed. (2002)

SYMPTOMS AND SIGNS OF CARDIOVASCULAR DISEASE

Dyspnea: Shortness of breath; labored breathing or increased awareness of the effort of breathing. Dyspnea can reflect hypoxemia (diminished oxygen tension in blood), hypercapnia (excessive carbon dioxide tension in blood), or both. When due to cardiovascular disease, these disturbances in blood gases can result directly from inadequacy of circulation (as in shock) or indirectly from congestion and edema of the lungs (as in congestive heart failure).

Dyspnea on exertion (or effort) (DOE): Shortness of breath that occurs only with increased activity such as stair-climbing or physical work.

Paroxysmal nocturnal dyspnea (PND): A sudden attack of labored breathing awakening the patient from sleep during the night.

Orthopnea: Shortness of breath in the recumbent position, relieved partly or completely by assuming an upright posture. Persons with orthopnea may be unable to sleep when lying flat. The number of pillows needed to ease breathing is a rough measure of the problem ("three pillow orthopnea").

Tachypnea: Rapid breathing.

Chest pain is a cardinal feature of myocardial ischemia (deficiency of blood flow) due to coronary artery disease. The pain of angina pectoris is a squeezing or crushing pain felt in the middle of the chest and often radiating to the neck, jaw, shoulder(s), arm(s), or back between the shoulder blades. The pain of myocardial infarction is similar but more prolonged and often more intense. Pericarditis usually causes substernal pain, sometimes radiating to the neck or back, that is aggravated by respiratory movements and by recumbency (lying down).

Pain in an extremity of circulatory origin may be caused by either ischemia (blocked artery) or vascular engorgement (blocked vein, arteriovenous fistula).

Palpitation: Any of various abnormal sensations accompanying heart action, and drawing attention to it: unduly rapid heartbeat, noticeably irregular beat, a feeling that some or all heartbeats are unusually strong, a sense of missed beats, or intermittent flip-flop sensations in the heart.

Edema: Local or diffuse swelling due to accumulation of fluid in tissues.

Dependent edema: Edema of the lower extremities, aggravated by the dependent (downward hanging) position.

Peripheral edema: Edema of the extremities.

Pitting edema: Edema that retains the impression of the examiner's fingers after pressure is released.

Ascites: Swelling of the abdomen due to effusion of fluid into the peritoneal cavity.

Lightheadedness or syncope (fainting) can result from inadequacy of blood flow to the brain, due to any severe impairment of systemic circulation.

Weakness, anorexia, nausea, hiccups. These may all be symptoms of cardiovascular disease.

Pallor, an abnormally pale skin, occurs in constriction of superficial blood vessels, as in shock.

Cyanosis, a bluish tinge of skin and mucous membranes, which may be particularly noticeable in the lips and nail beds, indicates an abnormally high concentration of reduced (unoxygenated) hemoglobin in the circulation. This can result from any disorder (circulatory, respiratory, metabolic, or toxic) that impairs the ability of the heart and lungs to replenish the oxygen supply of the blood.

DIAGNOSTIC PROCEDURES IN DISORDERS OF THE CARDIOVASCULAR SYSTEM

Vital Signs

Pulse: Heart rate and regularity, determined by palpation of arterial pulsations at the wrist (radial pulse) or another site or by auscultation of the heartbeat at the cardiac apex (apical pulse).

Blood pressure: The pressure of the blood in the arterial system is measured by a standard procedure involving application of an inflatable cuff (equipped with a pressure gauge) to an extremity (usually the arm) and auscultation over an artery just distal to the cuff. The cuff is inflated above the expected blood pressure and then the air is slowly released from it. The pressure in the cuff at which the blood can be heard squeezing through the compressed artery is taken as the maximum or systolic blood pressure (that is, the highest pressure attained by the blood during left ventricular contraction). The pressure in the cuff at which sounds of blood flow through the narrowed artery are no longer audible is taken as the minimum or diastolic blood pressure (that is, the lowest pressure to which the blood drops during left ventricular filling or diastole). Both pressures are recorded in torr (millimeters of mercury, mmHg) and written as a fraction, systolic over diastolic (for example, 120/80).

Pulse pressure is the difference between systolic and diastolic pressures (for example, 120 - 80 = 40).

Respiratory rate is increased in many cardiovascular disorders.

Jugular venous pulses, normally just visible in the neck, reflect fluctuations in the pressure within the superior vena cava during events in the cardiac cycle. They can be amplified and recorded by an instrument to detect abnormalities in right atrial and right ventricular function.

Auscultation of the Heart

Heart tones: Each beat of the heart normally produces two sounds or tones, the second following the first after an interval of less than 0.5 second. The

first heart sound (S1) corresponds to the beginning of ventricular systole and is due chiefly to closure of the mitral and tricuspid valves. It is lower in pitch, louder, and longer in duration ("lub") than the second heart sound ("dup").

The **second heart sound (S2)** corresponds to the beginning of ventricular diastole and is due chiefly to closure of the aortic and pulmonic valves. The physician notes the quality and loudness of sounds heard at the four valve areas (areas where valve sounds are best heard, not corresponding to the exact locations of the valves): aortic (A), mitral (M), pulmonic (P), and tricuspid (T).

- M2: The second heart sound as heard at the mitral valve area.
- A2 = P2: The second sounds as heard at the aortic and pulmonic valve areas are approximately equal in intensity.

A **third heart sound (S3)** may be heard immediately after the second, during ventricular diastole, in young patients or in older patients with cardiac disease.

A **fourth heart sound (S4)** may be heard immediately before the first heart sound. It is due to atrial systole and is seldom noted except in the presence of cardiac disease.

Gallop rhythm: An auscultatory finding that simulates the sound of a galloping horse, usually due to the presence of a third or a fourth heart sound, or both. Hence, diastolic gallop (lub-dup-ah), heard when there is a third heart sound; systolic gallop (ah-lub-dup), heard when there is a fourth heart sound.

Because each of the normal heart sounds represents the action of two valves, either sound may be split (heard as two distinct sounds) if the valves do not work in perfect synchrony.

Besides the normal heart tones, auscultation can reveal any of the following **abnormal sounds**:

Murmur: An abnormal sound, synchronous with the heartbeat, due to flow of blood through a valve or other passage in the heart. Murmurs are distinguished as to sound quality (for example, harsh, blowing, or high-pitched); timing (for example, systolic, mid-systolic, late diastolic, holosystolic = lasting throughout systole); loudness (graded from 1 to

4 in one system, and from 1 to 6 in another; 1/6 = grade 1 on a scale of 1 to 6, a barely audible murmur); where best heard (for example, left sternal border, aortic valve area); radiation (audibility of murmur in areas other than where it is best heard; for example, to cardiac apex, carotid arteries, left axilla); effect of position (squatting, standing, recumbency); and effect of respiratory movements (inspiration, expiration, breath-holding, Valsalva maneuver).

Snap, click: Abnormal valve sounds may be so designated.

Pericardial friction rub: A grating or creaking sound synchronous with heartbeat, due to friction between the surface of the heart and an inflamed pericardium.

Bruit: A humming or buzzing sound, detectable by auscultation, that is caused by the passage of blood through an artery (such as a carotid artery) whose caliber has been narrowed by arteriosclerosis, or through an abnormal vascular communication such as an arteriovenous fistula.

Palpation of the Chest

The examiner can learn something about the size and function of the heart by palpating the precordial chest wall.

Point of maximal intensity (PMI): The point on the chest wall where the impulse of the beating heart is most distinctly felt by the examiner's fingers. If the heart is enlarged, the PMI may be displaced downward or to the left from its normal location.

Precordial shock: An abnormally strong thrust applied to the chest wall by the beating heart, as detected by the examiner's fingers.

Thrill: An abnormal sensation felt by the examiner over the heart when blood jets through an anomalous orifice or narrowed valve.

Chest x-ray shows the size and shape of the heart and great vessels (venae cavae, aorta) and can detect pulmonary vascular congestion, pleural and pericardial effusions, abnormal calcifications, and other clues to cardiovascular disease.

Electrocardiography is the measurement and recording of the electrical activity of the heart. Electrodes placed at standard sites on the chest and extremities gather data that are then combined and processed by the instrument (electrocardiograph) to produce a linear tracing (electrocardiogram, ECG) on a strip of paper. The electrocardiogram permits precise determination of heart rate and rhythm, and can detect abnormalities of cardiac size, shape, conduction, and function as well as ischemia or infarction. (See Figure 6.)

Ambulatory (Holter) monitoring: Continuous recording of the ECG for 24 hours or longer by means of a miniaturized ECG machine and recording apparatus worn by the patient. Holter monitoring makes it possible to detect and analyze transitory and unpredictable periods of arrhythmia or ischemia.

Echocardiography: A form of ultrasound examination designed to provide information about the structure and function of the heart chambers and valves and adjacent structures. Doppler echocardiography: a modification in which ultrasound waves are bounced off flowing blood, whose velocity can then be calculated from the change in the frequency of the waves.

Stress testing: A standardized assessment of the effect of stress on cardiac function and myocardial perfusion. Stress may be induced by physical exercise on a motorized treadmill or bicycle ergometer, or by injection of a drug. Testing includes monitoring of pulse rate, blood pressure, and electrocardiogram before, during, and after the stress. Measurement of oxygen consumption, echocardiography, nuclear imaging, and cardiac catheterization may also be carried out during the testing period.

Angiography: Any imaging study of arteries involving injection of contrast medium into the circulation. Cineangiography is a recording of an angiographic examination on videotape.

Cardiac catheterization: Passage of a flexible catheter through a peripheral blood vessel and into the heart. Catheterization permits the measurement of pressures in the cardiac chambers, assessment of valve function, detection of septal defects and abnormal shunts, and sampling of blood for determination of oxygen concentration. Catheterization of a brachial or femoral vein allows passage of the catheter, in the direction of blood flow, into the right atrium and right ventricle. If equipped with a balloon tip (Swan-Ganz), the catheter may be further advanced into a pulmonary artery for determination of pulmonary artery pressure and pulmonary capillary wedge pressure (PCWP). Central venous pressure (CVP), valuable in assessment of shock, involves placement of a catheter in a major vein without advancement into the right heart. Catheterization of a peripheral artery (brachial or femoral) allows passage of the catheter, against the direction of blood flow, into the left ventricle.

Nuclear imaging involves injection of radioactive materials into the circulation and recording of its distribution with a gamma camera. A variety of techniques are in use to assess the adequacy of coronary circulation, the contracting ability of the myocardium, and the possibility of areas of necrosis or infarction.

CONGENITAL HEART DISEASE

A large and various group of structural abnormalities present at birth and involving the heart chambers, valves, associated great vessels, or some combination of these. Congenital heart disease can be genetically determined, or can result from interference with normal embryonic development by intrauterine exposure to maternal infections, medicines, drugs of abuse, or toxins. It can occur as an isolated problem or be part of a more extensive failure of normal development.

Some congenital heart disorders are incompatible with life; others cause few or no symptoms. Congenital heart diseases are divided into two large classes: cyanotic, causing obvious impairment of oxygenation of the blood in early life; and acyanotic, with delayed or absent symptoms. Cyanotic heart disease is a specialized topic within pediatric cardiology. Only a few types of acyanotic congenital heart disease can be discussed here.

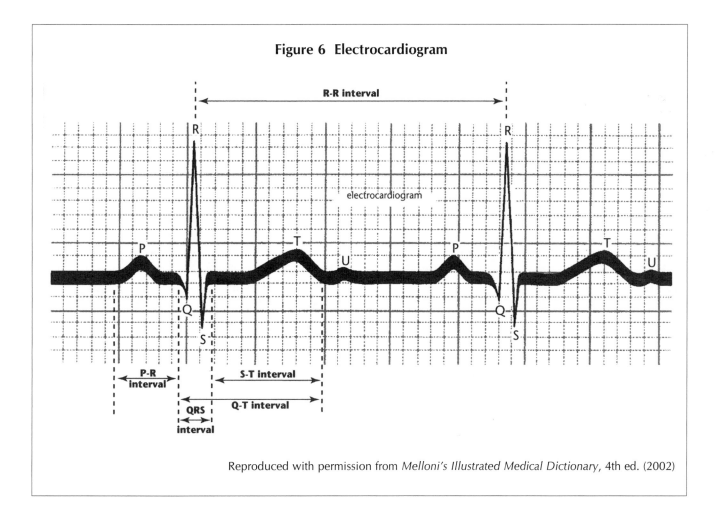

Figure 6 Electrocardiogram

Reproduced with permission from *Melloni's Illustrated Medical Dictionary*, 4th ed. (2002)

Coarctation of the Aorta

Narrowing of the aortic arch, just beyond the origin of the left subclavian artery, often associated with abnormality of the aortic valve.

History: Usually no symptoms until evidence of cardiac failure or consequences of hypertension become evident.

Physical Examination: Arterial pulses prominent in the neck, weak or absent in the lower extremities. Blood pressure elevated in the arms, normal or low in the legs. A systolic murmur at the site of narrowing.

Diagnostic Tests: Chest x-ray may show left ventricular hypertrophy (LVH) and notching of ribs by dilated collateral vessels. Electrocardiogram confirms LVH. Cardiac catheterization shows the pressure differential across the narrowing, and aortography depicts the narrowing.

Course: Congestive heart failure, early death due to hypertension, aortic rupture, or endocarditis.

Treatment: Surgical correction of the narrowing. Balloon dilatation is sometimes successful.

Patent Ductus Arteriosus (PDA)

Persistence of the fetal communication between the aorta and the pulmonary artery, which shunts blood around the (unexpanded and nonfunctioning) lungs until birth; clinical significance depends on the amount of shunting that persists after birth.

History: No symptoms, or symptoms only with development of left ventricular hypertrophy or failure.

Physical Examination: Widened pulse pressure, reduced diastolic pressure. Accentuated second heart sound; continuous "machinery" murmur along the left sternal border.

Diagnostic Tests: Chest x-ray may be normal or may show left ventricular hypertrophy and dilatation of the pulmonary and aortic silhouettes. ECG may show left ventricular hypertrophy.

Course: Depends on shunt size; may be benign or lead to heart failure.

Treatment: Intravenous indomethacin may induce closure of the ductus in infancy. Surgical ligation is effective; placement of a plug by catheter may be successful.

Atrial Septal Defect

Persistence of an opening through the interatrial septum (the wall between the right and left atria) after birth. Like the ductus arteriosus mentioned above, an opening between the atria permits the heart to function during fetal life even though full circulation through the pulmonary arteries and veins cannot occur until the lungs expand after birth. The defect may appear at various sites on the septum and may be associated with valvular anomalies. Symptoms and prognosis depend on the size of the shunt.

History: There may be few or no symptoms unless pulmonary hypertension or right ventricular failure occurs.

Physical Examination: Right ventricular pulsations may be prominent, with a right ventricular heave. A systolic murmur is heard at the left sternal border.

Diagnostic Tests: Chest x-ray may show right ventricular dilatation and prominence of pulmonary vasculature. ECG, echo Doppler, radionuclide studies, MRI, and especially cardiac catheterization confirm the diagnosis and measure the degree of cardiovascular functional impairment.

Course: No serious problems with small shunts. Large shunts may lead to pulmonary hypertension, cardiac arrhythmias, and heart failure in middle age.

Treatment: Surgical closure of the shunt, if necessary.

Ventricular Septal Defect (VSD)

Persistent communication between the right and left ventricle after birth, with shunting of blood from left to right. Symptoms, signs, and prognosis depend on the extent of the shunt.

History: There may be no symptoms unless pulmonary hypertension or right ventricular failure occurs.

Physical Examination: A precordial thrill and a holosystolic murmur heard along the left sternal border. Chest x-ray may show hypertrophy of one or both ventricles and increased pulmonary vascular markings. More precise and quantitative information may be provided by MRI, radionuclide scanning, and cardiac catheterization.

Course: The defect may close spontaneously. Progressive strain on the right and left ventricles may lead to cardiac failure; endocarditis may occur at the site of defect.

Treatment: Surgical closure, if necessary.

VALVULAR HEART DISEASE

Structural abnormality of one or more heart valves may be either congenital or acquired. Valvular defects consist of stenosis (abnormal narrowing of the valve opening), insufficiency (failure of the valve to prevent backflow during systole), or both.

Valvular stenosis causes reduction in the volume of blood ejected from the involved chamber when it contracts, and usually an audible murmur. Valvular insufficiency causes regurgitation of blood through the valve during diastole of the chamber involved, and usually an audible murmur. Either stenosis or insufficiency places an abnormal strain on the chamber affected, with the risk of dilatation and cardiac failure.

Cardiac catheterization is the definitive procedure for diagnosing valvular disease and measuring pressure gradients across defective valves at various points in the cardiac cycle. This discussion is limited to the most common types of valvular disease.

Mitral Stenosis

Abnormal narrowing of the mitral valve (between the left atrium and left ventricle).

Cause: Most cases are residuals of acute rheumatic fever, which is usually a childhood disease. Symptoms of mitral stenosis typically do not appear until the 30s or 40s.

History: Dyspnea, orthopnea, paroxysmal nocturnal dyspnea, fatigue, chronic cough, hemoptysis.

Physical Examination: The first heart sound at the mitral area (Ml) is accentuated. Early in (ventricular) diastole, a mitral opening snap may be heard, followed by an evanescent mid-diastolic rumble produced by passage of blood through the stenotic valve during left atrial systole.

Diagnostic Tests: Echocardiography and cardiac catheterization yield precise diagnostic information.

Course: Eventually, right ventricular failure. Atrial fibrillation frequently occurs, with risk of systemic arterial embolism.

Treatment: Supportive. Digitalis or other antiarrhythmic agents for atrial fibrillation, and anticoagulant to prevent arterial emboli. For severe disease, surgical commissurotomy (cutting of stenotic valve leaflets), balloon dilatation, or valve replacement.

Mitral Valve Prolapse

Abnormal bulging of mitral valve leaflets into the left atrium during left ventricular systole, due to structurally abnormal (floppy or billowing) valve leaflets.

Causes: May be inherited as an autosomal dominant trait. Often occurs in conjunction with other connective tissue abnormalities, particularly Marfan syndrome. Occurs in 1-5% of the general population, and is seen principally in women.

History: Usually there are no symptoms. A few patients experience nonspecific chest pain, palpitations with or without actual arrhythmia, dyspnea on exertion, fatigue, and syncope.

Physical Examination: Variable murmurs: usually midsystolic click and late systolic murmur. The patient may present other stigmata of connective tissue abnormality: thin body habitus, high palate, deformities of the chest wall (pectus excavatum, scoliosis).

Diagnostic Studies: Echocardiography confirms valve prolapse and indicates whether actual regurgitation occurs.

Course: Most patients have no symptoms and no complications. Rarely regurgitation may have serious hemodynamic consequences. Endocarditis may develop on the mitral valve. Atrial fibrillation may occur. Sudden death may result from ectopic ventricular rhythms (ventricular tachycardia).

Treatment: Antibiotic prophylaxis of endocarditis before dental work and surgery. Beta-blockers usually control chest pain and arrhythmias. Rarely, surgical valve replacement.

Aortic Stenosis

Abnormal narrowing of the aortic valve opening, with reduction of left ventricular ejection volume during systole.

Causes: May be a consequence of acute rheumatic fever, but usually results from calcification of the valve with aging. Most patients are men over 50.

History: Weakness, dyspnea, chest pain, palpitations, syncope.

Physical Examination: Carotid pulsations are reduced. A precordial thrill may be noted. The second heart sound is reduced or absent. A harsh "diamond-shaped" (crescendo-decrescendo) murmur is heard at the base of the heart and transmitted to the carotids and cardiac apex.

Diagnostic Tests: Chest x-ray may show left ventricular dilatation and calcification of the aortic valve. Electrocardiogram, Doppler echocardiogram, and cardiac catheterization provide more precise and quantitative information.

Course: Left ventricular failure, arrhythmias, angina, syncope.

Treatment: Surgical replacement of the valve. Balloon dilatation of the valve may be successful.

ENDOCARDITIS

Inflammation of the lining membrane of the heart (endocardium), particularly over cardiac valves, due to infection or as a complication of systemic disease (acute rheumatic fever, systemic lupus erythematosus). Only infective endocarditis will be discussed here.

Infective Endocarditis (Acute and Subacute Bacterial Endocarditis)

Bacterial infection of one or more heart valves.

Cause: Usually, the combination of pre-existing congenital or acquired valvular disease or abnormal communications (septal defects) and bacteremia (after dental or surgical procedures or in systemic infection or septicemia).

History: Fever, chills, dyspnea, cough, abdominal pain, muscle or joint pain.

Physical Examination: Fever, pallor. Audible cardiac murmur, or change in quality or loudness of a pre-existing murmur. Signs of peripheral embolization of infective material (vegetations) from heart valves: petechiae of the palate and conjunctivae, splinter hemorrhages under fingernails, Osler nodes (tender purplish lumps in fingers, toes), Janeway spots (painless red spots of palms and soles), Roth spots (retinal exudates). Splenomegaly.

Diagnostic Tests: Anemia, leukocytosis, hematuria, proteinuria. Blood cultures may permit identification of the organism. Chest x-ray, electrocardiogram, echocardiogram supply diagnostic information.

Course: Valve leaflets may ulcerate and slough, with severe impairment of cardiac function. Fragments of infectious material (septic emboli) may be carried to brain, heart, kidney, and other tissues, or to the lung, causing local infective vascular lesions (mycotic aneurysms).

Treatment: Intravenous antibiotics for several weeks. Surgery may be undertaken in very severe cases.

CARDIAC ARRHYTHMIAS AND CONDUCTION DEFECTS

Disturbance of the rate or rhythm of cardiac action due to abnormalities in the structure or function of the heart. Note the following terms pertaining to abnormalities of cardiac rate and rhythm:

Arrhythmia: Irregular rhythm of the heartbeat, with or without an abnormally slow or fast rate.

Bradyarrhythmia: A pulse that is both irregular and abnormally slow.

Bradycardia: Abnormal slowness of the heartbeat (pulse less than 60/min).

Tachyarrhythmia: A pulse that is both irregular and abnormally rapid.

Tachycardia: Rapid heart rate (over 100/min at rest).

The following is a useful classification of cardiac arrhythmias:

Disorders of Impulse Formation
- Failure of impulse formation (asystole).
- Ectopic focus (stimulus for heartbeat comes from an irritable or diseased zone of tissue rather than the normal pacemaker).
  - Supraventricular: (abnormal pacemaker in atrium):
    - Atrial fibrillation
    - Paroxysmal atrial tachycardia
  - Nodal: (pacemaker is in atrioventricular node)
  - Ventricular: (abnormal pacemaker in ventricle)
    - Ventricular tachycardia
    - Ventricular fibrillation

Disorders of Impulse Transmission
- Atrioventricular (AV) block (block between atria and ventricles)
  - First-degree block: delayed conduction, but all impulses get through.
  - Second-degree block: some impulses not conducted.
  - Third-degree block: no impulses transmitted.

- Bundle branch blocks (blockage in right or left bundle branch).
- Circus movement, reentry: Wolff-Parkinson-White syndrome.

Causes: Congenital anomalies in the impulse-forming or conducting system of the heart; coronary artery disease, including myocardial infarction, with ischemia of parts of the system; alcohol, tobacco, or drugs.

History: Intermittent or continuous palpitation, a sense of rapid, irregular, or violent heart action, dyspnea, heaviness in the chest, lightheadedness, syncope, diuresis.

Physical Examination: The pulse may be abnormally fast or slow, or irregular. The blood pressure is often below normal. Cardiac auscultation reveals irregularity in the rhythm or force of contractions, and there may be a difference between the apical and radial pulse rates (pulse deficit). Examination may disclose evidence of underlying or concomitant cardiac disease.

Diagnostic Tests: Electrocardiography delineates abnormalities of cardiac impulse formation, conduction, rhythm, and rate. Holter monitoring (ambulatory electrocardiography) may be useful in recording transitory arrhythmias. Electrophysiologic studies can often pinpoint the location and nature of electrical abnormalities.

Course: Risk of embolization from atrial fibrillation. Hemodynamic impairment may be mild or lethal.

Treatment: Correction of any underlying cardiac disorder and elimination of contributing factors (alcohol abuse, cigarette smoking, drug use or abuse) may suffice to correct a rhythm problem. Digitalis and calcium-channel blockers are used to treat supraventricular tachyarrhythmias. Ventricular arrhythmias are treated with quinidine, lidocaine, and other drugs related to local anesthetics. Ventricular fibrillation is treated with electric shock (defibrillation). Abnormal circuits in the conduction system (as in Wolff-Parkinson-White syndrome) can be interrupted with electrical or radiofrequency ablation. Complete heart block and other severe disorders of impulse formation are treated with a transvenous or implanted pacemaker.

CORONARY ARTERY DISEASE (ARTERIOSCLEROTIC HEART DISEASE, ISCHEMIC HEART DISEASE)

Angina Pectoris

Paroxysmal chest pain due to myocardial ischemia, without permanent damage to heart muscle.

Cause: The primary cause is narrowing of one or more coronary arteries by arteriosclerosis. Arteritis, congenital vascular anomalies, emboli, severe anemia, cardiac hypertrophy, and cocaine intoxication can also lead to signs and symptoms of inadequate coronary blood flow. Risk factors for development of coronary arteriosclerosis include a family history of the disease, male gender, hypertension, cigarette smoking, diabetes mellitus, overweight, a sedentary lifestyle, and elevation of total cholesterol, LDL cholesterol, homocysteine, lipoprotein(a), or C-reactive protein.

History: Angina pectoris is a syndrome of anterior chest pain coming on abruptly and resolving spontaneously in less than 30 minutes. Pain is typically precipitated by physical exertion, strong emotion, exposure to cold, or eating a meal, and is relieved by rest or by taking nitroglycerin. The pain is described as a tightness, squeezing, or pressure; the patient often expresses this by holding a clenched fist in front of the chest. The pain may radiate into the neck, jaw, or arm, particularly the left. A variant, Prinzmetal angina, occurs at rest and is more common in women and younger patients than typical angina.

Physical Examination: There may be no abnormal findings, but the blood pressure is often elevated by pain and anxiety. Examination may disclose signs of underlying cardiovascular or systemic disease.

Diagnostic Tests: The electrocardiogram may be normal during an attack, but usually shows ST segment depression and flattened or inverted T waves, indicating myocardial ischemia. There may also be evidence of conduction defects or ventricular hypertrophy. Holter monitoring allows recording of the ECG continuously for 24 hours. Stress testing records the electrocardiogram during standardized and closely supervised physical exertion. Angiography demonstrates narrowing of coronary vessels. Other studies (myocardial perfusion scintigraphy, radionuclide angiography, and echocardiography) can supply further information about the location and extent of coronary disease.

Course: Gradual progression to more severe disease (myocardial infarction, congestive heart failure) usually occurs, even with treatment. Unstable angina, which worsens with time despite treatment, has a less favorable prognosis.

Treatment: The standard treatment for an anginal attack is nitroglycerin sublingually (under the tongue), which promptly abolishes pain of coronary ischemia by producing dilatation in the coronary arteries. Nitroglycerin can also be taken prophylactically before physical exertion. Longer-acting nitrate preparations, beta-blocking agents, and calcium-channel blockers taken regularly can prevent or mitigate attacks. Most patients are advised to take aspirin daily for its effect in inhibiting platelet aggregation and reducing the risk of myocardial infarction. Coronary artery bypass graft (CABG) uses veins or other materials to conduct blood past narrowed places in coronary arteries. Percutaneous transluminal coronary angioplasty (PTCA, balloon angioplasty) dilates narrowed places with a balloon passed into the circulation through an arterial catheter.

Myocardial Infarction (Heart Attack, Coronary Thrombosis)

Damage to a segment of heart muscle by severe impairment of coronary blood flow.

Causes: The underlying causes are the same as for angina pectoris. Myocardial infarction is usually due to thrombosis in a coronary artery already narrowed by arteriosclerosis. Arteritis, vasospasm, embolism, sudden hypotension, or cocaine can also precipitate infarction.

History: Anterior chest pain, similar to angina but generally more severe and lasting more than 30 minutes. Pain often comes on at rest and is not relieved by nitroglycerin. Typically, men experience sweating, weakness, restlessness, shortness of breath, and nausea. Women may experience the same symptoms or may perceive jaw or shoulder discomfort and/or chest tightness or discomfort without actual crushing pain. Rarely, infarction occurs without pain (silent infarction).

Physical Examination: The pulse and blood pressure may be increased, normal, or decreased. Mild fever often develops after the first 12 hours. The heart sounds may be soft or distant. An atrial gallop (fourth heart sound) is often heard. A seagull murmur of mitral regurgitation indicates rupture of a papillary muscle. The cardiac rhythm may be abnormal. A pericardial friction rub is often heard. Jugular venous distention and rales of pulmonary edema are seen in heart failure.

Diagnostic Tests: The electrocardiogram shows ST segment elevation (changing later to depression) and inversion of T waves in leads pertaining to the area of infarction. Q waves indicate severe myocardial damage and a graver prognosis. The white blood cell count may be slightly elevated. Serial determination of the serum levels of the cardiac enzymes LDH (lactic dehydrogenase), CK-MB (the MB isoenzyme of creatine kinase), myoglobin, and troponins (C, I, and T) show characteristic rises. Fluoroscopy or other imaging techniques may show segmental wall motion at the site of infarction. Scintigraphy with technetium-99m pyrophosphate shows a hot spot at the site. Doppler echocardiography may also confirm the extent and location of infarction.

Course: About 20% of persons who sustain myocardial infarction die before reaching a hospital. With intensive therapy, the prognosis for the other 80% is good. During the acute phase, arrhythmia, shock, and congestive heart failure are serious possibilities. Other dangerous complications include rupture of a papillary muscle (one of the muscles in the ventricles that control movements of the mitral and tricuspid valves) with resulting serious valvular malfunction, cardiorrhexis (bursting of a ventricle), left ventricular aneurysm (extreme dilatation and thinning of the ventricle, with loss of contractile power), pericarditis, and formation of a mural thrombus (a localized clot adjacent to the infarcted area of ventricular wall).

Treatment: The standard treatment protocol includes hospitalization, administration of oxygen by inhalation and of narcotics for pain relief by injection, and continuous electrocardiographic monitoring. Thrombolytic agents (tissue plasminogen activator, streptokinase, or anistreplase) are administered intravenously to dissolve clots. Anticoagulants (aspirin, IV heparin) may also be administered. Beta-blocking agents are started early. In some centers, balloon angioplasty is performed during the acute phase of myocardial infarction.

DISORDERS OF CARDIAC (MYOCARDIAL) FUNCTION

Myocarditis

Local or generalized inflammation of heart muscle (myocardium).

Causes: Infection, drugs, chemical or biological toxins, autoimmune disorders. Infectious myocarditis may be due to viruses (coxsackievirus, Rocky Mountain spotted fever, HIV), parasites (Chagas disease, toxoplasmosis, trichinosis), or other organisms. Onset often follows an upper respiratory infection.

History: Chest pain, dyspnea, fatigue, palpitation.

Physical Examination: Tachycardia, sometimes gallop rhythm.

Diagnostic Tests: Chest x-ray shows cardiac dilatation. Electrocardiogram may indicate nonspecific electrical abnormalities. Scintigraphy and myocardial biopsy may provide more specific indications. Testing for antibodies in serum may identify a causative organism.

Course: Complete resolution often occurs spontaneously, but in other cases there is progressive deterioration of cardiac function and eventual circulatory failure.

Treatment: Largely supportive and symptomatic. Specific antimicrobial treatment may be available. Immunosuppressive agents may be used in autoimmune myocarditis. Heart transplant in end-stage (terminal) disease.

Congestive Heart Failure

A syndrome of impaired hemodynamics due to inability of the heart to maintain normal circulation.

Causes: Any condition that impairs the contractile force of the heart (ischemia due to coronary artery disease; myocarditis) or that overtaxes a normal heart (systemic or pulmonary hypertension, congenital or acquired valvular disease, hyperthyroidism). Right ventricular failure may be due to pulmonary hypertension or cor pulmonale. A distinction is sometimes made between forward failure (inability of the heart to pump blood at a volume that is adequate for the needs of tissues) and backward failure (inability of the heart to distend adequately during diastole, with resulting increase of pressure in the venous system). Purely mechanical inadequacy of heart function is complicated by inappropriate hormonal and biochemical responses,

including increase of peripheral vascular resistance due to sympathetic vasoconstriction and retention of sodium and water due to release of renin from kidneys whose blood flow is diminished.

History: Shortness of breath, particularly on exertion; orthopnea, paroxysmal nocturnal dyspnea, cough; fatigue, nocturia; anorexia and right upper quadrant fullness due to hepatic engorgement; ankle edema.

Physical Examination: Dyspnea, cyanosis, tachycardia, hypotension. Jugular venous distention. Left ventricular dilatation and hypertrophy. Diminished first heart sound. S3 gallop. Expiratory wheezes and rhonchi. Crepitant rales at bases; reduced breath sounds and dullness to percussion may indicate pleural effusion. Hepatomegaly, hepatojugular reflux (bulging of jugular veins when the liver is compressed, because of increased pressure in the venous system). Pitting edema of the lower extremities, ascites.

Diagnostic Tests: The red blood cell count may be diminished. The electrocardiogram may indicate myocardial infarction, arrhythmia, or left ventricular hypertrophy. Echocardiography gives more precise information about ventricular size and function. Chest x-ray shows cardiomegaly, signs of pulmonary venous congestion (fine lines at the periphery of the lungs due to edema of pulmonary alveolar septa, called Kerley B lines), and sometimes pleural effusion. Radionuclide angiography shows that the ventricular ejection fraction (the fraction of the blood contained in the ventricle that is expelled during systole) is reduced.

Course: Congestive heart failure indicates a serious impairment of cardiovascular dynamics, and even with treatment the course is often steadily downhill. The prognosis for long-term survival is poor, and death often occurs suddenly.

Treatment: Rest, salt restriction, and early correction of identifiable precipitating factors. Diuretics (thiazides, loop diuretics, potassium-sparing diuretics), ACE inhibitors, and beta-blockers are used to reverse biochemical imbalances and hormonal effects that lead to sodium retention and circulatory volume overload.

Acute Pulmonary Edema

An extreme form of left ventricular failure in which respiratory symptoms predominate. It can be precipitated by acute myocardial infarction or by any factors that increase the severity of existing cardiac failure. There are severe dyspnea, cough, and wheezing, with frothy pink sputum. The pulse is rapid and weak, the lips and nail beds cyanotic. Auscultation reveals rales and rhonchi in the lungs. The arterial oxygen is low. Chest x-ray shows cardiomegaly, increased vascular markings, Kerley B lines, pleural effusion. Treatment includes oxygen by inhalation, morphine, and intravenous diuretics.

PERICARDITIS

Inflammation of the pericardium. Acute pericarditis can result from numerous causes but is often idiopathic. In pericarditis with effusion, fluid within the pericardium threatens to impair cardiac function. Constrictive pericarditis is scarring or calcification of the pericardium as a late consequence of inflammation, with the risk of hemodynamic compromise. Only the first two will be discussed here.

Acute Pericarditis

Causes: Often occurs after a viral respiratory infection. Frequently the exact cause cannot be determined. Infection can spread from the lungs or pleura in bacterial pneumonia and pulmonary tuberculosis. Pericarditis may complicate acute myocardial infarction. Systemic diseases that can cause pericarditis include acute rheumatic fever, systemic lupus erythematosus, uremia, malignancy, and myxedema. Exposure to radiation and certain drugs and toxins can also cause pericarditis.

History: The onset is often sudden. Sharp, dull, or intermittent anterior chest pain, aggravated by coughing or deep inspiration and relieved by sitting up or leaning forward. Fever. Dyspnea, weakness.

Physical Examination: Fever, tachycardia. A pericardial friction rub, often faint, transitory, or changing, may be heard along the left sternal border with the patient leaning forward.

Diagnostic Tests: The white blood cell count is elevated. The ECG shows widespread elevation of ST segments; later sometimes flattening or inversion of T waves.

Course: Spontaneous resolution usually occurs in 1-3 weeks. Recurrences are common after recovery.

Treatment: Rest and supportive therapy. Aspirin may be prescribed to combat pain; in severe cases, adrenal steroids. The underlying disease must be treated as well.

Pericarditis with Effusion

Causes: Same as for acute pericarditis.

History: In addition to symptoms of pericarditis, other symptoms include severe dyspnea, orthopnea, palpitations, cough, and difficulty swallowing.

Physical Examination: Pallor, diaphoresis, tachycardia, hypotension, pulsus paradoxus (drop in systolic blood pressure of 10 mm or more during inspiration), distention of neck veins. Heart tones distant, cardiac borders indistinct on percussion.

Diagnostic Tests: Chest x-ray and MRI confirm the effusion. The electrocardiogram shows reduced voltage and sometimes T wave inversion.

Course: Spontaneous resolution may occur. A large effusion carries the risk of cardiac tamponade (compression of the heart chambers, with failure of circulatory function).

Treatment: With a substantial effusion, pericardiocentesis (puncture of the pericardium with a needle or catheter and withdrawal of fluid). Any underlying disease must be treated.

DISORDERS OF BLOOD PRESSURE: SHOCK AND HYPERTENSION

Shock

A condition in which the systemic blood pressure is too low to maintain adequate tissue perfusion.

Causes: Hypovolemia (reduced blood volume due to hemorrhage, dehydration, severe burns, ascites); cardiogenic (impairment of cardiac function by arrhythmia, myocardial infarction, myocarditis, acute valvular failure); vascular obstruction (pericardial tamponade, pulmonary embolism); dilatation of the circulatory system (septic shock, anaphylactic shock, toxic shock syndrome, neurogenic shock, drugs).

History: Weakness, palpitations, thirst, sweating, anxiety, loss of consciousness.

Physical Examination: The blood pressure is low and the pulse rapid. Peripheral pulses are weak or absent. The tilt test is positive (rise in pulse and drop in blood pressure when patient is moved from recumbent to erect position). In hypovolemic shock the skin is pale, cold, and clammy. In septic shock there may be high fever and flushing. Agitation, confusion, and deteriorating level of consciousness.

Diagnostic Tests: Procedures used during early treatment to assess the degree of shock include blood tests (complete blood count, electrolytes, arterial blood gases), measurement of urine flow, cardiac monitoring, and central venous pressure or pulmonary wedge pressure with Swan-Ganz catheter.

Course: Without treatment shock may lead to irreversible damage: cerebral ischemia and infarction, myocardial infarction, renal failure.

Treatment: Vigorous treatment is required to maintain tissue perfusion and prevent irreversible consequences. The patient is placed in the Trendelenburg position (head lower than feet), and oxygen is administered. Morphine sulfate is given for pain (unless there is respiratory depression or head injury). Volume replacement with blood, plasma, or artificial plasma expanders in hypovolemic shock. Treatment of underlying conditions. Compression of the arms, legs, and abdomen by an inflatable garment (military antishock trousers, MAST) can maintain cerebral, coronary, and renal blood flow until bleeding or other underlying condition is controlled and blood volume restored. Dopamine, adrenal steroids, and other drugs may be administered.

Hypertension

Sustained elevation of arterial blood pressure above 140 mmHg systolic or 90 mmHg diastolic.

Cause: Unknown in more than 90% of cases, which are thus called essential hypertension. Essential hypertension shows a genetic pattern, running in families and being much commoner in African-Americans. Its development may depend on environmental factors, excessive dietary salt, sodium retention by the kidney, abnormalities of the renin-angiotensin system, obesity, alcohol abuse, and use of NSAIDs. Secondary hypertension is due to a demonstrable cause: renal parenchymal disease, renal ischemia, Cushing disease, primary aldosteronism, pheochromocytoma, or estrogen use in the form of oral contraceptives.

History: There may be no symptoms until complications develop.

Physical Examination: Elevated blood pressure and accentuation of the second heart sound at the aortic valve area; otherwise there may be no findings. Retinopathy is indicated by detection of Keith-Wagener-Barker changes on ophthalmoscopic examination. Left ventricular hypertrophy may be indicated by precordial heave or by a systolic ejection murmur.

Diagnostic Tests: Laboratory studies may be normal. The search for a cause of secondary hypertension includes testing blood and urine for signs of renal disease. In pheochromocytoma, a tumor of the adrenal medulla that raises blood pressure by secreting epinephrine and norepinephrine, urine levels of catecholamines and vanillylmandelic acid (VMA). In malignant carcinoid syndrome, in which hypertension is due to serotonin secreted by one or more neoplasms, the urine level of 5-hydroxy-indoleacetic acid (5-HIAA) is elevated.

Course: Some hypertensive patients experience a return of blood pressure to normal after a few weeks, months, or years. In most, however, elevation of blood pressure remains throughout life. Hypertension causes several forms of damage to the cardiovascular system (hypertensive cardiovascular disease), including left ventricular hypertrophy and dysfunction, arteriosclerosis, dilatation and dissecting aneurysm of the aorta, hypertensive encephalopathy, and hypertensive renal disease. In accelerated or malignant hypertension there is sustained high blood pressure responding poorly to treatment, and rapid progression of cardiovascular damage.

Treatment: Therapy of essential hypertension ideally includes lifestyle modification (reduction of alcohol intake, increased physical exercise), restriction of dietary salt, and control of overweight. Drug therapy is tailored to the severity of the disease, and typically starts with a single drug (a thiazide diuretic or a beta-blocker), others being added as needed: ACE inhibitors, angiotensin II receptor inhibitors, calcium channel blockers, methyldopa, alpha-receptor antagonists, and drugs of other classes.

PERIPHERAL ARTERIAL DISEASE

Atherosclerosis

Hardening and even calcification of arterial walls, with narrowing of their lumens.

Cause: Degeneration of arterial walls, with diffuse or plaque-like deposition of cholesterol crystals in the tunica intima (inner lining) of systemic arteries. Various inborn metabolic abnormalities in lipoproteins may predispose to abnormal elevation of serum cholesterol level and abnormal deposition of cholesterol in arterial walls. (Involvement of coronary and cerebral arteries in the same process is a principal cause of coronary artery disease and cerebral vascular disease.)

History: Intermittent claudication: cramping muscle pain in calves, thighs, buttocks (depending on site of arterial obstruction) that is brought on by walking and relieved by rest. Erectile dysfunction.

Physical Examination: Weakness or absence of femoral, popliteal, or pedal pulses. Bruit over aorta, iliac or femoral arteries. Trophic changes (loss of hair, thinning of skin, pigmentation).

Diagnostic Tests: Evidence of reduced blood flow can be obtained by Doppler ultrasonography, transcutaneous oximetry, or other measures.

Treatment: Physical therapy and treatment with cilostazol, pentoxifylline, or other agents may improve blood flow and exercise tolerance slightly. Surgical treatment (endarterectomy or arterial grafting) yields much better results. Percutaneous transluminal angioplasty (balloon dilatation) is effective in selected cases.

Aneurysm

A local dilatation of an artery due to congenital anomaly, degenerative disease, or trauma.

Aneurysm in a systemic artery can produce local swelling and pain with reduction of distal blood flow, manifested by pallor, cyanosis, pain, numbness, or intermittent claudication. Treatment is by surgical excision and insertion of a graft. Aortic aneurysm usually results from degenerative disease; surgical grafting is performed to avoid aortic rupture, which can be rapidly fatal.

Dissecting Aneurysm

Burrowing of blood between layers of the aorta.

Cause: Hypertension and abnormality or degeneration of the aorta (as in Marfan syndrome).

History: Sudden onset of severe chest pain radiating to the back, abdomen, or extremities; weakness, paralysis, collapse.

Physical Examination: The blood pressure is elevated despite clinical appearances of shock. Peripheral pulses are reduced or unequal. There may be loss of reflexes in the extremities.

Diagnostic Tests: Electrocardiogram may show left ventricular hypertrophy as a reflection of chronic hypertensive cardiovascular disease. Chest x-ray may show an abnormal aortic silhouette. CT scan, MRI, and angiography can provide more specific information.

Course: About 20% of patients die within the first 24 hours. More than 90% will eventually die without treatment.

Treatment: Reduction of blood pressure with IV nitroprusside, beta-blockers, or other agents, followed by surgical repair of the dissection.

Raynaud Phenomenon

A vasomotor disorder of the circulation affecting principally the fingers.

Causes: Various connective tissue disorders (rheumatoid arthritis, CREST syndrome, systemic lupus erythematosus), drugs. When no underlying cause can be found, the disorder is called Raynaud disease. Most patients are young women.

History: Sudden attacks of pallor, coldness, numbness, stiffness, and pain in 1-8 fingers, precipitated by exposure to cold or emotional upset. The thumbs are rarely involved. Pallor resolves spontaneously after a few minutes, and is succeeded by rebound erythema, warmth, throbbing, and swelling.

Physical Examination: During attacks, pallor and coldness of fingers; at other times, no abnormalities.

Course: Generally benign. When severe, Raynaud phenomenon may lead to atrophy of finger tissue, ulceration, or gangrene.

Treatment: Avoidance of cold exposure. Nifedipine to prevent vasospasm. In severe cases, cervical sympathectomy to block autonomic impulses causing vasospasm.

THROMBOSIS AND EMBOLISM

Thrombosis is the formation of a clot (thrombus) within the circulatory system. Thrombosis is usually due to injury of a blood vessel, prolonged immobilization with reduction of blood flow through a part, increased coagulability of the blood, or some combination of these. Most thrombi of medical importance form in veins of the pelvis and lower extremity. A mural thrombus is a clot adherent to the wall of a heart chamber; this may occur in myocardial infarction or chronic atrial fibrillation. A thrombus may completely obstruct the vessel in which it develops. Eventually most thrombi are reabsorbed and replaced by scar tissue, usually with reestablishment of a passage (recanalization).

While venous obstruction is of some concern in thrombosis, a far greater danger is that of embolization—release of a clot from its point of origin, and travel to a remote site in the circulation where it can obstruct a large capillary zone. An embolus originating in a systemic vein can travel through the right atrium and right ventricle to block a portion of the circulation of a lung (pulmonary embolism, discussed in Chapter 10). An embolus released into the systemic arterial system from the left atrium or left ventricle can block the blood supply to part of the brain, kidney, a limb, or any other tissue. Any foreign substance in the circulatory system (air, fat, amniotic fluid, injected material) can act as an embolus.

THROMBOPHLEBITIS

Inflammation in the wall of a vein associated with clotting of blood within the vein. Thrombophlebitis generally affects the superficial or deep veins of the lower extremities.

Superficial Thrombophlebitis

Causes: Local trauma, venous catheter, venous stasis (pregnancy, varicose veins). Rarely, pancreatic carcinoma.

History: Soreness, redness, and swelling along the course of a vein, usually at the site of injury or recent venipuncture.

Physical Examination: Erythema, edema, induration, tenderness along the course of a superficial vein. No edema distal to the site of inflammation.

Diagnostic Tests: Doppler ultrasonography with compression, impedance plethysmography, and contrast venography confirm, localize, and quantify venous obstruction.

Course: Spontaneous resolution generally occurs. There is a very small risk of thrombo-embolism.

Treatment: Elastic wrapping of the leg and thigh, elevation, application of warm compresses, nonsteroidal anti-inflammatory medicines.

Deep Thrombophlebitis

Causes: Congestive heart failure, recent surgery or immobilization, oral contraceptives, malignancy.

History: Pain or tightness in the calf or thigh, with edema distally. There may be no symptoms until pulmonary embolism occurs.

Physical Examination: Distal edema may be the only objective sign. There may be pain or tenderness on calf rocking, or a positive Homans sign (calf pain or tightness on passive dorsiflexion of the foot).

Diagnostic Tests: As for superficial thrombophlebitis; MRI, radionuclide scintigraphy.

Course: There is considerable danger of pulmonary embolism. Healing may be followed by deep venous insufficiency, with chronic edema.

Treatment: Hospitalization. The same measures as for superficial thrombophlebitis. In addition, intravenous or low-dose intramuscular heparin.

QUESTIONS FOR STUDY AND REVIEW

1. Trace the path of a drop of blood from the aorta through the circulatory system and back to its point of origin (using outside research as necessary). How many cardiac chambers did it pass through? How many cardiac valves?

_____

_____

_____

_____

_____

_____

_____

_____

2. Shock and congestive heart failure are both forms of circulatory failure. In what ways are they similar and in what ways different?

_____

_____

_____

_____

_____

_____

3. Define or explain these terms:
   a. arrhythmia
   b. embolism
   c. hypertension
   d. infarction
   e. thrombosis

4. Name three preventable or controllable risk factors for coronary artery disease:

   a. _____

   _____

   b. _____

   _____

   c. _____

   _____

5. Name three noncontrollable risk factors for coronary artery disease:

   a. _____

   b. _____

   c. _____

6. List five potentially serious cardiac disorders in which the pulse rate and rhythm may be normal:

   a. _____

   b. _____

   c. _____

   d. _____

   e. _____

CASE STUDY: YOU'RE THE DOCTOR

Ernest Marks, a 47-year-old white male high school science teacher, is referred to you, a general cardiologist, by his primary care physician because of a history of chest pain. Mr. Marks states that he began having spells of a pressure or squeezing sensation across his chest about 5 months ago. Because these spells often occur after a heavy meal, he attributed them at first to indigestion. But lately he has had similar pain while walking his dog up a long, steep sidewalk near his home. The pain is diffuse, unrelated to swallowing, breathing, or body position, and lasts up to 10 minutes, never longer. Sometimes it goes away within a minute or two. Other times it lasts longer, gets quite severe ("a good solid eight on a scale of one to ten"), and radiates into the jaw and to the area between the shoulder blades. There is no associated shortness of breath or cardiac palpitation, but his skin sometimes feels clammy after the pain goes away.

1. What is the medical term for the symptom complex Mr. Marks is describing?

   _____

   _____

   _____

The review of systems is essentially negative except for pain in the hips and knees attributed by the patient to arthritis and "getting old." He has a mild chronic cough which he attributes to smoking. About 3 years ago he was turned down as a blood donor because of elevated blood pressure, but he never saw his doctor about that. He has smoked about one package of cigarettes and drunk 1-3 beers daily for about the past 20 years. He takes no medicine regularly. His father died of a heart attack at age 56. His mother is living and well except for severe hearing loss at age 71. There is no family history of diabetes mellitus.

2. What risk factors does Mr. Marks have for coronary artery disease?

_____

_____

_____

3. Which of the above risk factors are susceptible to modification?

_____

_____

_____

The patient is a pleasant, voluble, well-groomed man appearing his stated age, normally developed, and about 50 lb overweight, with predominantly truncal obesity. His temperature and pulse are normal, blood pressure 195/104. Pupils are equal and react to light. Funduscopic examination shows narrowing of retinal arterioles but no hemorrhages or exudates. Examination of ears, nose, throat is unremarkable. Carotid pulsations are full and equal, without bruits. The thyroid is not enlarged and there are no cervical masses. The heart tones are somewhat distant; no murmurs, clicks, rubs, or gallop rhythm. The lungs are clear to auscultation. The abdominal examination is unremarkable. There are no renal artery bruits. Neurologic and musculoskeletal exams are normal except for some restricted range of motion in the hip and knee joints. Peripheral pulses are strong and bilaterally equal. The lower limbs show no edema or evidence of venous thrombosis.

4. In the light of these findings, do you now believe that, after all, Mr. Marks's chest pain may be due to indigestion or muscular soreness in the chest wall? Justify your response.

_____

_____

_____

5. Is it appropriate to perform further diagnostic testing? Why or why not?

_____

_____

_____

6. What kind of testing should be done?

_____

_____

_____

> An electrocardiogram shows nonspecific ST segment and T wave changes compatible with mild diffuse coronary artery disease. Chest x-ray is unremarkable. Blood studies show a 2-hour postprandial glucose of 214 mg/dL (normal <200), total cholesterol of 377 mg/dL (normal <180), low-density lipoprotein cholesterol of 260 mg/dL (normal <180). An echocardiogram yields essentially normal results, with an ejection fraction of 60% and normal ventricular wall thickness and motion.

7. What additional risk factors for coronary artery disease have now come to light?

_____

_____

_____

_____

8. How important is lifestyle modification going to be for Mr. Marks in dealing with his medical problems?

_____

_____

_____

_____

9. What further diagnostic testing might be appropriate?

_____

_____

_____

_____

10. What kinds of therapy might be recommended?

_____

_____

_____

_____

SUGGESTIONS FOR ADDITIONAL LEARNING ACTIVITIES

1. Cardiovascular disease is the leading cause of death for men and women in the United States. It is likely that this disease has affected someone in your life. Write a short report on the cardiovascular condition with which you are most familiar, without relying on your textbook or any outside research. Include only what you already know, and limit your report to no more than one page. After you have completed this task, prepare a second report relying only on outside research. Use your textbook, medical journals, or other official sources of information. You may not include any information in the second report that you used in the first one.

2. Obtain three pastel colored highlighters or marking pens, in pink, yellow, and blue, or choose crayons of similar shade. Go through the chapter and highlight in pink the name of every cardiovascular disease. Highlight in yellow the name of every diagnostic test, including both laboratory and imaging studies. Highlight in blue every distinct treatment modality, including the names of medications, surgical procedures, and so on. Rely on the highlighted text when reviewing for a test.

3. Watch an episode of a television medical drama, capturing it on videotape, if possible, so you can pause it during playback. Make notes for every patient encountered, paying particular attention to any dialogue regarding the treatment of cardiovascular conditions or the cardiovascular status of patients with noncardiovascular conditions. Don't overlook blood pressures, pulses, or ECG readings. Afterwards, look up any unfamiliar terms or laboratory values. Imagine that you are the head nurse and need to make a report of everything that occurred on your shift. Prepare an outline that gives the diagnosis and current cardiovascular status for each patient whose care you observed.

Diseases of the Ear, Nose, and Throat

(Outline continued on next page)

LEARNING OBJECTIVES

Upon completion of this chapter, you should be able to

- describe the basic anatomy and physiology of the ears, nose, and throat;

- explain diagnostic procedures and treatments used for diseases of the ears, nose, and throat;

- classify common diseases of the ears, nose, and throat by their signs, symptoms, and treatment.

DISEASES OF THE EAR, NOSE, AND THROAT
(continued)

THE THROAT: ANATOMY AND PHYSIOLOGY

DIAGNOSTIC PROCEDURES IN DISORDERS
OF THE THROAT
Acute Pharyngitis (Sore Throat)
Obstructive Sleep Apnea (OSA)

QUESTIONS FOR STUDY AND REVIEW

DISEASES OF THE EAR, NOSE, AND THROAT

The ears, nose, and throat are adjacent to one another anatomically, similar in histologic structure, and subject to many of the same diseases. Diseases, injuries, and abnormalities of the ear, nose, and throat (ENT) are the special field of the otorhino-laryngologist. This chapter briefly surveys the more common disorders to which these parts of the body are subject. If you encounter unfamiliar terms, look them up in the Glossary or the Index.

THE EAR

ANATOMY AND PHYSIOLOGY

Each ear has three parts (See Figure 7):

1. The **outer ear**, consisting of the pinna (the cartilaginous appendage on either side of the head, which collects sound waves like a funnel) and the external auditory meatus (a tube that conducts sound waves from the pinna to the middle ear). The meatus is lined with skin that secretes cerumen (ear-wax), a mildly antimicrobial substance that traps dust and other particulate foreign material.

2. The **middle ear**, a cavity in the temporal bone separated from the external auditory meatus by the tympanic membrane, which vibrates in response to sound waves and imparts the vibration to a series of very small bones (malleus, incus, and stapes), which in turn transmit them to the inner ear.

3. The **inner ear**, consisting of the cochlea (an organ shaped like a snail shell, in which sound vibrations are converted to nerve impulses to be sent through the eighth cranial, or vestibulocochlear,

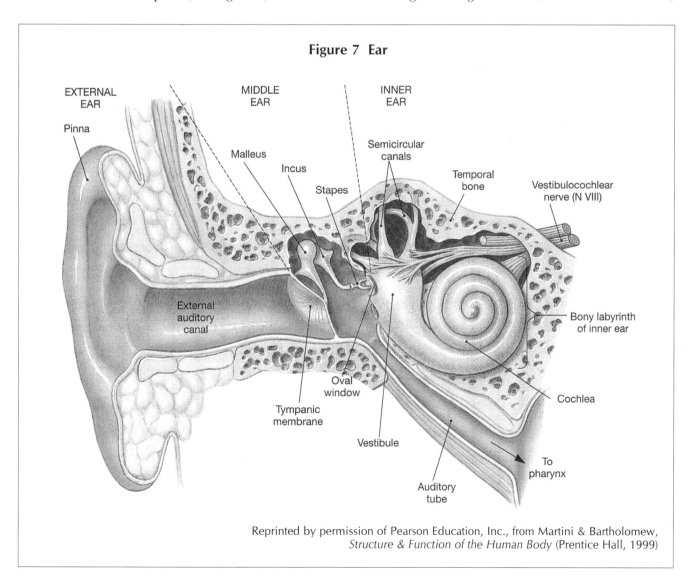

Figure 7 Ear

EXTERNAL EAR

MIDDLE EAR

INNER EAR

Pinna

Malleus

Incus

Stapes

Semicircular canals

Temporal bone

Vestibulocochlear nerve (N VIII)

External auditory canal

Oval window

Bony labyrinth of inner ear

Tympanic membrane

Vestibule

Cochlea

Auditory tube

To pharynx

Reprinted by permission of Pearson Education, Inc., from Martini & Bartholomew, *Structure & Function of the Human Body* (Prentice Hall, 1999)

nerve) and the vestibular system (the organ of balance, containing minute position sensors in a fluid medium, which send information about head position to the balance center in the brain, also through the eighth cranial nerve).

The middle ear communicates with the pharynx by a minute passage called the auditory (eustachian) tube, which serves to equalize air pressure between the middle ear and the atmosphere (see box). It also communicates with epithelium-lined air cells within the skull, called mastoid air cells.

The auditory tube between the middle ear and the pharynx was discovered by Bartolomeo Eustachio (1524-1574), an Italian anatomist who also made important studies of the heart, the kidney, and the nervous system.

It has been suggested that when William Shakespeare wrote *Hamlet,* he had in mind the then recent discovery of this passage. In Act I, Scene 5, the ghost of Hamlet's father tells Hamlet how he was murdered by his brother Claudius, who poured "juice of cursed hebona . . . in the porches of my ears."

According to Nomina Anatomica (NA) and Terminologia Anatomica (TA), the name of this tube is *tuba auditoria* (or *auditiva*), usually rendered *auditory tube* in English.

Many health professionals nonetheless cling to the traditional name, **eustachian tube**, and most of them pronounce it with the soft French *ch* sound (as in champagne) rather than the more appropriate hard Italian *ch* (as in Chianti).

DIAGNOSTIC PROCEDURES IN DISORDERS OF THE EAR

Inspection and palpation of the pinna.

Otoscopy: Inspection of the external auditory meatus and tympanic membrane with an otoscope, an instrument that directs light into the ear through a conical speculum, and is equipped with a magnify-ing lens; mobility of the tympanic membrane can be assessed when the subject swallows or performs the Valsalva maneuver (or when, in children, the examiner blows a puff of air into the ear with a rubber bulb attached to the otoscope).

Measurements of hearing: (1) simple tests with ticking watch or tuning fork; (2) audiography, a precise measurement of the faintest loudness (in decibels) that the subject can hear, each being ear tested separately at each of several pitches (for example, 250, 500, 1000, 2000, 3000, 4000, 6000, and 8000 Hz); this can be performed by a technician with carefully calibrated testing equipment, or by automated machinery activated by the subject; (3) more elaborate testing of the subject's ability to discriminate spoken words.

Weber test: A vibrating tuning fork placed firmly against a bony surface of the head at the midline sends vibrations through the bones of the skull. These should be heard equally in the two ears; if there is hearing loss due to blockage of the external auditory meatus or to injury or disease of the middle ear, the tone of the fork will be heard louder in the affected ear; in hearing loss due to damage to the inner ear or acoustic nerve, however, the tone will be heard louder in the more normal ear.

Rinne test: The sound of a vibrating tuning fork positioned so that the tines are near the pinna (air conduction) should be heard by the subject even after the sound sensed when the shank of the tuning fork is placed on the mastoid process behind the ear (bone conduction) can no longer be heard; when bone conduction is heard longer than air conduction in an ear with reduced hearing, the hearing loss is due to obstruction of the meatus or disease of the middle ear.

Tympanocentesis: Puncture of the tympanic membrane and withdrawal of fluid from the middle ear for examination, including culture.

Pneumotympanometry: Assessment of the mobility of the tympanic membrane by applying pressure to its outer surface with a device fitting tightly in the external meatus.

INFECTIONS OF THE OUTER AND MIDDLE EAR

Otitis Externa (Swimmer's Ear)

Infection of the external auditory meatus.

Causes: Infection with bacteria (*Proteus, Pseudomonas*) and sometimes fungi (*Aspergillus*). Predisposing causes include water exposure (swimming, showering), excessive cerumen, mechanical trauma (probing with paperclip), foreign body (cotton, pencil eraser), diabetes mellitus, and immune compromise.

History: Earache, itching in the external auditory meatus, purulent discharge. Hearing loss if the meatus is occluded by swelling or exudate.

Physical Examination: Redness and swelling of the meatus, sometimes with complete occlusion; purulent exudate, perhaps with excessive cerumen or foreign body visible. Tenderness on manipulation of the pinna.

Course: Generally benign, but in diabetes mellitus and AIDS an external ear infection may resist conservative treatment and become chronic, perhaps invading the skull or brain, with resulting neurologic damage.

Treatment: After gentle cleansing and removal of any foreign material, cerumen, or exudate, topical antibiotics (ear drops), often with hydrocortisone to combat local inflammation, are instilled several times a day. Sometimes a gauze wick is inserted to facilitate penetration of ear drops when edema of the meatus is extreme. In invasive infections, intravenous antibiotics and even surgery may be required.

Otitis Media

Bacterial infection of the middle ear and adjoining mastoid air cells.

Cause: Infection by *Streptococcus pneumoniae, Haemophilus influenzae, Streptococcus pyogenes,* and other bacteria. Otitis media commonly occurs as a sequel to a viral upper respiratory infection. Obstruction of the auditory tube by edema leads to pressure changes within the middle ear and secretion of mucus and serous fluid, which becomes infected by bacteria already present in the tissues. Otitis media is often bilateral. It is commoner in infants and small children than in adolescents and adults, accounting for one-third of all pediatric office visits.

History: Pain and pressure in one or both ears, hearing loss, sometimes fever.

Physical Examination: Redness of the tympanic membrane, sometimes with formation of bullae. Immobility of the tympanic membrane, reflecting malfunction of the auditory tube. Occasionally bulging of the membrane. If spontaneous rupture occurs, blood or purulent exudate in the external auditory meatus.

Course: It is estimated that 20-80% of all cases of otitis media will resolve spontaneously without treatment. When there is fever or severe pain, antibiotic treatment is usually prescribed because of the risk of serious complications in a few patients. Neglect of the infection, its failure to respond to standard initial treatment, or a series of recurrent infections can lead to chronic otitis media, typically due to different organisms (*Proteus, Pseudomonas,* staphylococci) than acute infection. Complications of chronic otitis media include spontaneous rupture of the tympanic membrane, with chronic purulent drainage; destruction of the bones within the middle ear that transmit sound; invasion of mastoid air cells (mastoiditis), skull bones, and even the central nervous system by infection; formation of cholesteatoma, a benign but locally invasive growth of the tympanic membrane caused by prolonged negative pressure (partial vacuum) in the middle ear. Chronic otitis media can lead to permanent conductive hearing loss and, in small children, speech defects because of inability to hear speech sounds properly.

Treatment: In the absence of fever and severe pain in patients over age 2, analgesics and observation are preferred to antibiotic treatment. For selected patients, systemic antibiotics (amoxicillin with or without clavulanic acid, erythromycin, trimethoprim-sulfamethoxazole), decongestants, analgesics. If tympanic membrane rupture threatens, myringotomy (surgical puncture of the membrane, with release of pus). In children with recurrent or refractory infections, polyethylene tubes may be placed in the tympanic membrane(s) to aerate the middle ear(s) and allow for escape of purulent secretion. Cholesteatoma and mastoiditis are treated surgically. Chronic perforation of the tympanic membrane requires surgical repair (tympanoplasty).

DISORDERS OF THE INNER EAR

Tinnitus

Perception of abnormal sounds in the ear(s) or head. When pulsatile (simultaneous with heartbeat), it may result from vascular disease (arterial stenosis, aneurysm). Tinnitus is generally a humming or squealing noise heard constantly or intermittently in one or both ears, especially at night when external sounds are at a minimum. It is generally due to degenerative disease of the inner ear, and frequently accompanies sensorineural hearing loss (discussed below). Common causes are excessive noise exposure and certain medicines. Aspirin and other salicylates at higher doses cause tinnitus lasting only as long as they remain in the body. Other drugs (certain antibiotics) can cause permanent tinnitus. Treatment of tinnitus is generally unsatisfactory but includes masking with other sounds (music, "static" on a radio).

Vertigo

A sense of motion (spinning, falling, floor tipping) when no such motion is occurring.

Causes: Labyrinthitis, often following respiratory infection and hence often called viral. Degenerative changes in the balance-sensing mechanism of the inner ear. Increased pressure within the endolymphatic sac (Ménière disease). Vascular or neoplastic disease of the inner ear or temporal lobe of the cerebral cortex. Diplopia, head injury, multiple sclerosis, drugs, alcohol.

History: A feeling of spinning or falling to one side, or a sense that the floor is tipping or rotating, coming on suddenly, often with head movement, and lasting seconds, minutes, hours, days, weeks, or months. When severe, vertigo may make it impossible for the patient to stand or walk, and may be accompanied by nausea and vomiting. There may also be tinnitus and hearing loss.

Physical Examination: May be essentially normal. The Romberg test (patient standing with eyes closed) may indicate inability to maintain equilibrium. Eyes may show nystagmus.

Treatment: May be limited to treatment of the underlying cause. In Ménière disease, salt restriction and diuretic therapy may help by reducing the pressure of the endolymph. Medicines such as meclizine and dimenhydrinate may diminish or abolish vertigo temporarily. In some cases of positional vertigo, head manipulation can reduce symptoms by promoting reorientation of the balance mechanism.

Hearing Loss

Reduction, often permanent, in the acuity of hearing in one or both ears. Hearing loss is divided into three types depending on the location of the abnormality.

Conductive hearing loss due to disease or abnormality in the outer or middle ear: cerumen impaction, otitis media with effusion, hardening of the tympanic membrane (otosclerosis), injury or disease of the ossicles.

Sensory hearing loss due to disease of the cochlea: acoustic trauma, ototoxicity (aminoglycosides, loop diuretics, cisplatin), aging.

Neural hearing loss due to eighth nerve lesions or cerebrovascular disease.

Hearing loss is assessed by audiometry and the Weber and Rinne tests. Treatment is that of the underlying cause, if possible.

Generally no treatment is effective.

THE NOSE

ANATOMY AND PHYSIOLOGY

The external nose is supported by a framework of cartilage and covered by skin. The nostrils (anterior nares) open into paired passages lined with mucous membrane, which is rich in serous and mucous glands and blood vessels. The lining membrane of these passages is closely attached to convoluted ridges of bone called turbinates (three on each side), which increase the surface area of membrane that is exposed to inspired air. Adjacent to the nasal passages, and communicating with them by narrow orifices, are the paranasal sinuses. These are cavities within the bones of the skull, somewhat variable in size and shape, and lined with mucosa like that of the nose. The nasal passages end at the choanae, or posterior nares, where they enter the nasopharynx, the uppermost part of the pharyngeal cavity. The nasal passages warm and moisturize inspired air, and the mucus film lining them traps particulate matter in the air.

DIAGNOSTIC PROCEDURE IN DISORDERS OF THE NOSE

Direct inspection with nasal speculum or rhinoscope.

Posterior rhinoscopy: Inspection of posterior nares with angled mirror placed in the oropharynx.

Nasal smear: Examination of a stained smear of scrapings from the nasal mucosa for evidence of infection (neutrophilic leukocytes) or allergy (eosinophilic leukocytes).

Culture of nasal secretions to identify bacterial pathogens.

Diseases of the Nose

Coryza (Common Cold)

A common, mild rhinitis caused by viruses.

Causes: Any of numerous viruses, which can be spread readily from person to person. Risk of catching cold may be heightened by exposure to severe winter weather (especially whole-body chilling), drying of indoor air by heating systems, or crowding indoors during the winter.

History: Headache, nasal stuffiness, runny nose, sneezing, throat irritation, malaise. Occasionally fever, chills, anorexia, and muscle aching.

Physical Examination: Erythema and edema of nasal mucosa. Temperature may be slightly elevated.

Course: Generally self-limited. Sometimes complicated by sinusitis, otitis media, pharyngitis, bronchitis.

Treatment: Purely symptomatic. Oral decongestants are moderately effective. Aspirin, acetaminophen, or ibuprofen relieve discomfort. Rest, fluids. Antihistamines do not decongest, antibiotics do not kill cold viruses, and nasal decongestant sprays cause rebound congestion worse than the disease.

Allergic Rhinitis (Hay Fever)

A recurrent, often seasonal, inflammation of the nasal mucous membrane caused by allergy to inhaled materials.

Causes: Sensitivity to pollens, grasses, mold spores, dust mites, animal dander, second-hand cigarette smoke, and other inhalant allergens.

History: Recurrent or constant nasal congestion and irritation, with copious watery discharge, itching, sneezing (often many times in a row), and itching and watering of the eyes. Symptoms may occur consistently at certain seasons (spring, fall) or, especially when due to house dust, may be perennial.

Physical Examination: Watery, red eyes. Pale or bluish, markedly swollen nasal mucosa. Nasal polyps (massive overgrowths of chronically inflamed mucosa) may be present.

Diagnostic Tests: Nasal smear shows eosinophils. Skin testing or RAST (radioallergosorbent testing) can identify causative allergens.

Treatment: Decongestants, antihistamines, nasal corticosteroid spray. Avoidance of known allergens when possible. Use of air filters as appropriate. Continued administration of desensitizing antigens often markedly reduces symptoms.

Sinusitis (Rhinosinusitis)

Infection of one or more paranasal sinuses.

Cause: Involvement of the paranasal sinuses often occurs along with any type of rhinitis, including particularly the common cold. Swelling of the nasal mucosa leads to blockage of the sinus openings, with accumulation of secretions within the sinuses affected. Persons with allergic rhinitis may be subject to recurring episodes of sinusitis due to chronic blockage of sinus openings (ostia). Acute sinusitis is nearly always viral. Recurrent or persistent obstruction to sinus drainage can lead to chronic sinusitis with secondary bacterial infection.

History: Pressure or pain in one or more sinus cavities, often aggravated by bending forward. Pain may be manifested as a severe headache or may radiate into the teeth. Purulent or bloody nasal or postnasal discharge may be present. Occasionally fever, chills, and malaise.

Physical Examination: Edema and erythema of nasal mucosa. Purulent discharge in nasal passages or oropharynx (postnasal drip).

Diagnostic Tests: In chronic sinusitis, x-ray or other diagnostic imaging shows thickening of sinus membranes and often presence of fluid within cavities.

Treatment: Decongestant, analgesic. A short course of nasal decongestant spray may help to open and drain sinuses. Control of allergic component if present. When symptoms (severe, persistent pain) or clinical picture (fever, bloody discharge) suggests bacterial infection, an oral antibiotic (amoxicillin, trimethoprim-sulfamethoxazole) is prescribed. Chronic sinusitis may respond to prolonged antibiotic therapy. Surgical procedures can be used to correct anatomic lesions predisposing to sinusitis, or to improve drainage of a chronically infected sinus.

Epistaxis (Nosebleed)

Bleeding from the nose may be due to nasal trauma, irritation of the mucosa by dust or dry air, upper respiratory infection or allergic rhinitis, or coagulation defect. Treatment of acute nosebleed is by application of direct pressure and, if necessary, topical vasoconstrictor. If bleeding persists or recurs, cautery with silver nitrate or anterior nasal packing may be necessary. Rarely bleeding comes from the posterior nares (usually in middle-aged or elderly patients with hypertension or arteriosclerosis) and requires a posterior nasal pack. Prevention of further nosebleeds may include use of lubricating applications to the mucosa, humidification of air, and avoidance of dusts and other irritants.

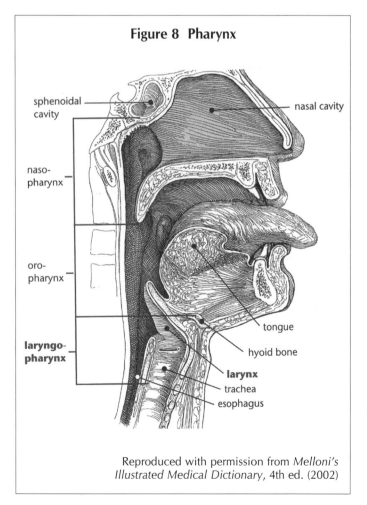

Figure 8 Pharynx

sphenoidal cavity — nasal cavity

naso-pharynx

oro-pharynx

laryngo-pharynx

tongue

hyoid bone

larynx

trachea

esophagus

Reproduced with permission from *Melloni's Illustrated Medical Dictionary*, 4th ed. (2002)

THE THROAT

ANATOMY AND PHYSIOLOGY

The throat, or pharynx, is a cavity lined with mucous membrane that conducts air from the nose and mouth into the trachea, and food and drink from the mouth into the esophagus. It consists of three portions: the nasopharynx, on a level with the nasal passages and communicating with them; the oropharynx, on a level with the mouth and communicating with it; and the hypopharynx or laryngopharynx, which lies below the oropharynx and gives entry to the esophagus and the larynx. (See Figure 8.)

The tonsils and adenoids are masses of lymphoid tissue surrounding the zone between the mouth and the oropharynx. At the boundary between the oropharynx and the hypopharynx lies the epiglottis, a flexible valve that closes the respiratory passage during swallowing of food or drink.

The lining of the pharynx secretes mucus, which keeps the surface moist, traps inhaled particles, and supplements the saliva as a lubricant for food. Lymph glands in the front and back of the neck receive lymphatic drainage from the throat and adjacent structures.

DIAGNOSTIC PROCEDURES IN DISORDERS OF THE THROAT

Inspection of the throat with a focused light, often with the aid of a tongue depressor (tongue blade) to press the tongue out of the field of vision.

Palpation of cervical lymph glands and of masses, swellings, or other structures within the throat.

Throat culture to identify bacterial pathogens.

Strep screen (faster than culture, but detects only group A beta-hemolytic streptococci).

Biopsy of masses or lesions suspected of being malignant.

X-ray or other imaging to identify foreign bodies, masses, or abnormalities of the airway due to injury or disease.

Acute Pharyngitis (Sore Throat)

Acute inflammation of the throat due to infection.

Cause: Usually viruses, including the Epstein-Barr virus, which causes infectious mononucleosis (discussed in Chapter 3). Occasionally bacteria such as *Streptococcus pneumoniae* and Group A beta-hemolytic *Streptococcus pyogenes* ("strep throat"), or fungi such as *Candida*. Infection with cold viruses may predispose to bacterial infection. Sore throat is more prevalent in cold weather.

History: Pain, irritation, or a sense of fullness or swelling in the throat, accentuated by swallowing and often radiating to the ears. Fever, painful glandular swelling in the neck.

Physical Examination: May be essentially normal. Fever is often present. Edema and erythema of the oropharynx, often involving the tonsils, soft palate, and uvula, occur in most bacterial and many viral throat infections. Severe infections, including streptococcal pharyngitis (strep throat) and infectious mononucleosis, cause formation of white or gray exudate (consisting of dead tissue, white blood cells, and bacteria) on pharyngeal walls and especially on the tonsils. A firmly adherent exudate is characteristic of *Candida* infection (thrush). The presence of vesicles or ulcers suggests viral infection (herpes simplex virus, coxsackievirus). Severe pain and swelling may cause a hollow or "hot potato" voice, and may make swallowing virtually impossible, so that the patient drools to avoid swallowing saliva, and becomes dehydrated from lack of fluid intake. Extreme swelling may compromise the airway. Cervical lymph glands may be swollen and tender. Some strains of beta-hemolytic streptococci cause a widespread red rash (scarlet fever, scarlatina).

Diagnostic Tests: Throat culture or strep screen may identify the causative organism. Blood studies (white blood cell count and differential, antistreptolysin O titer, heterophile antibodies) help to diagnose strep throat and infectious mononucleosis. Smears or scrapings of exudate can confirm presence of *Candida*.

Course: Viral sore throat runs its course within a week or two. Occasionally it becomes complicated by streptococcal infection, which may lead to acute rheumatic fever. It may also progress to otitis media, acute or chronic tonsillitis, or lower respiratory infection. Peritonsillar abscess (quinsy) is a severe bacterial infection developing above and behind one tonsil and causing extreme pain and swelling, with deviation of the uvula away from the affected side.

Treatment: Acute viral pharyngitis requires no treatment except analgesics, gargles, soothing lozenges, and perhaps a soft diet. Adrenal corticosteroid may be administered orally or by injection for severe pain and swelling. If streptococcal infection is diagnosed, a 10-day course of an antibiotic known to be able to eradicate streptococci (such as penicillin V, erythromycin, or cephalexin) is mandatory. Candidal oropharyngitis (thrush) is treated with topical or systemic antifungal medicine. The treatment of peritonsillar abscess is surgical drainage.

Obstructive Sleep Apnea (OSA)

A disorder in which breathing is repeatedly interrupted during sleep by intermittent obstruction of the airway.

Cause: Lax, excessively bulky, or malformed pharyngeal tissues (soft palate, uvula, and sometimes tonsils). Obesity, hypothyroidism, cigarette smoking, alcohol, and some medicines (particularly benzodiazepines) are predisposing factors. The swallowing reflex may be impaired during sleep. The condition is twice as common in men. Incidence increases with advancing age.

History: Loud snoring and recurrent episodes of apnea (respiratory arrest) during sleep followed by gasping inspiration with partial or complete arousal. The period of apnea may last for 10-120 seconds, and may be accompanied by sinus bradycardia or atrioventricular block.

Physical Examination: The shape and caliber of upper respiratory passages may be abnormal.

Diagnostic Tests: Polysomnography (continuous monitoring of heart rate, respiratory action and air flow, eye movements, and electroencephalogram during sleep), supplemented by recording of chin movements and arterial oxygen saturation.

Course: Nocturnal hypoxemia (deficiency of oxygen in blood) and shallow, non-refreshing sleep may lead to daytime lethargy, difficulties with memory and concentration, and even personality change and accident-proneness. About 15% of persons with OSA develop sustained pulmonary hypertension.

Treatment: Weight loss, smoking cessation, avoidance of alcohol and benzodiazepines. An appliance worn inside the mouth may reduce symptoms by holding the lower jaw in a forward position. The nightly use of continuous positive airway pressure (CPAP), which provides a steady flow of room air at low pressure through the nose to overcome intermittent upper respiratory obstruction, is often effective. Surgical trimming and reshaping of the uvula and soft palate can be performed by laser or radiofrequency ablation under local anesthesia. A more elaborate procedure is mandibular osteotomy with genioglossus muscle advancement.

QUESTIONS FOR STUDY AND REVIEW

1. List and classify several reasons for hearing loss:

    _____

    _____

    _____

    _____

    _____

    _____

2. List some common causes of nosebleed:

    _____

    _____

    _____

    _____

    _____

3. Define or explain these terms:

    a. audiography_____

    _____

    b. auditory tube_____

    _____

    c. cerumen_____

    _____

    d. coryza_____

    _____

    e. epistaxis _____

    _____

    f. mastoiditis _____

    _____

    g. pharyngitis_____

    _____

    h. pinna _____

    _____

    i. vertigo _____

    _____

4. Point out some ways in which the ear, nose, and throat are related anatomically, physiologically, and with respect to diseases affecting two or more of them.

_____

_____

_____

_____

_____

5. Discuss the inappropriate treatment of viral respiratory infections with antibiotics. State some objections to this practice. What share of the blame would you assign to patients, pharmaceutical manufacturers, and physicians respectively?

_____

_____

_____

_____

_____

_____

_____

_____

_____

_____

_____

CASE STUDY: YOU'RE THE DOCTOR

Rashid Rahman is a 37-year-old computer programmer from Pakistan who has been in the United States for a year and a half as part of a cultural exchange program. He visits an urgent care clinic where you are on duty because of a "sinus infection."

1. Approximately one-third of adults queried report that they have had a sinus infection during the past year. What do you think is the likelihood that Mr. Rahman has bacterial rhinosinusitis requiring antibiotic treatment?

_____

_____

_____

The patient states that he began having nasal congestion and rhinorrhea yesterday, associated with pain and pressure in the frontal and maxillary areas. His nasal discharge is thick and yellow. He denies sore throat, cough, eye or ear symptoms, and fever. He sneezes often, sometimes four or five times in a row. He began taking pseudoephedrine and acetaminophen as soon as the symptoms appeared, but has had no relief yet. When closely questioned, he admits that his facial pain is really more of a stuffiness or pressure than a pain, and that it seems to wax and wane, being worst when he bends forward to tie or untie his shoes.

2. Which, if any, of these historical points favor a diagnosis of bacterial rhinosinusitis?

_____

_____

_____

Mr. Rahman gives a long history of recurrent sinus infections, for which he has had numerous x-ray examinations in his own country. He states that his infections invariably progress to the point of disabling pain and fever unless treated with an antibiotic, and he tells you which antibiotic consistently works for him. His general health is good. He does not smoke or drink alcohol and he takes no prescription medicines. He is allergic to cats and some plants but not to any foods or medicines.

3. Does this additional history change your view as to the likelihood of bacterial infection? How?

_____

_____

_____

On examination the patient appears alert, normally oriented, and in no distress. He is afebrile and his pulse and blood pressure are normal. His voice is somewhat nasal and he is breathing predominantly through his mouth, but there is no dyspnea, hoarseness, or cough. He sneezes repeatedly into a facial tissue during the consultation. The conjunctivae are slightly injected. Both nares show edema and pallor of the mucosa, with scant glairy secretion. There is slight tenderness to palpation above and below the eyes. The pharyngeal mucosa is normally hydrated and not injected. A thin postnasal discharge is evident on the posterior pharyngeal wall. The ear canals are clear and the tympanic membranes are not injected. The neck is supple, without masses. The lungs are clear to auscultation.

4. Do you now have grounds for agreeing with Mr. Rahman that he needs an antibiotic? Explain your rationale.

_____

_____

_____

You advise Mr. Rahman that his condition has not yet progressed to the point where antibiotic treatment is appropriate. In fact, there are indications (staccato sneezing, pale nasal mucous membranes, absence of fever, history of inhalant allergies) that his symptoms may be due partly or entirely to respiratory allergy. He vigorously resists the idea of allergic rhinitis, since he hasn't been around any animals or flowering plants. He also says that since he knows from prior experience that he will eventually need an antibiotic, and since he doesn't want to spend the time and money to make a second visit to the clinic, your clear medical duty is to prescribe an antibiotic now.

5. Will you agree? Why or why not?

_____

_____

_____

SUGGESTIONS FOR ADDITIONAL LEARNING ACTIVITIES

1. Role-play a physician office visit with you as the doctor. Ask your patient (another student or family member) to choose a condition from this chapter and assume the history and symptoms of that condition. Ask relevant questions of your patient in order to elicit the information you need to formulate a differential diagnosis. Order lab tests by asking the patient to give you the results from those described in the chapter. If you order a lab test that isn't discussed, the patient should not tell you this but instead just say the results of that particular test were within normal limits. Make your final diagnosis and ask your patient to tell you if you were right.

2. Starting at the beginning of the chapter, make a list of all the anatomical terms that are discussed, including the structures of the ear, nose, and throat. Organize them down the left side of one or more sheets of paper, but don't number them. Label this list "A." Then starting with a separate sheet of paper but beginning at the back of the chapter and working in reverse, list all the diseases and symptoms that are associated with the ears, nose, and throat. Number the items in this list beginning with the number 1. Label this list "B." Starting with the first item on list A, write down the numbers of all the diseases or symptoms associated with that structure from list B. Continue through all the items on list A. When you are finished, make sure that you have used every number from list B.

3. You have been asked to be part of an expert panel on obstructive sleep apnea at the annual meeting of the American Academy of Otolaryngology–Head and Neck. You will give a 5-minute summary on the latest findings in the treatment of this condition. Use medical journals, the library, or the Internet for your research. Prior to your presentation, prepare questions on slips of paper and distribute them to your audience (class members, study group participants, or family members). After your presentation, "field" the planted questions. In the classroom, form multiple expert panels, three students to a group, assigning each panel a topic.

Diseases of the Respiratory System

LEARNING OBJECTIVES

Upon completion of this chapter, you should be able to

- describe the basic anatomy and physiology of the respiratory system;

- explain diagnostic procedures and treatments used for respiratory diseases;

- classify common diseases of the respiratory system by their signs, symptoms, and treatment.

DISEASES OF THE RESPIRATORY SYSTEM

ANATOMY AND PHYSIOLOGY OF THE RESPIRATORY SYSTEM

The respiratory system comprises all the organs and tissues that serve to deliver oxygen to circulating blood and to remove carbon dioxide from it. The respiratory system consists of the nose, mouth, pharynx, larynx, trachea, bronchi, lungs, pleura, diaphragm, and chest wall (ribs and muscles).

Inspiration occurs when the diaphragm moves downward and the chest wall moves outward. This creates a slight vacuum within the chest cavity, causing the lungs to expand and draw air inward through the airway (mouth and nose, throat, trachea, and bronchi) into the lung tissue proper. At the end of inspiration, the diaphragm and chest wall relax, so that the lungs passively contract and expel air. This is known as expiration. During both phases of respiration, blood in pulmonary vessels takes up oxygen from the inspired air and releases carbon dioxide into the air that is about to be exhaled. Respiration is under involuntary control from a center in the brain stem. Respiratory rate varies with changes in the oxygen and carbon dioxide levels in the blood as well as in the composition and pH (alkalinity vs. acidity) of the serum.

The airway is lined by mucous membrane, which contains glands producing both mucous and serous secretions. The walls of the trachea and bronchi are reinforced by partial rings of cartilage, which prevent their collapse under negative pressure.

Lung tissue proper consists of numerous microscopic air sacs or alveoli (singular, alveolus), through whose extremely thin epithelial walls the respiratory gases can readily diffuse between the air within them and the blood in adjacent pulmonary capillaries. The lungs are protected by a delicate serous membrane called the pleura. The visceral layer of the pleura is closely applied to the external surfaces of the lungs; the parietal layer lines the chest cavity. Normally the two layers are in contact, with a minute amount of serous fluid between them to serve as a lubricant as the lungs move with respect to the chest wall during respiration.

SYMPTOMS AND SIGNS OF RESPIRATORY DISEASE

Cough (dry or productive) or choking.

Production of sputum (watery, viscous, or purulent).

Hemoptysis (coughing up blood from respiratory passages).

Dyspnea (shortness of breath), tachypnea (increased respiratory rate).

Audible wheezing with respirations (inspiratory or expiratory).

Chest pain (constant, intermittent, or synchronous with breathing). Pleuritic chest pain, the pain of pleurisy (pleuritis), is sharp, localized, and closely related to chest wall movement with breathing.

Cyanosis (bluish color of skin, particularly lips and nail beds, due to presence of excess unoxygenated blood in the circulation).

Respiratory distress, indicated by increased effort to breathe, pursing of lips, use of accessory muscles of respiration (neck and upper chest muscles not needed for normal breathing), intercostal retractions (sucking in of muscles between ribs on inspiration).

Percussion of the chest may disclose hyperresonance due to a cavity within lung tissue or air in the pleural space; or dullness due to consolidation of lung tissue by infection, or neoplasm, or to fluid in the pleural space.

Auscultation may detect rales (crackling or bubbling sounds due to passage of air through fluid in respiratory passages); rhonchi (singular, rhonchus; whistling or honking sounds due to passage of air through respiratory passages narrowed by edema, secretions, or neoplasm); a pleural friction rub (due to inflammation or scarring of adjacent surfaces of visceral and parietal pleura); or reduction or absence of breath sounds (due to pulmonary consolidation, pleural air or fluid, collapse of a lung, or neoplasm).

Digital clubbing (enlargement of fingertips with elevation of proximal parts of nails, due to chronic pulmonary disease).

DIAGNOSTIC PROCEDURES IN RESPIRATORY DISEASE

History and physical examination, with particular attention to skin color, respiratory effort, the fullness and symmetry of chest expansion during inspiration, respiratory noises heard with or without a stethoscope, and findings on percussion.

Examination of sputum for pathogenic organisms (by smear and culture), neoplastic cells, or other abnormal findings.

Pulmonary function tests, which measure the rate and volume of air exchange in the respiratory system by means of finely calibrated instruments.

Arterial blood gas determination (measurement of partial pressures of oxygen and carbon dioxide in arterial blood).

Bronchoscopy (inspection of the interior of the trachea and main bronchi with a fiberoptic instrument). Specimens and biopsies can be taken through the instrument, and bronchoalveolar lavage (BAL; obtaining material from lung tissue by washing) can be performed.

Imaging studies: Standard PA (posteroanterior) and lateral chest x-rays, oblique or tomographic studies as needed; fluoroscopy; CT and MRI for various specialized diagnostic investigations; ventilation-perfusion scan (comparison of distribution of inspired radioactively tagged gas with distribution of injected radioactively tagged albumin, particularly useful in the diagnosis of pulmonary embolism).

Pleural or lung biopsy, either by percutaneous (needle) or open procedure.

DISEASES OF RESPIRATORY PASSAGES

Acute Bronchitis

Acute, self-limited inflammation of the bronchial passages.

Cause: Usually viral in origin, as a complication of an upper respiratory infection. Sometimes due to bacterial secondary infection. Can also be due to irritation by smoke or dust.

History: Cough, usually productive, occurring as a complication of a respiratory infection. When severe it may be accompanied by fever, shortness of breath, and wheezing. Cough may be worsened by the recumbent position and may keep the patient awake at night.

Physical Examination: Often no physical findings other than frequent or spasmodic coughing. The breath sounds may be bronchial, or rhonchi may be heard, chiefly on inspiration.

Diagnostic Tests: Blood studies are normal. Smear and culture of sputum may indicate bacterial

infection but usually do not. Chest x-ray may show increased bronchial markings.

Course: Cough may continue for weeks or months but resolution is eventually complete. Cough may result in rib fracture or other complications. Bronchitis lasting for three months and occurring in two successive years is termed chronic bronchitis.

Treatment: Largely symptomatic, with hydration, expectorants, and cough suppressants, at least for nighttime use. Most patients experience improvement when taking bronchodilator drugs either orally or by inhaler. Many patients are treated with antibiotics (clarithromycin, trimethoprim-sulfamethoxazole, tetracyclines), even though the vast majority of cases of bronchitis are due to viral infection.

Chronic Bronchitis

Chronic productive cough lasting for at least three months in each of two successive years. Chronic bronchitis is one form of chronic obstructive pulmonary disease, the other being emphysema. The two forms may be combined in varying proportions.

Cause: Most cases occur in smokers. Air pollution, allergy, and infection may play a part in some cases. Obesity is a risk factor.

History: Severe, persistent cough with copious production of bronchial mucus, particularly on arising in the morning.

Physical Examination: Wheezes and inspiratory rhonchi on auscultation of the chest. When bronchitis is severe, cyanosis may be noted.

Diagnostic Tests: The hematocrit may be slightly elevated, reflecting polycythemia (increase in number of circulating red blood cells) in response to diminished oxygen exchange in the lungs. Arterial blood shows reduction of oxygen and increase of carbon dioxide. Chest x-ray shows increased bronchopulmonary markings. Electrocardiogram may show evidence of strain on the right side of the heart: right axis deviation indicating right ventricular hypertrophy and P pulmonale, an abnormal P wave suggesting right atrial hypertrophy.

Course: Progressive deterioration of pulmonary function and heightened susceptibility to bacterial infection.

Treatment: Cessation of smoking and avoidance of respiratory irritants and infections are essential. Bronchodilators orally or by inhaler may improve bronchial air flow. Ipratropium by inhaler is particularly effective. Hydration, exercise, and postural drainage may assist in freeing the tract of secretions. When hypoxia is severe, home oxygen may be useful.

Bronchiectasis

An irreversible dilatation of large bronchi, due to chronic infection, obstruction, or autoimmune disease. About half of cases occur in persons with cystic fibrosis. Symptoms include chronic cough, production of copious purulent sputum, and hemoptysis. Most patients suffer weakness, weight loss, and recurrent pneumonia. Rales are heard at the lung bases, and x-ray, particularly CT scan, may show lung cysts and fibrous cuffing around affected bronchi. Treatment is with careful personal hygiene, postural drainage of chest secretions, antibiotics selected on the basis of sputum culture and sensitivity, and bronchodilators.

Asthma (Reactive Airways Disease, RAD)

A chronic or recurrent inflammatory disease of the trachea and bronchi characterized by reversible narrowing of air passages with wheezing, shortness of breath, and cough.

Cause: Abnormal sensitivity of respiratory passages to a wide variety of triggering factors: emotional stress, airborne irritants (dust, cigarette smoke) and allergens (pollen, animal dander, dust mite protein), physical exertion (exercise-induced asthma), respiratory infection, and drugs. Asthma affects about 5% of the population; there may be a genetic predisposition.

History: Paroxysms of wheezing, dyspnea, cough, and tightness in the chest. Severe asthma may result in physical exhaustion and symptoms of hypoxemia (deficiency of oxygen in circulating blood).

Physical Examination: Tachypnea; labored, noisy respirations with prolongation of the expiratory phase. Sibilant (whistling) or sonorous (humming) rhonchi may be heard throughout the chest, particularly on expiration. In severe asthma, retraction of intercostal muscles may be noted on inspiration. The chest may be hyperresonant to percussion, and cyanosis may indicate hypoxemia.

Diagnostic Tests: Pulmonary function tests indicate significant reduction in measures of air flow, particularly FEV_1 (forced expiratory volume in the first second of exhalation) and peak flow (maximum flow at the beginning of forced expiration). When the diagnosis is in doubt, a provocative test (challenge of an asymptomatic patient with

methacholine or histamine) will lead to reduction in air flow. During an asthmatic attack, administration of bronchodilator by injection or inhalation leads to marked improvement in air flow measurements. In severe asthma, the blood level of oxygen may be reduced. The eosinophil count may be increased in allergic asthma, and eosinophils may be detected in sputum. Chest x-ray may show hyperinflation of the thorax.

Course: Many cases of childhood asthma are "outgrown." Asthma may persist and progress throughout life, depending on its underlying cause and triggering factors. Infection, cor pulmonale, and acute respiratory distress syndrome are possible complications.

Treatment: Avoidance of known inciting factors; smoking cessation. For intermittent symptoms and exercise-induced asthma, aerosolized bronchodilator administered by inhalation usually suffices to control symptoms. More severe or chronic disease is better treated with aerosolized corticosteroid, with bronchodilator treatment during exacerbations. The patient may be instructed to adjust the dosage of these agents on the basis of measurements made with a simple, portable peak flow meter. Other treatments include oral theophylline, mast-cell stabilizers (cromolyn, nedocromil), leukotriene antagonists (montelukast, zafirlukast), and the atropine-like drug ipratropium. In severe, refractory asthma (status asthmaticus), oxygen is administered by inhalation and bronchodilators and corticosteroids are administered by injection.

DISEASES OF THE LUNGS

Pneumonia (Pneumonitis)

Inflammation of lung tissue, usually due to infection.

Cause: Infection by a variety of microorganisms, including *Streptococcus pneumoniae* (pneumococcus), *Klebsiella pneumoniae, Mycoplasma pneumoniae, Chlamydia pneumoniae, Legionella pneumophila, Staphylococcus aureus, Pneumocystis carinii*, and various viruses. Symptoms, signs, and clinical course depend on the infecting agent. Predisposing causes are debility, impaired immunity, cigarette smoking, chronic pulmonary or bronchial disease, and advanced age. Pneumonia often occurs as a complication or extension of upper respiratory infection.

History: Fever, chills, cough, purulent or bloody sputum, pleuritic chest pain (stabbing, sharply localized pain with respiratory movements), dypsnea, myalgia, malaise.

Physical Examination: Most patients have fever. The pulse and respiratory rate may be markedly increased. Examination of the lungs reveals rales or evidence of consolidation (reduced or absent breath sounds, flat percussion note). In mycoplasmal or viral pneumonia, physical findings may be minimal.

Diagnostic Tests: The white blood cell count may be elevated. Examination of stained sputum shows white blood cells and the infecting organism, if bacterial. Sputum culture yields growth of bacterial agents. Bronchoscopy and bronchoalveolar washings may be necessary to obtain satisfactory sputum for examination. Chest x-ray shows evidence of pulmonary infiltrates or consolidation, atelectasis, pleural effusion.

Course: Some pneumonias, including most viral and mycoplasmal infections, resolve spontaneously. Lobar pneumonia due to *Streptococcus pneumoniae*, staphylococcal pneumonia, or (in immunocompromised hosts) *Pneumocystis carinii* pneumonia frequently progresses to a fatal termination, even with treatment. Pneumonia ranks sixth as a cause of death in the U.S.

Complications: Pleural effusion, empyema, septicemia, endocarditis, arthritis, respiratory failure.

Treatment: Oral antibiotics may suffice in mild disease. Penicillins, cephalosporins, and erythromycin are the agents usually chosen. In more severe disease, hospitalization, intravenous antibiotics, and oxygen by inhalation may be necessary.

A vaccine against pneumococcus is recommended for adults over 65 and others at increased risk of acquiring pneumococcal pneumonia because of immune compromise, chronic renal failure, or other factors.

Pulmonary Tuberculosis

Cause: Infection of lungs and other tissues and organs by Mycobacterium tuberculosis. Person-to-person spread by respiratory droplets is the usual route of infection. Primary infection may be asymptomatic but leaves a focus of infective organisms in the lung and induces a state of hypersensitivity to the infecting organism. Postprimary infection, which may result from breakdown of a primary focus

or from a new dose of organisms from without, typically leads to significant and chronic clinical disease. The infection can also be transmitted by unpasteurized milk from infected cows. Other species, notably those of the M. avium-intracellulare complex (MAI, MAC) may also cause tuberculosis, typically acquired through the gastrointestinal tract. Persons with AIDS are at particular risk of tuberculosis, including MAI tuberculosis.

History: Cough, purulent or bloody sputum, fever, night sweats, weakness, anorexia, weight loss.

Physical Examination: Fever, cachexia (wasting), evidence of rales, consolidation, or cavitation in the lungs.

Diagnostic Tests: The tuberculin skin test is positive. Sputum contains acid-fast organisms, and sputum culture is positive for *M. tuberculosis*. Chest x-ray may show a calcified primary focus, hilar lymphadenopathy, upper lobe infiltrates, pleural effusion, or cavitation.

Course: Prognosis with treatment is good. Complications include phthisis (wasting) and hemorrhage.

Treatment: Simultaneous treatment with three or four drugs (isoniazid, rifampin, pyrazinamide, streptomycin, ethambutol) for a protracted period is the standard.

Pneumoconiosis

A chronic fibrosis of lung tissue caused by prolonged inhalation of mineral dusts, including coal, silicates, and asbestos.

Cause: Chronic pulmonary exposure, usually occupational, to finely divided mineral materials.

History: Many patients have few or no symptoms. When lung damage is severe, particularly in asbestosis, there may be progressive shortness of breath.

Physical Examination: Auscultation of the chest may reveal crackling rales on inspiration. Severe disease may lead to digital clubbing and cyanosis.

Diagnostic Tests: Chest x-ray shows diffusely scattered fibrotic changes in the lungs. In anthracosis (due to inhalation of coal dust), nodular opacities are seen particularly in the upper lung fields. In silicosis (due to inhalation of silicates, particularly from sand and hard coal) there are also rounded densities in lung tissue, and egg-shell calcification may be noted in hilar lymph nodes. Asbestos causes interstitial fibrosis, with linear and nodular markings in lung tissue, pleural thickening, and calcified pleural plaques. Pulmonary function tests show reduced vital capacity and flow rates. Arterial oxygen is reduced, and so is arterial carbon dioxide because of hyperventilation.

Course: Although many persons are free of symptoms despite x-ray evidence of fibrosis, others experience progressive and disabling impairment of lung function. Pneumoconioses, especially asbestosis, tend to be worse in cigarette smokers. There is an increased incidence of pulmonary tuberculosis in persons with silicosis. Asbestos exposure can lead to a malignant tumor of the pleura (pleural mesothelioma). In addition, the risk of bronchogenic carcinoma in smokers is greatly increased by concomitant asbestosis.

Treatment: Purely supportive and symptomatic.

Adult (also Acute) Respiratory Distress Syndrome (ARDS)

Acute respiratory failure induced by severe respiratory or systemic illness.

Causes: Respiratory: pneumonia, inhalation of smoke or toxic gases, pulmonary injury, near-drowning, hanging, pulmonary embolism, aspiration of gastric contents. Systemic: septicemia, severe trauma (particularly burns and head injuries), shock, repeated blood transfusions, drugs, toxins.

History: Abrupt onset of severe dyspnea within 24-48 hours after the inciting event or condition.

Physical Examination: Obvious respiratory distress, tachypnea, intercostal retractions, coarse rales on auscultation. Signs of underlying disease are usually evident.

Diagnostic Tests: The arterial oxygen level is depressed. Chest x-ray shows diffuse infiltrates in both lungs.

Course: Most cases progress to multiple organ system failure. The mortality rate is over 50% and average survival time is about 2 weeks. Survivors usually regain full health eventually.

Treatment: Largely supportive. Identification and treatment of underlying condition. Oxygen, antibiotics, diuretics, and other agents as appropriate.

Emphysema

An abnormal and irreversible enlargement of air spaces in lung tissue due to breakdown of walls of air sacs.

Cause: Cigarette smoking is a principal cause. Some cases are due to infection, allergy, or respiratory

irritants. In some patients, emphysema is linked to an inherited deficiency of alpha$_1$-antitrypsin in respiratory epithelium and other tissues.

History: The onset is usually after age 50. Shortness of breath, growing progressively worse, is the dominant symptom. Some patients experience weakness and weight loss.

Physical Examination: Tachypnea and dyspnea may be evident, with activity of the accessory respiratory muscles and pursed lips. The anteroposterior diameter of the chest is increased (barrel chest). There is hyperresonance of the thorax on percussion, and the breath sounds are reduced on auscultation. Weakness and wasting of the muscles of the extremities are often noted.

Diagnostic Tests: Chest x-ray typically shows hyperinflation of the chest cavity (low diaphragm, heart in vertical position) and hyperlucency (reduced resistance to passage of x-rays) of lung tissue. X-ray may also show bullae or blebs (air-filled cavities). Blood gas studies are usually normal but may show diminished partial pressure of oxygen. Pulmonary function tests show increased total lung capacity but reduced vital capacity and rate of air exchange.

Course: Recurrent respiratory infections, congestive heart failure (right ventricular failure, cor pulmonale), progressive respiratory failure.

Treatment: Smoking cessation, bronchodilators, oxygen inhalation, antibiotics as needed, physical therapy. For cardiac failure, sodium restriction and diuretics.

Pulmonary Embolism and Infarction

Obstruction of parts of the pulmonary arterial circulation by one or more emboli.

Cause: Thromboemboli from the deep veins of the lower extremities or pelvis passing through the right ventricle are the principal cause. Emboli may also consist of tumor material, amniotic fluid, fat, air, or injected foreign material. Predisposing causes of pulmonary thromboembolism are prolonged immobilization, surgery, childbirth, injury to venous endothelium, hypercoagulable state (cancer, oral contraceptives), congestive heart failure, obesity, and advanced age. Trapping of an embolus in a pulmonary artery results in both reflex vasoconstriction, with extensive compromise of pulmonary circulation, and reflex bronchoconstriction, with impairment of pulmonary gas exchange.

History: Sudden onset of dyspnea, chest pain, anxiety, diaphoresis, collapse. If infarction occurs, chest pain may be pleuritic and there may be hemoptysis.

Physical Examination: Tachycardia, tachypnea, crackling rales or wheezes, pleural friction rub, cyanosis, fever.

Diagnostic Tests: The arterial oxygen tension is diminished. The electrocardiogram may show right axis deviation or right heart strain. Chest x-ray in acute pulmonary embolism may show an infiltrate or atelectasis. If infarction occurs, a wedge-shaped zone of opacification may be apparent. A ventilation-perfusion scan shows an area of lung tissue that are normally ventilated (normal air flow) but not normally perfused (impeded blood flow). Pulmonary angiogram confirms and localizes pulmonary arterial obstruction. The source of the embolus may be discovered by venography, ultrasonography, impedance plethysmography, or other diagnostic modality.

Course: About 10% of patients die within the first hour, and the overall mortality rate is about 30%. Fatal outcome is usually due to right ventricular failure or cardiogenic shock.

Treatment: Vigorous supportive efforts, including oxygen and treatment for shock and cardiac failure. Thrombolytic therapy with streptokinase, urokinase, or tissue plasminogen activator (TPA) is often successful in dissolving the embolus. Intravenous heparin and oral warfarin are administered to prevent further thrombosis of deep veins. Passage of further emboli through the inferior vena cava may be prevented by surgical plication, ligation, or insertion of a filter. Prevention of pulmonary embolism includes use of compressive stockings in surgical and other bedfast patients, early ambulation after surgery, and use of low-dose heparin in selected medical and surgical patients.

DISEASES OF THE PLEURA

Pleural Effusion

Presence of fluid in the pleural space as a result of local or systemic disease.

Causes: Pleural transudates (fluid relatively low in protein) occur in congestive heart failure, cirrhosis with ascites, nephrotic syndrome, myxedema, and obstructive disorders of the pulmonary circulation (superior vena cava obstruction, pulmonary embolism, constrictive pericarditis). Pleural exudates (fluid higher in protein and also containing LDH) are due to pneumonia and other pulmonary or pleural infections including tuberculosis, malignant disease, and uremia.

History: There may be no symptoms. With large effusions, dyspnea. With local inflammation, pleuritic chest pain.

Physical Examination: Reduced breath sounds, dullness to percussion, reduced tactile fremitus (transmission of vocal vibrations to the examiner's hand on the chest wall) over the effusion. In the presence of pleural inflammation, a pleural friction rub may be heard.

Diagnostic Tests: Chest x-ray, particularly lateral decubitus films (taken with patient lying on side), shows the effusion. Fluid obtained by thoracentesis (needle puncture of chest wall with aspiration of fluid by syringe) is examined for protein and LDH (lactic dehydrogenase) to distinguish between transudate and exudate, and for white blood cells, pathogenic microorganisms, and malignant cells to establish an underlying cause for the effusion. Pleural biopsy, closed (needle) or open, may be required for definitive diagnosis.

Treatment: Correction of the cause of effusion, if possible.

Spontaneous Pneumothorax

Sudden leakage of air from a lung into the pleural space.

Cause: Rupture of a bleb or bulla, which may be solitary or part of a generalized process. The condition is commoner in males and in smokers.

History: Sudden onset of chest pain and dyspnea, which may occur at rest or during sleep.

Physical Examination: Tachycardia; reduced breath sounds, hyperresonance, and reduced tactile fremitus over the pneumothorax.

Diagnostic Tests: Chest x-ray (inspiratory and expiratory films) shows pneumothorax.

Course: A small pneumothorax resolves spontaneously. Larger ones may severely compromise cardiopulmonary dynamics. The recurrence rate is 50%.

Treatment: Thoracostomy tube connected to a water seal bottle and suction, to withdraw air from the pleural space. Thoracotomy (open surgery) may be required for a continuing leak, or for recurrent pneumothorax.

QUESTIONS FOR STUDY AND REVIEW

1. List five pulmonary disorders that cause cough and shortness of breath:

    a. _____

    b. _____

    c. _____

    d. _____

    e. _____

2. Explain the results of arterial gas studies and pulmonary function tests in the following:

    a. asthma _____

    _____

    _____

    b. acute respiratory distress syndrome _____

    _____

    _____

    c. pneumoconiosis _____

    _____

    _____

    _____

3. Define or explain these terms:

    a. (pulmonary) alveolus _____

    _____

    b. asthma _____

    _____

    c. bronchiectasis _____

    _____

    d. bronchoalveolar lavage_____

    _____

    e. cyanosis _____

    _____

    f. hemoptysis _____

    _____

    g. pleura _____

    _____

   h. pneumoconiosis _____

_____

   i. rhonchus _____

_____

4. In what diseases might bronchoscopy be of help in diagnosis?

_____

_____

_____

_____

5. In what diseases might sputum smear and culture be of help in diagnosis?

_____

_____

_____

_____

6. In what diseases might a ventilation-perfusion scan be of help in diagnosis?

_____

_____

_____

_____

7. What is the single most important preventable cause of respiratory disease and death?

_____

_____

_____

CASE STUDY: YOU'RE THE DOCTOR

Lily Domstra is a 55-year-old married custodial supervisor at a motel. She is referred to you, a specialist in pulmonary disease, by her primary care physician because of a chronic cough of 2-3 months' duration.

1. What diagnostic considerations come to mind, given just this much history?

_____

_____

_____

Ms. Domstra states that about 3 months ago she began to notice a recurrent dryness or tickling sensation in her throat that made her want to cough. Her throat has not been swollen or painful and she has had no fever, but at times she is somewhat hoarse. She denies any nasal symptoms such as sneezing, nasal congestion, or rhinorrhea. Her cough is seldom if ever productive of any sputum. It seems worse in the morning and evening but doesn't keep her awake. She has had no shortness of breath, wheezing, or pain in the chest. Over-the-counter cough drops and cough syrups seem to have little or no effect on the cough. Her family physician has prescribed benzonatate, a prescription cough suppressant, and more recently an inhaler containing an anticholinergic and a bronchodilator, without any impact on her symptom.

2. List the questions you would ask to elicit additional historical information you need:

_____

_____

_____

_____

_____

Ms. Domstra has never smoked, but her husband smokes a pipe. She has no history of asthma, bronchitis, or respiratory allergy. She has not noted any problems with exposure to dust or cleaning products at work, and her cough is no worse on days when she is at work than when she is at home. Her appetite, weight, sleeping pattern, and energy level seem normal. Her general health is good except for mild hypertension, for which she is being treated by an internist with a pill whose name she can't remember.

3. Of the three most common causes of chronic non-productive cough in the absence of lower respiratory tract infection, which is suggested by the history elicited thus far from Ms. Domstra?

____ a. postnasal drip

____ b. asthma

____ c. gastroesophageal reflux

____ d. none of the above

Your examination reveals an alert, normally developed and nourished adult woman who is eupneic and in no distress. She is not coughing or hoarse. She is afebrile and her blood pressure is 128/80. The skin shows no pallor, flushing, or cyanosis. The nares, pharynx, and ears are normal to examination. There are no cervical masses. The thorax is symmetrical with a normal AP diameter and respiratory excursions are full and equal. Auscultation of the lungs reveals no rales, rhonchi, or pleural friction rubs. A peak-flow meter reading performed in the office shows a normal rate of expiratory flow. A PA chest x-ray is read by you as showing no pulmonary infiltrate, pleural thickening or fluid, or space-occupying lesion.

4. Check all of the following measures that would now be appropriate:

  ___ a. tuberculin skin test

  ___ b. bronchoscopy with lung biopsy

  ___ c. CT scan of the lungs

  ___ d. sputum smear and culture

  ___ e. esophageal pH probe to detect acid reflux

  ___ f. allergy skin testing,

  ___ g. obtaining more history

You call the office of Ms. Domstra's internist and learn from her receptionist that the patient has been taking captopril, an ACE inhibitor, for hypertension, for the past 4 months. The receptionist also remarks that this patient's ophthalmologist prescribed timolol eye drops for glaucoma about 3 months ago. Both of these drugs are known to cause a dry cough in some patients.

---

5. Evaluate each of the following courses of action:

  a. Stop taking all medicines for a month or two to see if the cough goes away.

  _____

  _____

  _____

  b. Keep taking her medicine but also take a codeine cough syrup regularly to suppress the cough.

  _____

  _____

  _____

  c. Check with her internist and her ophthalmologist to discuss the best way to assess the possibility that one or both of her prescription medicines are making her cough and to explore alternative treatments for her hypertension and glaucoma.

  _____

  _____

  _____

SUGGESTIONS FOR ADDITIONAL LEARNING ACTIVITIES

1. Make a list of the names of diseases, diagnostic tests, and treatments discussed in this chapter. Use a medical dictionary to find the definition for each term. If there are terms in your list that do not appear in a medical dictionary, draft your own definition from the context presented in your textbook.

2. Contact the American Lung Association using your telephone directory, library resources, or the Internet. Obtain statistics on the prevalence of several lung diseases over the last 10 years. Make a graph with years listed across the bottom and the number of patients affected in thousands along the left margin. On your graph, plot the statistics you obtained, placing a dot for the number of cases for each disease in each year. Connect the dots for each disease. Does your graph demonstrate that the occurrence of these diseases is increasing, decreasing, or staying relatively constant?

3. You are a researcher for the scriptwriting department of the popular television drama, Crime Scene Investigation. You have been asked to find information on a respiratory disease that will be used in an upcoming episode. From the diseases discussed in this chapter, choose one that could result in death and where some aspects of the cause, history, and physical findings, might not be chalked up to natural causes. For a real creative challenge, draft a possible storyline yourself.

11

Diseases of the Digestive System

(Outline continued on next page)

LEARNING OBJECTIVES

Upon completion of this chapter, you should be able to

- describe the basic anatomy and physiology of the digestive system;

- explain diagnostic procedures and treatments for digestive disorders and hepatobiliary disease;

- classify common diseases of the digestive system by their signs, symptoms, and treatment.

DISEASES OF THE DIGESTIVE SYSTEM
(continued)

DISORDERS OF THE RECTUM AND ANUS
Hemorrhoids
Anal Fissure

DISORDERS OF THE PERITONEUM
Acute Peritonitis

ABDOMINAL HERNIA

DISEASES OF THE LIVER
Hepatitis A
Hepatitis B
Hepatitis C
Hepatitis D (Delta Hepatitis)
Hepatitis Cirrhosis (Portal Cirrhosis,
    Laënnec Cirrhosis)

DISEASES OF THE GALLBLADDER
AND BILIARY TRACT
Cholelithiasis (Gallstones)
Acute Cholecystitis

DISEASES OF THE PANCREAS
Acute Pancreatitis
Chronic Pancreatitis

QUESTIONS FOR STUDY AND REVIEW

DISEASES OF THE DIGESTIVE SYSTEM

ANATOMY AND PHYSIOLOGY OF THE DIGESTIVE SYSTEM

The digestive system includes all those structures concerned with the ingestion of solids and liquids, their mechanical and chemical breakdown into usable nutrients, the absorption of these into the circulation, and the excretion of solid wastes. The alimentary canal is a coiled but unbranched tube extending from the lips to the anus and divided into mouth, oropharynx, esophagus, stomach, small intestine (duodenum, jejunum, ileum), and large intestine (colon, rectum). (See Figure 9.)

Numerous microscopic glandular structures occur in the walls of the digestive tract (gastric glands, intestinal glands), and in addition larger secretory organs (salivary glands, liver, pancreas)

pour their products through ducts into parts of the tract. These secretions serve to liquefy and lubricate food and to break down fats, proteins, and carbohydrates to fatty acids, amino acids, and simple sugars, respectively.

SYMPTOMS AND SIGNS OF DIGESTIVE DISORDERS

Dysphagia (difficulty in swallowing), **odynophagia** (pain on swallowing).

Anorexia (loss of appetite), nausea, vomiting.

Hematemesis (vomiting of blood).

Constipation (firm, difficult stools), **obstipation** (total inability to pass stool).

Diarrhea (abnormal frequency, urgency, and looseness of stools), **lientery** (passage of undigested food in stools).

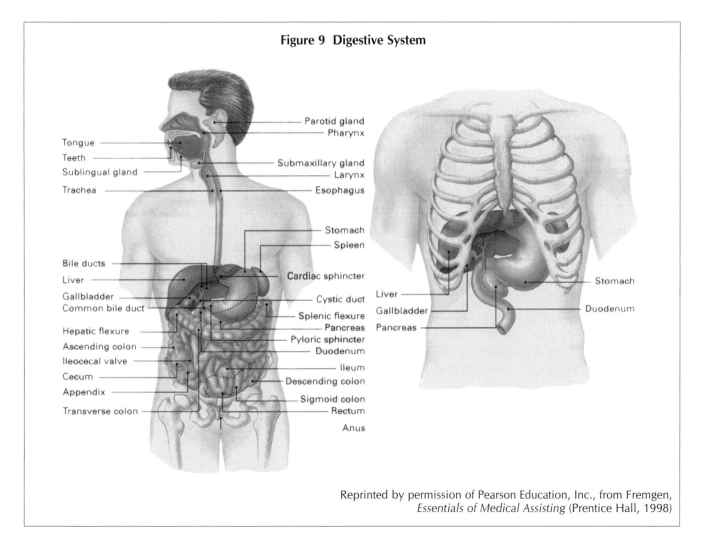

Figure 9 Digestive System

Reprinted by permission of Pearson Education, Inc., from Fremgen, *Essentials of Medical Assisting* (Prentice Hall, 1998)

Hematochezia (passage of blood from the rectum), **melena** (black stools, often due to the presence of blood), pale or white stools (due to absence of bile flow into the intestine), **steatorrhea** (passage of bulky, greasy stools due to nonabsorption of dietary fat).

Tenesmus (painful, often ineffectual straining to defecate).

Abdominal pain (diffuse or localized; intermittent or constant; random or affected by body position, meals, certain foods, bowel movement, medicine). Sharp, crampy pains are often referred to as colicky. Burning pain in the epigastrium or chest due to digestive disorders may be called heartburn.

Abdominal tenderness (local or generalized), rebound tenderness (additional stab of pain when pressure on abdomen is released, often indicating peritoneal irritation), spasm of abdominal wall, palpable abdominal mass, enlargement of abdominal organs, abnormal bulge of abdominal wall.

Bloating, belching, flatulence (excessive intestinal gas). **Tympanites** (hollow percussion note due to distention of underlying digestive tract with gas).

Borborygmi (singular, borborygmus) (audible rumbling and gurgling sounds in the digestive tract).

Hyperactive bowel sounds on auscultation (due to diarrhea, mechanical obstruction), **diminished or absent bowel sounds** ("silent abdomen") due to intestinal spasm or ileus, often reflecting local or generalized peritonitis.

Anal pain, itching, swelling, or bleeding.

Muscle wasting, pallor, fatigue.

Jaundice (discoloration of skin and whites of eyes by excessive bile pigment).

DIAGNOSTIC PROCEDURES IN DIGESTIVE DISORDERS

History and physical examination: Observation of abdomen for surgical or traumatic scars, swellings, discolorations, asymmetry; palpation of abdomen for masses, palpable organs, tenderness, spasm, hernia; percussion for hyperresonance (indicating excessive or displaced gas or air), flatness or dullness (indicating an abnormal mass, enlargement or consolidation of an organ, or impacted stool); auscultation for diminished, hyperactive, or high-pitched bowel sounds.

External anal examination, digital rectal examination.

Examination of stool for occult blood, fat, pathogens (bacteria, fungi, parasites), abnormal constituents.

Absorption tests, to assess the ability of the digestive tract to absorb certain nutrients or other materials, based on the determination of blood or stool levels of substances that have been ingested in measured amounts.

Imaging studies: Flat, upright, and (usually left) lateral decubitus films of the abdomen to assess distribution of gas and fluid in the stomach and bowel, identify free air in the peritoneal cavity, and detect other abnormalities (masses, calcifications, foreign bodies); fluoroscopic studies with swallowed or injected barium or other contrast medium (barium swallow, upper GI series, small bowel series, barium enema); percutaneous transhepatic cholangiography (PTC, injection of contrast material into biliary tract via catheter inserted through skin), endoscopic retrograde cholangiopancreatography (ERCP, endoscopically guided injection of contrast material into biliary and pancreatic ducts); CT, MRI, or ultrasound for specific indications (for example, to assess gallbladder, masses); hepatobiliary iminodiacetic acid (HIDA) scan with radioactive technetium.

Endoscopy: Esophagoscopy, gastroscopy, gastroduodenoscopy, anoscopy, sigmoidoscopy, colonoscopy; biopsy specimens, washings, cultures, and other materials can be obtained through endoscopes.

Laparoscopy (inspection of abdominal cavity through an endoscope inserted through an incision in the abdominal wall), exploratory laparotomy (inspection of the abdominal and pelvic cavities through an incision in the abdominal wall).

Liver biopsy (with biopsy needle inserted through skin of abdomen).

DISEASES OF THE ESOPHAGUS

Gastroesophageal Reflux Disease (GERD)

Backflow of gastric juice into the esophagus.

Cause: Structural or functional incompetence of the lower esophageal sphincter (LES), associated with disordered gastric motility and prolonged gastric emptying time. In a few cases, reflux of gastric juice may be facilitated by esophageal hiatus hernia (weakness or dilatation of the opening in the diaphragm where the esophagus passes through, with herniation of part or all of the stomach into the thorax; often asymptomatic). Reflux of acid gastric juice into the esophagus causes inflammation because the esophageal mucosa is not adapted to resist acid and digestive enzymes.

History: Recurrent epigastric and retrosternal distress, usually described as heartburn; belching, nausea, gagging, cough, hoarseness in varying proportions. There is a strong association with asthma, obesity, and diabetes mellitus. Symptoms are triggered or aggravated by recumbency (especially after a meal), vigorous exercise, smoking, overeating, caffeine, chocolate, alcohol, and certain drugs.

Physical Examination: Unremarkable.

Diagnostic Tests: Imaging studies confirm reflux of swallowed barium from the stomach and may identify ulceration or stricture. Twenty-four-hour monitoring of esophageal pH with a swallowed electrode confirms a sustained abnormal acid state in the esophagus. Endoscopy gives direct visual proof of inflammation and may identify a zone of Barrett esophagus (cellular change due to chronic inflammation).

Course: The underlying disorder of the LES and of gastric motility is irreversible. Severe reflux disease can lead to peptic ulceration of the esophagus, with eventual stricture due to scarring. Barrett esophagus, a metaplasia (transformation) of normal squamous esophageal epithelium into columnar epithelium, can progress to adenocarcinoma.

Treatment: Avoidance of smoking, alcohol, caffeine, and large meals. Over-the-counter antacids may suffice to control symptoms. Otherwise acid production may require suppression by H_2 antagonists (cimetidine, ranitidine, famotidine, nizatidine) or proton pump inhibitors (omeprazole, lansoprazole). Prokinetic drugs (bethanechol, metoclopramide) may improve sphincter function and gastric motility.

DISEASES OF THE STOMACH AND INTESTINE

Peptic Ulcer Disease and Gastritis

Inflammation and ulceration of the stomach, duodenum, or both by acid gastric juice.

Cause: Most commonly, infection of the gastric mucosa by *Helicobacter pylori*, a motile bacterium that survives in the acid environment of the stomach by secreting urease, an enzyme that converts urea to ammonia and bicarbonate, thus providing itself with a protective alkaline medium. *H. pylori* infection, which is spread from person to person by the fecal-oral route, results ultimately in a marked increase of acid production. Peptic ulceration can also result from regular use of prostaglandin-inhibiting drugs: adrenal corticosteroids and nonsteroidal anti-inflammatory agents such as ibuprofen and aspirin. In rare cases it is part of Zollinger-Ellison syndrome, in which a tumor of the pancreas produces excessive amounts of the hormone gastrin and thus causes hypersecretion of gastric acid. Severe stress, head injuries, and burns are sometimes complicated by peptic ulcer. Most peptic ulcers occur in the duodenum, but the stomach may be involved as well or instead.

History: Burning epigastric pain that comes on within an hour after meals and is relieved by taking antacids or food. Night pain is common. Tobacco, alcohol, caffeine, and certain foods aggravate symptoms, apparently by stimulating acid production. With complications: hematemesis, melena, early satiety (feeling that the stomach is full after only one or two mouthfuls of food), weight loss, severe abdominal pain, collapse.

Physical Examination: Unremarkable. Abdominal tenderness is variable and may be absent. With hemorrhage: pallor and tachycardia. With perforation: boardlike rigidity of the abdomen due to chemical peritonitis.

Diagnostic Tests: Upper GI studies with barium contrast medium can show ulceration, scarring, obstruction, or perforation. Endoscopy visualizes ulcers, bleeding sites, and scarring, and is important to rule out carcinoma in gastric lesions. Infection by *H. pylori* can be confirmed by culture, biopsy, serologic testing, or breath-testing for evidence of urease activity on orally administered, radioactively tagged urea.

Course: Without treatment, peptic ulcer disease tends to persist, with remissions and exacerbations, for many years. The most serious complications are hemorrhage (the principal cause of ulcer mortality), obstruction due to scarring, perforation of the digestive tract with release of gastric juice into the peritoneal cavity, and penetration into the retroperitoneal space.

Treatment: Smoking cessation, avoidance of alcohol and caffeine. Acidity may be adequately controlled by over-the-counter antacids, H_2 antagonists (cimetidine, ranitidine, famotidine, nizatidine) in over-the-counter or prescription strength, or proton pump inhibitors (omeprazole, lansoprazole). Proven *H. pylori* infection is treated with a course of therapy including bismuth subsalicylate and two antibiotics: tetracycline or amoxicillin, and metronidazole or clarithromycin.

Gastroenteritis

Inflammation of the stomach and intestine, manifested by abdominal pain, vomiting, and diarrhea; usually acute, infectious, and self-limited.

Causes: Infection with viruses (adenovirus, echovirus, coxsackievirus, rotavirus), bacteria (*Escherichia coli* H157:O7 and other virulent strains, *Campylobacter, Yersinia, Salmonella, Shigella, Clostridium*), protozoa (*Entamoeba histolytica, Giardia lamblia*), fungi (*Candida albicans*). Most of these infections are acquired by the fecal-oral route. Some are much more likely to occur in immunocompromised persons. Outbreaks are usually due to contaminated food or water. "Food poisoning" is due to toxins produced by staphylococci, *Salmonella, Clostridium,* or other organisms. Gastroenteritis can also be a reaction to medicines, foods, poisonous plants, toxic chemicals.

History: Usually abrupt onset of abdominal distress or cramping, anorexia, nausea, vomiting, and diarrhea. Chills, fever, malaise. Hematemesis and bloody diarrhea are ominous signs. In severe or protracted disease, or in children or the elderly, dehydration and electrolyte depletion can lead to prostration, vascular collapse, and death.

Physical Examination: May be unremarkable. Abdominal tenderness, tympanites (hollow percussion note due to distention of bowel with gas), hyperactive bowel sounds. In severe disease, signs of dehydration and electrolyte depletion include dryness of mucous membranes, decreased skin turgor (loss of normal consistency and fullness), tachycardia, hypoactive deep tendon reflexes, and decreased urine output.

Diagnostic Tests: Stool examination for white blood cells and organisms, with culture for pathogenic bacteria. Blood studies may show hematologic abnormalities or fluid and electrolyte imbalance.

Course: Most cases of gastroenteritis, even those caused by bacteria such as *Salmonella, Campylobacter,* and *Yersinia*, resolve spontaneously without specific treatment. However, cholera (due to *Vibrio cholerae,* rare in the U.S.), bacillary dysentery (due to *Shigella* species), typhoid fever (due to *Salmonella typhi*), and pseudomembranous enterocolitis (due to toxin-producing *Clostridium difficile*, often following treatment with antibiotics that kill normal intestinal flora) are all severe and potentially fatal infections requiring prompt, aggressive antimicrobial treatment. Any case of gastroenteritis in small children or in elderly or debilitated persons can lead to dangerous electrolyte and water depletion and vascular collapse.

Treatment: Largely symptomatic and supportive. Over-the-counter products may suffice to control nausea, cramping, and diarrhea. Water and electrolytes may be replaced orally or intravenously as indicated. Antibiotic treatment is indicated only in certain specific infections. Trimethoprim-sulfamethoxazole or ciprofloxacin are effective in bacillary dysentery (shigellosis), typhoid fever, and cholera; pseudomembranous enterocolitis is treated with metronidazole or vancomycin.

Appendicitis

Acute inflammation of the appendix.

Cause: Obstruction of the appendiceal lumen by a fecalith (stonelike mass of hardened feces), seed, or parasite, or by swelling due to infection or neoplasm. Obstruction is followed by inflammation, impairment of blood supply, necrosis, and rupture.

History: Gradual onset of generalized abdominal distress gradually becoming more severe and steady and localizing in the right lower quadrant. Anorexia, nausea, vomiting, fever, chills, constipation. Sudden spontaneous relief of pain suggests perforation.

Physical Examination: Slight fever and tachycardia, tenderness and rebound tenderness over McBurney point (about one-third of the distance from the right anterior superior iliac spine to the umbilicus), tenderness and rebound tenderness in the same area on rectal or pelvic examination. Diminished bowel sounds. After perforation, boardlike rigidity of the abdomen indicating peritonitis, signs of toxicity, vascular collapse. In infants, the elderly, and pregnant women the findings may be atypical or deceptively mild.

Diagnostic Tests: Moderate elevation of the white blood cell count, with left shift (increase of band or immature forms). Abdominal imaging (focused CT) may show a mass, ileus or other signs of peritonitis, or an opacity in the appendiceal lumen; barium injected by rectum fails to fill the appendix.

Course: Without treatment the condition has a mortality rate over 90%. Most cases progress to perforation within 12-36 hours, followed by generalized peritonitis, septicemia, and collapse.

Treatment: Surgical removal of the appendix (by open procedure or laparoscopy) is the only effective treatment. Perforation requires surgical repair, intravenous fluids, and antibiotics.

Irritable Bowel Syndrome (IBS)

Intermittent or chronic abdominal distress and bowel dysfunction without any demonstrable organic lesion.

Cause: Unknown. A derangement of the normal interaction between the brain and the bowel is postulated. IBS is more likely to occur with emotional stress, dietary irregularities, and heavy intake of caffeine. Lactose intolerance and abuse of antacids or laxatives may be partly responsible. The disorder is more common in women and in persons under 65. As many as 50% of patients report a history of verbal or sexual abuse.

History: Intermittent lower abdominal pain, often relieved by having a bowel movement; alternating diarrhea and constipation; a sense of inadequate evacuation after bowel movement; excessive mucus in stools; flatulence.

Physical Examination: Essentially negative.

Diagnostic Tests: Stool examinations, barium enema, colonoscopy, and blood studies are all negative. X-ray does not confirm distention of bowel with gas.

Course: Symptoms tend to wax and wane for many years, with intervals of complete remission.

Treatment: Regular eating habits, avoidance of coffee and other triggering factors. Antispasmodics may be prescribed to reduce bowel motility and cramping.

INFLAMMATORY BOWEL DISEASE

Crohn Disease (Regional Enteritis, Regional Ileitis)

A chronic inflammatory disease of the bowel that can lead to intestinal obstruction, abscess and fistula formation, and systemic complications.

Cause: Unknown. The disease shows a familial pattern of incidence.

History: Recurrent crampy or steady abdominal pain, nausea, diarrhea, steatorrhea (excessive fat in stool), hematochezia (blood in stool), weakness, weight loss, and fever.

Physical Examination: Abdominal tenderness, signs of complications.

Diagnostic Tests: The white blood cell count and erythrocyte sedimentation rate are elevated. There may be mild anemia and reduction of serum levels of potassium, calcium, magnesium, and other substances because of excessive bowel losses. Barium enema shows regional narrowing of the lumen ("string sign") alternating with areas of normal caliber. Sigmoidoscopy and colonoscopy show local inflammation with skip areas (intervening zones of normal mucosa). On biopsy, all layers of the bowel are seen to be involved, not just the mucosa as in ulcerative colitis.

Course: Complications include intestinal obstruction, formation of abscesses and fistulas, perforation of the bowel.

Treatment: Low-fiber diet, drugs to reduce intestinal motility, specific anti-inflammatory drugs (azathioprine, sulfasalazine, olsalazine). Surgery may be necessary to deal with perforation or fistula formation. In severe disease, segmental resection of the bowel, or colectomy (removal of the colon) with ileostomy (formation of an artificial opening from the small bowel through the anterior abdominal wall), may be necessary.

Ulcerative Colitis

A chronic inflammatory disease of the colon, chiefly the left colon, causing superficial ulceration.

Cause: Unknown.

History: Bloody diarrhea, abdominal cramps, tenesmus, anorexia, malaise, weakness, hemorrhoids or anal fissures. Bowel movements may occur more than 20 times a day, and may awaken the patient at night.

Physical Examination: Fever, abdominal tenderness, signs of complications.

Diagnostic Tests: The white blood cell count and erythrocyte sedimentation rate are elevated. Anemia may be present. Stool examination reveals mucus, blood, and pus, but no bacteria or parasites. Serum electrolytes and protein may be depleted. Sigmoidoscopy and colonoscopy show erythematous, friable mucosa with superficial ulceration and sometimes polyp formation. Biopsy shows chronic inflammation and microabscesses of the crypts of Lieberkühn.

Course: The course is intermittent, with spontaneous remissions and exacerbations. Physical and emotional stress and dietary irregularities may increase symptoms. Possible complications include colonic hemorrhage, perforation, toxic dilatation (extreme dilatation of the colon, compounded by effect of bacterial toxins), polyp formation with progression to carcinoma, arthritis, spondylitis, iritis, oral ulcers.

Treatment: General supportive treatment and control of diet (high protein, low milk) are crucial to long-term control of the disease. Sulfasalazine, mesalamine, and corticosteroids suppress colonic inflammation and reduce symptoms. In severe disease, hospitalization with intravenous alimentation and fluid replacement and antibiotic treatment to combat sepsis may be necessary. In intractable disease, colectomy and ileostomy may be necessary.

OTHER INTESTINAL DISORDERS

Diverticulosis and Diverticulitis

A diverticulum (plural, diverticula) is a blister- or bubble-like outpouching of a hollow or tubular organ. Diverticulosis of the colon is the formation of one or more such outpouchings of the colon. Diverticulitis means inflammation and infection of colonic diverticula.

Cause: Unknown; more common in middle-aged and elderly.

History: Most patients with diverticulosis have no symptoms. The diverticula may be discovered incidentally on routine examination (barium enema, colonoscopy). A few patients may experience irregular bowel habits or abdominal pain. Diverticulitis can cause acute abdominal pain, nausea, vomiting, constipation, and sometimes fever or blood in the stools.

Physical Examination: There may be mild fever, abdominal tenderness, and even the sensation of a mass, most often in the region of the sigmoid colon (left lower quadrant of the abdomen).

Diagnostic Tests: The white blood cell count and sedimentation rate may be slightly elevated. The stool may be positive for occult blood. Barium

enema, sigmoidoscopy, or colonoscopy may be performed to identify and localize the lesion, but are contraindicated in the presence of acute inflammation because of the danger of perforation of the bowel. X-ray studies may be used to identify free air in the peritoneal cavity due to perforation, and CT scan to detect abscess formation. Diagnostic evaluation needs to be particularly thorough to rule out malignancy.

Course: Diverticulitis may lead to hemorrhage, perforation of the bowel, obstruction due to fibrous scarring, fistula formation, or abscess formation.

Treatment: Patients with mild or no symptoms may require no treatment, but are often advised to follow a high-fiber diet. During the acute phase of diverticulitis, patients are kept at bed rest, with nothing by mouth, intravenous fluids and nutrition, and, if necessary, a nasogastric tube. Usually antibiotic treatment is used because of the risk of peritonitis and abscess formation. Metronidazole, ciprofloxacin, and trimethoprim-sulfamethoxazole are the drugs usually used. As many as one-third of patients with diverticulitis will need surgery to drain an abscess or to resect a segment of badly diseased colon.

Adenocarcinoma of the colon and rectum is discussed in Chapter 5.

Intestinal Obstruction

Blockage of the flow of digestive fluids through the small or large intestine.

Causes: Surgical adhesions, hernia, neoplasms, gallstones, volvulus (twisting of a loop of intestine), intussusception (passage of a segment of intestine into the segment distal to it), foreign body, fecal impaction. Obstruction due to causes outside the bowel (volvulus, hernia) are often complicated by strangulation (ischemia of the involved portion of bowel).

History: Crampy abdominal pain, nausea, vomiting, obstipation. Obstruction of the small intestine causes more severe and rapidly progressing symptoms than obstruction of the colon.

Physical Examination: Abdominal distention, borborygmi (gurgling sounds due to intestinal activity); increased bowel sounds, often high-pitched or in peristaltic rushes (urgent-sounding series of squeaking or gurgling sounds occurring with overactive peristaltic movements). A fullness or mass may be palpated at the site of obstruction. Tenderness, if strangulation has occurred. The rectum is empty of stool unless fecal impaction is the cause of obstruction.

Diagnostic Tests: The white blood cell count is elevated, particularly in the presence of strangulation. Blood chemistries may show electrolyte imbalance and dehydration due to vomiting and sequestration of fluid above the obstruction. Abdominal x-rays show dilated loops of bowel containing fluid levels, and may demonstrate the cause (volvulus, gallstone). Barium enema may be necessary to identify an obstruction in the colon.

Treatment: A nasogastric tube with suction to decompress the bowel proximal to the obstruction. Intravenous fluids to correct dehydration and electrolyte imbalance. Surgery is often necessary to relieve obstruction and to resect infarcted areas of bowel in cases of strangulation.

Adynamic Ileus

Failure of normal flow of materials through the digestive tract because of atony or paralysis of the bowel.

Causes: Recent abdominal surgery, peritonitis, mesenteric ischemia or infarction, medicines (opiates, anticholinergics).

History: Nausea, vomiting, obstipation, abdominal distention. Pain mild or absent.

Physical Examination: Abdominal distention, little or no tenderness, bowel sounds diminished or absent.

Diagnostic Tests: X-ray of the abdomen shows distended loops of small intestine with fluid levels.

Treatment: Nasogastric tube and suction, intravenous fluids, correction of the underlying cause if possible.

DISORDERS OF THE RECTUM AND ANUS

Hemorrhoids

Dilated veins just above or just below the anus.

Cause: Unknown. Constipation with straining at stool, prolonged sitting, and local infection have been implicated.

History: Anorectal discomfort or pain, swelling or protrusion, and bleeding.

Physical Examination: Dilated veins externally or internally, as seen by external inspection or endoscopy. Sigmoidoscopy or colonoscopy and barium enema may be performed to rule out malignancy.

Course: Symptoms are typically mild and intermittent. Bleeding is occasionally significant. Thrombosis of a hemorrhoid results in acute pain and swelling, but the problem resolves spontaneously in a few weeks.

Treatment: High-fiber diet, stool softeners, hot sitz baths, soothing applications or suppositories. With severe pain or bleeding, surgery is indicated. Band ligation is used for internal hemorrhoids; external hemorrhoids are treated by excision or cryosurgery.

Anal Fissure

A superficial longitudinal ulceration of the anal canal.

Cause: Probably trauma from a hard stool or hard, sharp material in stool. Chronic fissure may result from infection.

History: Anorectal pain and bleeding, chiefly with bowel movements.

Physical Examination: Fissure in anal canal. With chronic fissure a tag of anoderm (sentinel pile) may form below the fissure. Digital examination demonstrates anal tenderness and spasm.

Course: Acute fissures heal spontaneously in a few days. Chronic fissure may persist for weeks or months.

Treatment: High-fiber diet, stool softeners, hot sitz baths, anesthetic or anti-inflammatory ointments or suppositories. Severe chronic fissure occasionally requires surgical excision.

DISORDERS OF THE PERITONEUM

The peritoneum is a delicate serous membrane that lines the abdominal and pelvic cavities (parietal peritoneum) and also covers the stomach, small intestine, and colon (except for the distal part of the rectum), as well as the liver, spleen, uterus, ovaries, ureters, and dome of the bladder (visceral peritoneum). Structures such as the pancreas and kidneys that lie behind the peritoneal cavity are called retroperitoneal.

Acute Peritonitis

Acute inflammation of the peritoneum.

Causes: Infection (penetrating abdominal wounds, surgery, peritoneal dialysis for renal failure, spread from digestive or urinary tract or from a systemic site); chemical irritation (leakage of gastric or intestinal contents, bile, or pancreatic secretions from an injured, diseased, or perforated structure); systemic disease, neoplasm.

History: Fairly abrupt onset of severe local or generalized abdominal pain, nausea, vomiting, fever.

Physical Examination: Elevated temperature and pulse. Boardlike rigidity of abdomen, tenderness, and rebound tenderness. Diminished or absent bowel sounds and abdominal distention due to ileus.

Diagnostic Tests: The white blood cell count is elevated. Blood studies may also show electrolyte imbalances due to peritoneal effusion, vomiting, and dehydration. Anemia may occur. Fluid obtained by abdominal paracentesis (entry of peritoneal cavity with a needle passed through the abdominal wall) may show amylase or lipase (indicating leak of intestinal contents or pancreatic juice), significant cellular abnormalities, or infecting microorganisms. Various types of imaging may be of use in confirming and identifying intra-abdominal catastrophe.

Course: Without treatment the outlook is poor. Septicemia and vascular collapse often occur within a few hours of onset. In some patients, peritonitis becomes localized, with abscess formation, particularly subphrenic (just below diaphragm) or pelvic. Peritonitis often results in eventual formation of fibrous adhesions that may produce intestinal obstruction.

Treatment: Hospitalization, nothing by mouth, gastrointestinal suction to decompress the bowel and draw off secretions, intravenous fluids, narcotics for pain, antibiotics for infection, surgery to repair underlying abnormality.

ABDOMINAL HERNIA

A localized weakness in the musculoaponeurotic wall of the abdomen, with protrusion of abdominal contents. Abdominal hernias are classified according to position as:

Umbilical (at the navel): Often congenital, seldom requiring surgical repair because it resolves during infancy.

Inguinal (in the groin):
• Direct inguinal: Due to thinning and stretching of the lower abdominal wall, often with aging.
• Indirect inguinal (usually congenital): Weakness and bulging in the inguinal canal, the passage through which, in the male fetus, the testicle descends from the abdominal cavity to the scrotum; a similar potential passage exists in women.

Femoral: Herniation into the femoral canal, through which the femoral artery and vein pass from the pelvis into the thigh.

Cause: Congenital weakness or malformation; thinning of the abdominal musculature by aging. Herniation may be precipitated or aggravated by vigorous or repeated straining of the abdominal wall (chronic constipation, urinary obstruction, heavy lifting, chronic cough).

History: A tender bulge in the abdominal wall that enlarges with straining. Intestinal obstruction may occur, with severe abdominal pain, nausea, vomiting, weakness, shock, and collapse.

Physical Examination: A fluctuant bulge in the abdominal wall that enlarges with straining and can be reduced with manipulation or recumbency unless incarceration has occurred. A defect in the abdominal wall at the site of the hernia can be palpated. Visible or palpable mass, tenderness. There may be evidence of strangulation or bowel obstruction.

Diagnostic Tests: Barium enema and other studies may be done to rule out obstructive disease of the bowel or urinary tract.

Complications: Strangulation (compromise of blood supply), incarceration (inability to reduce hernia), bowel obstruction.

Treatment: Surgical repair of the defect, sometimes with implantation of reinforcing mesh.

DISEASES OF THE LIVER

The liver, the largest gland in the body, lies in the right upper quadrant of the abdomen just below the diaphragm and is largely covered by peritoneum. The portal vein carries nutrients and other substances from the digestive tract to the liver. The liver performs numerous vital functions and is intimately concerned with carbohydrate and nitrogen metabolism and with removal of certain waste products. Bile, the secretory product of the liver, passes through a duct into the duodenum. Bile contains bile salts, which help in the digestion of fats, and bilirubin, a breakdown product of hemoglobin. Bile does not flow steadily into the duodenum, but is stored in the gallbladder, a bulb or pouch connected by the cystic duct to the common bile duct. Ingestion of a fatty meal stimulates contraction of the gallbladder and increased flow of bile into the intestine.

Hepatitis A

Cause: Hepatitis A virus. Transmission is by the fecal-oral route. Contaminated food and water are important means of infection.

History: Anorexia, nausea, vomiting, malaise, upper respiratory or flulike symptoms, fever, joint pain, aversion to tobacco, abdominal discomfort, diarrhea or constipation. Infection may be asymptomatic in children.

Physical Examination: Fever, jaundice, enlargement and tenderness of the liver, splenomegaly, cervical lymphadenopathy.

Diagnostic Tests: The serum bilirubin is elevated, and liver function tests are abnormal. Atypical lymphocytes may appear in the blood. Anti-HAV (IgM) antibody appears early in the course of the disease and disappears after recovery. IgG antibody develops later and persists indefinitely, indicating past history of, and immunity to, the disease.

Course: Symptoms characteristically resolve within 2-3 weeks. The mortality is very low.

Treatment: Supportive and symptomatic.

Hepatitis B

Cause: Hepatitis B virus. Transmission is by blood (shared needles, needlestick injury in health-care workers) or sexual contact. Maternal transmission to neonates also occurs.

History: Fever, anorexia, nausea, vomiting, malaise, joint pain and swelling, rash, aversion to tobacco, abdominal pain, bowel irregularities.

Physical Examination: Fever, jaundice, enlargement and tenderness of liver. Splenomegaly, cervical lymphadenopathy.

Diagnostic Tests: The serum bilirubin is elevated, and liver function tests are abnormal. Atypical lymphocytes may appear in the blood. Hepatitis B surface antigen (HB_SAg) appears early in the disease and indicates presence of infection and infectivity of the patient. Antibody to surface antigen ($AntiHB_S$) indicates recovery, immunity to future infection, and lack of infectivity. Presence of HB_SAg after the acute phase suggests chronic infection.

Course: The incubation period may be 6-12 weeks or longer, and acute illness may persist for as long as 16 weeks. The mortality rate is somewhat higher than that of hepatitis A. Some patients become carriers of the disease, able to transmit infection months or years after recovery. In some, a chronic phase occurs. Chronic persistent hepatitis is mild and generally asymptomatic, while chronic active hepatitis leads to gradual deterioration of liver function, cirrhosis, and an appreciable risk of hepatocellular carcinoma.

Treatment: Chiefly supportive. Chronic hepatitis is treated with interferon alfa-2b and lamivudine.

Hepatitis C

Cause: Hepatitis C virus (HCV). Transmission is by sharing of needles among drug-abusers (60% of all cases), contaminated blood or blood products, transplanted organs, sexual contact, and from mother to fetus.

History: Malaise, weakness, anorexia, fever, jaundice. Symptoms of acute infection are typically mild and occur in only one-third of patients. About 85% of patients eventually develop chronic disease, with unpredictable progression toward hepatic failure.

Physical Examination: May be unremarkable until signs of hepatic failure or cirrhosis appear.

Diagnostic Tests: Antibody to HCV is present in serum. Polymerase chain reaction (PCR) or other methods allow quantitative determination of viral DNA in serum. Liver function tests and liver biopsy to assess degree of hepatocellular damage.

Course: Progressive decline of hepatic function in chronic disease. Complications include hepatic cirrhosis (20%), hepatocellular carcinoma (5%), arthritis, glomerulonephritis, autoimmune syndromes.

Treatment: Interferon alfa, ribavirin. Liver transplantation.

Hepatitis D (Delta Hepatitis)

Hepatitis due to a defective virus; it occurs only in persons already infected with hepatitis B, and is common among IV drug users. In itself a relatively mild illness, it may add to the severity of hepatitis B.

Hepatic Cirrhosis (Portal Cirrhosis, Laënnec Cirrhosis)

A chronic disorder of the liver characterized by inflammation of secretory cells followed by nodular regeneration and fibrosis.

Causes: The principal cause is chronic alcohol abuse. About 20% of persons with hepatitis C eventually develop cirrhosis. Other toxic, metabolic, nutritional, and infectious factors may play a part in the genesis of this disorder. The cirrhotic liver contains various combinations of fatty change and fibrosis forming small and large nodules.

History: Usually gradual onset of anorexia, nausea, weakness, weight loss, abdominal swelling due to ascites (accumulation of fluid in the abdominal cavity), and often jaundice. Disturbance of sex steroid hormone metabolism causes impotence in men and amenorrhea in women.

Physical Examination: Fever, muscle wasting, pleural effusion, ascites, peripheral edema. The liver is usually enlarged and may be firm or even hard. The spleen may also be enlarged. Jaundice appears relatively late. Elevation of estrogen level causes gynecomastia in men, spider angiomas (spider nevi) on the face and upper trunk, and palmar erythema. The tongue may appear smooth, shiny, and inflamed. With advanced disease there may be coarse, flapping tremors (asterixis) and delirium due to hepatic failure, which may progress to hepatic coma.

Diagnostic Tests: Laboratory tests show elevation of bilirubin and enzymes such as transaminases, lactic dehydrogenase, and alkaline phosphatase, which rise in the presence of liver cell damage. Anemia may be present, and coagulation studies may yield abnormal results. Liver biopsy confirms presence of typical histologic changes. Imaging studies including radioactive liver scans provide further information. Esophagoscopy may show esophageal varices.

Course: Symptoms may wax and wane over a period of years, often in response to varying levels of alcohol consumption. Progressive hepatic failure often occurs. Fibrosis within the liver typically shuts off branches of the portal circulation and increases the pressure in the portal vein (portal hypertension). (See Figure 10.) In consequence, other vessels (particularly the lower esophageal venous plexus) dilate and become varicose (bulging) or tortuous (coiled, twisted). Hemorrhage from bleeding esophageal varices is often life-threatening, particularly when hepatic disease causes a coagulation disorder. There is an increased incidence of hepatocellular carcinoma in persons with cirrhosis.

Treatment: Abstinence from alcohol, attention to nutrition, particularly carbohydrate, protein, vitamins. Rest, sodium restriction, and diuretics for edema and ascites. Severe ascites may require abdominal paracentesis (removal of peritoneal fluid with a needle passed through the abdominal wall). Patients with portal hypertension and bleeding esophageal varices may need a portacaval shunt (surgical procedure allowing portal vein blood to bypass the liver and empty directly into the inferior vena cava).

DISEASES OF THE GALLBLADDER AND BILIARY TRACT

Cholelithiasis (Gallstones)

The formation of gallstones is a common disorder, generally due to some disturbance in the flow of bile from the gallbladder or in the composition of bile. Gallstones are more common in women and in elderly persons. Risk factors include pregnancy, diabetes mellitus, high serum cholesterol, Crohn disease, and sickle cell anemia. In the latter condition, stones consist primarily of bilirubin from broken-down red blood cells. In the other conditions, gallstones are composed primarily of cholesterol.

Gallstones are often asymptomatic ("silent"), but about 90% of persons with cholecystitis (inflammation of the gallbladder) have pre-existing cholelithiasis. Stones may be demonstrated on plain abdominal films, but ultrasound and imaging after injection of opaque medium are more sensitive and specific. Potential serious complications are blockage of the common bile duct by a stone with ensuing obstructive jaundice, blockage of the cystic duct with ensuing cholecystitis, and passage of a stone into the intestine with the potential for causing bowel obstruction (gallstone ileus). Treatment of symptomatic gallstones is surgical removal (along with the gallbladder), usually through a laparoscope. Stones can also be crushed and flushed out with instruments passed through an endoscope inserted through the mouth and threaded into the common bile duct. Oral bile salts (chenodeoxycholic acid, ursodeoxycholic acid) and extracorporeal shockwave lithotripsy (ESWL) sometimes dissolve stones.

Figure 10 Portal Circulation

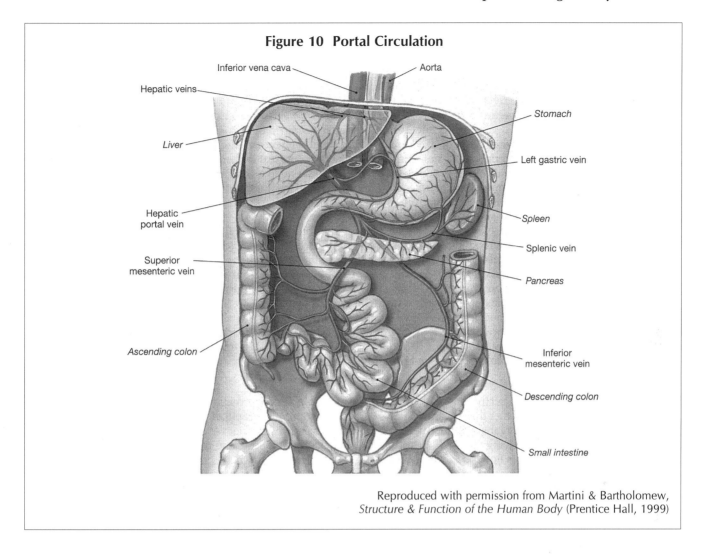

Inferior vena cava
Aorta
Hepatic veins
Liver
Stomach
Left gastric vein
Hepatic portal vein
Spleen
Splenic vein
Superior mesenteric vein
Pancreas
Ascending colon
Inferior mesenteric vein
Descending colon
Small intestine

Reproduced with permission from Martini & Bartholomew,
Structure & Function of the Human Body (Prentice Hall, 1999)

Acute Cholecystitis

Acute inflammation of the gallbladder.

Causes: As mentioned above, most patients with cholecystitis have pre-existing cholelithiasis. Impaction of a stone in the cystic duct leads to obstruction of the flow of bile from the gallbladder, with ischemia, acute inflammation, and sometimes abscess formation or perforation.

History: Fairly acute onset of severe epigastric and right upper quadrant pain, nausea, and vomiting.

Physical Examination: Fever and jaundice may be present. In the right upper quadrant of the abdomen, there are tenderness, rebound tenderness, and involuntary guarding (spasm of abdominal muscles on palpation). Bowel sounds are reduced or absent. Occasionally a mass can be felt below the liver edge, representing a distended gallbladder.

Diagnostic Tests: The white blood cell count, bilirubin, and levels of serum enzymes reflecting hepatic damage may all be elevated. Imaging studies (plain abdominal x-ray, ultrasound, scans with radiotagged media) may precisely identify the problem.

Course: Acute cholecystitis may resolve spontaneously. Often relapses occur, with gradual development of chronic cholecystitis. Inflammation may culminate in gangrene (tissue death due to compromise of blood supply) or perforation of the gallbladder, or may ascend into the liver via the biliary tract (ascending cholangitis).

Treatment: Chiefly supportive, with narcotics for pain, intravenous fluids, and close observation. Impending or actual perforation is treated by surgical (laparoscopic) decompression (drainage) of the gallbladder or, preferably, by removal of the gallbladder (cholecystectomy).

DISORDERS OF THE PANCREAS

The pancreas is a flat retroperitoneal organ lying behind and below the stomach, with its right end (head) embraced by the C-shaped curve of the duodenum. (See Figure 11.) It is composed of two types of glandular tissue: groups of cells that secrete enzymes for the digestion of carbohydrate, protein, and fat, which are poured through a duct into the duodenum near the orifice of the common bile duct; and other groups of cells that secrete hormones (insulin, glucagon, somatostatin) and release them directly into the blood-stream. The endocrine function of the pancreas is discussed in Chapter 15.

Acute Pancreatitis

Acute inflammation of the pancreas.

Causes: Most cases occur in alcoholics or in persons with chronic biliary tract disease (cholelithiasis, cholecystitis). In these instances, obstruction of the pancreatic duct by edema, or backflow of bile from the duodenum into the pancreatic duct, causes release of pancreatic enzymes into the substance of the gland, with resulting intense inflammation, necrosis, and often hemorrhage. Other causes are hypercalcemia (abnormally high level of calcium in the blood), hypertriglyceridemia (abnormally high level of triglycerides in the blood), abdominal trauma or surgery, certain medicines, and viral infection including mumps. An acute attack of pancreatitis is often precipitated by excessive alcohol consumption or by eating a large meal.

History: Abrupt onset of severe, persisting epigastric pain, worse on lying flat, and radiating to the flanks and back. Nausea, vomiting, sweating, prostration, restlessness.

Physical Examination: Pallor, tachycardia, fever, epigastric tenderness, reduced or absent bowel sounds. Jaundice or hypotension may occur. In the presence of severe pancreatic hemorrhage, a bluish discoloration of the skin may appear over the left flank (Turner or Grey Turner sign). There may be evidence of ascites or a left pleural effusion.

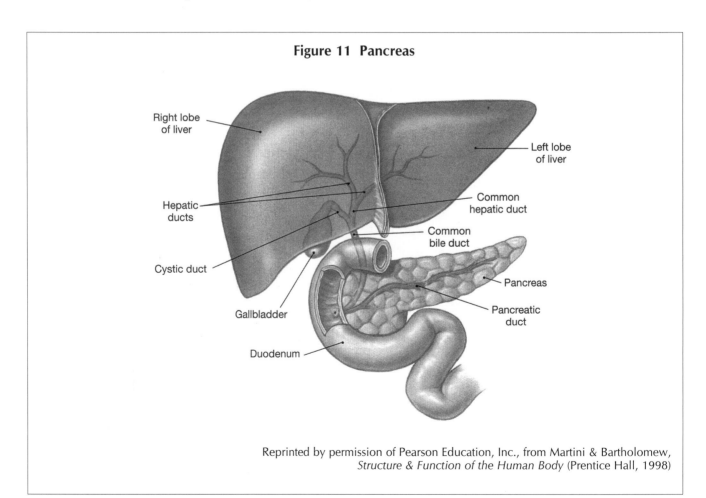

Figure 11 Pancreas

Reprinted by permission of Pearson Education, Inc., from Martini & Bartholomew, *Structure & Function of the Human Body* (Prentice Hall, 1998)

Diagnostic Tests: Blood studies may show leukocytosis, hyperglycemia, anemia, and hypocalcemia (drop in serum calcium). Blood levels of pancreatic enzymes (amylase, lipase) are typically elevated. Imaging studies may show gallstones, a mass representing the swollen pancreas, left atelectasis (collapse of part of left lung caused by shallow breathing at site of pain), or left pleural effusion (inflammatory fluid in pleural cavity).

Course: Acute pancreatitis has a high mortality rate and, among survivors, a high recurrence rate. Possible outcomes include abscess formation, splenic vein thrombosis, ileus, shock, renal failure, adult respiratory distress syndrome, severe hypocalcemia with tetany, formation of pseudocysts (pockets of inflammatory fluid and debris between the pancreas and surrounding tissues), and progression to chronic disease.

Treatment: Hospitalization, narcotics for pain relief, nasogastric suction, intravenous fluids with attention to water balance, nutritional needs, and replacement of calcium. Surgery may be required to control hemorrhage, correct underlying disease, or drain pseudocysts.

Chronic Pancreatitis

Chronic inflammation of the pancreas.

Causes: Essentially the same as for acute pancreatitis. With recurrent or chronic disease, fibrosis of the pancreas and its ducts leads to worsening disease, with loss of both endocrine and exocrine pancreatic function.

History: Recurrent bouts of left upper quadrant pain, anorexia, nausea, vomiting. Weight loss, flatulence, and steatorrhea (greasy stools) because of deficiency or absence of pancreatic enzymes.

Physical Examination: Epigastric and left upper quadrant tenderness, involuntary guarding, ileus.

Diagnostic Tests: Sugar may appear in the urine and blood sugar may be elevated as a result of diabetes mellitus due to destruction of pancreatic endocrine tissue. The serum levels of pancreatic amylase and lipase may be elevated. The proportion of fat in the composition of the stools is increased because of deficiency of lipase in the intestine. Abdominal x-ray may show widening of the curve of the duodenum due to pancreatic edema. Retrograde injection of opaque medium into the pancreatic duct with a catheter placed endoscopically can clearly outline anatomic conditions (dilatation vs. narrowing of duct, stone formation).

Course: Without treatment, progressive deterioration of pancreatic function, with nutritional deficiencies, flatulence, steatorrhea, and diabetes mellitus. Pseudocyst formation.

Treatment: Avoidance of alcohol and fatty foods, oral supplementation of pancreatic enzymes. Surgery may be required to improve pancreatic drainage or remove pseudocysts.

QUESTIONS FOR STUDY AND REVIEW

1. Name three gastrointestinal disorders that are due to infection:

    a. _____

    b._____

    c. _____

2. Name three gastrointestinal disorders that may be precipitated or aggravated by alcohol abuse:

    a. _____

    b._____

    c. _____

3. Name three gastrointestinal disorders that may be precipitated or aggravated by smoking:

    a. _____

    b._____

    c._____

4. Name three gastrointestinal disorders that can be complicated by life-threatening hemorrhage and result in intestinal obstruction:

    a. _____

    b._____

    c._____

5. Define or explain these terms:

    a. anorexia _____

    _____

    b. Crohn disease _____

    _____

    c. dysphagia _____

    _____

    d. flatulence_____

    _____

    e. GERD _____

    _____

    f. hematochezia_____

    _____

    g. ileus_____

    _____

h. melena _____

_____

i. pancreas_____

_____

j. peritoneum_____

_____

6. Name three kinds of gastroenteritis that must generally be treated with antibiotics:

a. _____

b. _____

c. _____

7. Name three kinds of gastroenteritis that do not respond to antibiotics:

a. _____

b. _____

c. _____

8. State three important differences between Crohn disease and ulcerative colitis:

a. _____

b. _____

c. _____

9. State three important differences between hepatitis A and hepatitis B:

a. _____

b. _____

c. _____

CASE STUDY: YOU'RE THE DOCTOR

Ezra Toldt, a 57-year-old homeless white male, is brought by an ambulance crew to the hospital emergency department where you are on duty. He was found by custodial workers around 10 p.m. in a public park vomiting, confused, and "doubled over with pain." He has no known address and no known family. Past medical history and information about insurance coverage are unavailable.

1. What types of health problems does this background suggest?

_____

_____

_____

_____

Mr. Toldt is unkempt, unshaven, and unwashed. His clothing smells of urine and vomitus, and in addition there is a strong smell of liquor on his breath. He is moaning and holding his abdomen. He cries out in pain when rescue personnel transfer him to a gurney. He responds to some commands but not others. He answers questions incoherently or not at all.

2. To what extent do you expect his inability to give a clear history to impair your ability to diagnose and treat him appropriately? What reasons support your position?

_____

_____

_____

_____

Rectal temperature is 100.8, pulse 116, blood pressure 114/54. The skin is sallow, warm, damp, and of reduced turgor. Bruises and abrasions of various ages are noted over the chest and extremities. There is no evidence of head trauma. Examination of the eyes shows conjunctival injection, scleral icterus, and lateral nystagmus. The pupils are equal and sluggishly reactive. The pharyngeal mucosa appears dry and beefy red. The teeth are in poor repair. There are no cervical masses. The ribs are not tender. The heart is regular without murmurs, rubs, or third or fourth heart sound. The lungs are clear. The abdomen is slightly distended and shows no scars. Palpation of the abdomen reveals marked guarding, tenderness, and rebound tenderness in all four quadrants. A firm, smooth liver edge is palpated four fingerbreadths below the right costal margin. The spleen is not palpable. No abdominal masses are felt. No bowel sounds are heard. Rectal examination is performed with difficulty because of the patient's pain and confusion. The prostate is symmetrically enlarged, slightly boggy, and apparently slightly tender. The rectal pouch contains soft dark stool that is positive for occult blood.

3. What diagnostic possibilities do these findings raise?

_____

_____

_____

_____

4. What further procedures will you use to narrow the diagnosis?

_____

_____

_____

_____

5. What forms of treatment are indicated immediately while you proceed with your evaluation?

_____

_____

_____

_____

SUGGESTIONS FOR ADDITIONAL LEARNING ACTIVITIES

1. Write a history and physical examination report for a patient admitted to the hospital with a digestive disorder discussed in this chapter. Include a chief complaint, history of present illness, past medical history, family and social histories, review of systems, and complete physical examination. Describe the laboratory data ordered and obtained upon admission. Your differential diagnosis should include other possible conditions that need to be ruled out as the cause of the patient's problem. Draft a treatment plan. For an additional challenge, remove the diagnosis and treatment plan sections from your H&P and exchange reports with another student. Write a differential diagnosis and treatment plan for this new report and then compare your conclusions.

2. Make a 3-D (three-dimensional) model of the digestive system using modeling clay or any household objects (cardboard paper towel holders, small boxes, and so on). Assemble your model and label the individual structures, including explanations of the role of each structure in the function of the digestive system.

3. Medications are commonly prescribed for the treatment of gastrointestinal conditions. Compile a list of all the types of medications described in this chapter. Consult a drug reference book and locate several brand names for each type of drug mentioned. Write down the indications, usual dosage, and form for each drug.

12

The Excretory System, the Male Reproductive System, and Sexually Transmitted Diseases

Chapter Outline

LEARNING OBJECTIVES

Upon completion of this chapter, you should be able to

- describe the basic anatomy and physiology of the excretory and male genitourinary systems;

- explain diagnostic procedures and treatments for the male reproductive and genitourinary systems;

- classify common diseases affecting the male reproductive and genitourinary systems by their signs, symptoms, and treatment;

- give examples of some of the more common sexually transmitted diseases.

173

Chapter Outline

THE EXCRETORY SYSTEM, THE MALE REPRODUCTIVE SYSTEM, AND SEXUALLY TRANSMITTED DISEASES
(continued)

SEXUALLY TRANSMITTED DISEASES
Syphilis (Lues)
Gonorrhea
Chlamydial Infection

QUESTIONS FOR STUDY AND REVIEW

THE EXCRETORY SYSTEM, THE MALE REPRODUCTIVE SYSTEM, AND SEXUALLY TRANSMITTED DISEASES

DISORDERS OF THE EXCRETORY SYSTEM

ANATOMY AND PHYSIOLOGY

The excretory or urinary system consists of the kidneys, the ureters, the bladder, and the urethra. (See Figure 12.) The kidneys are paired, bean-shaped organs lying behind the abdominal cavity on either side of the aorta. The kidneys produce urine by filtering the blood through numerous microscopic units called glomeruli and then further processing the filtrate in the renal tubules. Most of the water that passes through the glomeruli is reabsorbed in the renal tubules. Other substances are reabsorbed as well, while still others are actively excreted by the tubules. The principal functions of the kidney are the excretion of water, waste materials (particularly nitrogenous wastes such as urea and creatinine), and other substances (potassium, extraneous chemicals including medicines), and the maintenance of water and electrolyte balance.

Urine formed by the glomeruli and tubules passes into the renal pelvis, a funnel-shaped collecting cavity, from which it flows downward through the ureter and into the bladder. The urethra, the outflow tract of the bladder, differs in the two sexes. The female urethra is short, emptying near the vestibule of the vagina but otherwise independent of the female reproductive system. The male urethra passes through the penis and in addition to its function in emptying the bladder it serves as the channel for the ejaculation of semen.

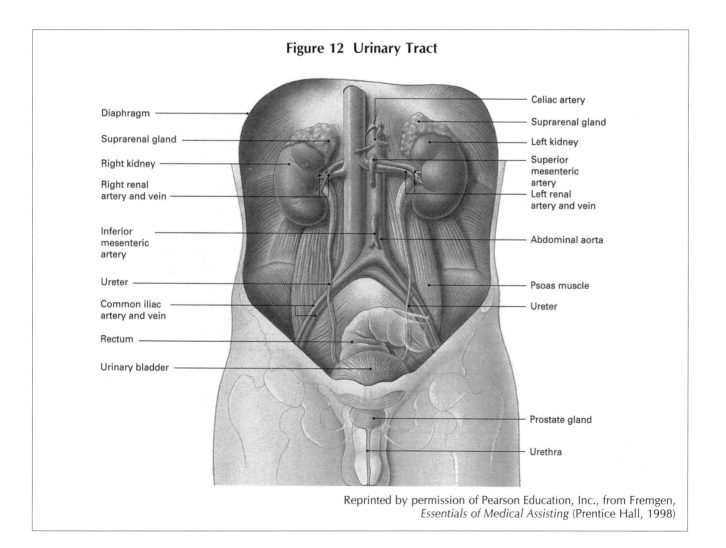

Figure 12 Urinary Tract

Reprinted by permission of Pearson Education, Inc., from Fremgen, *Essentials of Medical Assisting* (Prentice Hall, 1998)

SYMPTOMS AND SIGNS OF URINARY DISORDERS

Pain, constant or intermittent, generally located at or near the site of disease.

Flank or costovertebral angle (CVA) pain (pain at the angle formed by the lowermost rib and the spinal column), usually accompanied by tenderness, suggests disease within the kidney (pyelonephritis).

Ureteral pain (ureteral colic) is intense pain, generally intermittent or with intermittent exacerbations, that originates in the flank or abdomen and radiates into the groin; it suggests ureteral obstruction by a stone.

Suprapubic pain, overlying the site of the bladder, suggests bladder distention or infection (cystitis).

Perineal pain (in the male) suggests prostatic disease.

Pain with voiding (dysuria) indicates urethritis or cystitis.

Urinary Abnormalities

Anuria: Total or nearly total cessation of urine excretion by the kidney (sometimes defined as less than 100 mL/day of urine production).

Decreased force or caliber of the urinary stream.

Dribbling: Uncontrollable passage of drops of urine, particularly just after voiding.

Hematuria: Blood in the urine (gross hematuria is visible to the naked eye; microscopic or occult hematuria can be detected only by microscopic or chemical examination of the urine).

Hesitancy: Difficulty in initiating urine flow.

Incontinence: Involuntary passage of urine.

Oliguria: Marked reduction in the volume of urine excreted in 24 hours (sometimes defined as urine output between 100 and 400 mL/day).

Pollakiuria: Increased frequency of urination, without an increase in the total volume of urine excreted in 24 hours.

Polyuria: Increase in the 24-hour excretion of urine.

DIAGNOSTIC PROCEDURES IN EXCRETORY DISORDERS

History and physical examination, with special attention to the external genitalia and abdominal, rectal, and pelvic examinations.

Urinalysis: A group of standard laboratory examinations of the urine, including determination of pH and specific gravity, chemical testing for sugar (normally absent), albumin (protein, normally absent), occult blood, leukocyte esterase (an enzyme indicating the presence of white blood cells), nitrite (a product of bacterial action), acetone, bilirubin, and other substances, and microscopic examination for red and white blood cells, renal tubular epithelial (RTE) cells, crystals, casts (abnormal plugs of material formed in renal tubules), and other materials.

Quantitative determination of protein in a 24-hour specimen of urine can detect microalbuminuria (passage of smaller amounts of protein that can be detected by routine qualitative tests), which is a sign of diabetic nephropathy.

Assessment of kidney function by determination of blood levels of substances normally removed by the kidney: blood urea nitrogen (BUN), creatinine. Creatinine clearance compares blood and urine levels of creatinine.

Urine culture, usually with colony count and sensitivity studies, to identify urinary pathogens.

Catheterization of the bladder: Insertion of a flexible or rigid tube into the bladder through the urethra to withdraw urine; its principal diagnostic application is determination of residual volume (amount of urine remaining in the bladder after normal voiding).

Cystoscopy: Insertion of an endoscope through the urethra and into the bladder to inspect its inner surfaces, including the ureteral orifices.

Imaging studies: Plain or KUB (kidney, ureters, bladder) film; ultrasound or MRI studies to identify stones, neoplasms, cysts; intravenous pyelogram (IVP) (x-ray examination of urinary tract after intravenous injection of radiopaque contrast medium that is quickly excreted in the urine); voiding cystourethrogram (film of the act of voiding with contrast medium in the urine).

Renal biopsy: Removal of a sample of kidney tissue through a needle passed through the skin or through a surgical incision.

DISORDERS OF THE KIDNEY

Polycystic Kidney

A hereditary abnormality of both kidneys transmitted in an autosomal dominant pattern. Both kidneys are enlarged and cystic, and some patients also have hepatic cysts or cerebral aneurysms. Symptoms include abdominal or flank pain, hematuria, and a tendency to urinary tract infections and stones. On examination the kidneys are large and palpable through the abdominal wall. Ultrasound examination or CT scan confirms enlargement and cystic malformation. The urine contains protein and red blood cells. Progression to renal failure is the usual outcome. Many patients develop renal hypertension (high blood pressure due to disease of kidney cells). Treatment includes monitoring of renal function, vigorous treatment of infection and hypertension, and, with advancing failure of kidney function, renal dialysis or renal transplant.

Acute Renal Failure

An abrupt, severe decline in kidney function, with retention of nitrogenous waste products of protein metabolism (azotemia, uremia)

Cause: The abnormality may be prerenal (impaired blood supply to kidney), renal (also called parenchymal or intrinsic: disease of the kidney proper), or postrenal (obstruction of the outflow of urine from the kidney). Prerenal azotemia can result from renal artery stenosis, hypotension, or the effects of certain drugs (NSAIDs, ACE inhibitors) on renal blood flow. Renal azotemia can result from any severe disease of kidney tissue, including acute glomerulonephritis, vasculitis affecting the intrinsic renal circulation, or acute tubular necrosis.

History: Malaise, weakness, anorexia, nausea, reduced urine volume (oliguria). In advanced disease, vomiting, hematemesis, diarrhea, drowsiness, seizures, pruritus, cardiac arrhythmias, peripheral edema, dyspnea.

Physical Examination: Essentially negative. A pericardial friction rub may be heard in uremic pericarditis. In advanced disease, pallor, peripheral edema, pulmonary edema, congestive heart failure, coma.

Diagnostic Tests: Blood levels of BUN and creatinine are markedly increased. The serum pH is low (metabolic acidosis). Serum potassium and phosphorus levels are elevated and calcium is depressed. Anemia may be severe.

Course: The case mortality rate is 20-50% depending on the cause and underlying diseases. If the inciting cause is reversible, the renal failure itself may completely resolve. Most patients with reversible

disease recover completely within six weeks. Typically there is an oliguric acute phase, followed by copious diuresis (increased urine formation) as renal function improves, and at length a return to normal urine volume. Infection is a common complication.

Treatment: Largely supportive. Restriction of water, protein, and potassium intake, with high carbohydrate diet and vitamin supplementation. Close monitoring of water and electrolyte balance. Renal dialysis or intravenous administration of glucose, insulin, and sodium bicarbonate, and oral sodium polystyrene sulfonate, to reduce serum potassium.

Acute Glomerulonephritis

Acute inflammation of renal glomeruli, with failure to excrete nitrogenous wastes.

Causes: Poststreptococcal glomerulonephritis is an autoimmune disease that follows infection (usually pharyngitis) with group A beta-hemolytic streptococci, type 12. In Berger disease (IgA nephropathy), immune complexes form in the glomerulus, often after a respiratory or gastrointestinal infection or a flu-like illness.

History: Sudden appearance of tea-colored or Coca-Cola-colored urine, with reduction in urine volume and possibly peripheral edema.

Physical Examination: Blood pressure elevation (in poststreptocccal glomerulonephritis); peripheral edema.

Diagnostic Tests: The urine contains red blood cells, white blood cells, renal tubular epithelial cells, casts, and protein. Creatinine clearance and urinary sodium are reduced, and the 24-hour urinary excretion of protein is increased. In poststreptococcal disease, the ASO titer is elevated. Serum protein electrophoresis and antibody studies may indicate the presence of antibody to glomerular protein. Renal biopsy allows precise identification of tissue changes.

Course: Most patients with poststreptococcal glomerulonephritis recover without sequelae, but in a few the renal damage is rapidly progressive. About half of patients with Berger disease suffer progressive loss of kidney function.

Treatment: Largely supportive. Antibiotic to eradicate streptococci. Fluid restriction. Diuretics to reverse fluid retention. Attention to nutrition and control of hypertension. Renal dialysis if renal failure becomes severe.

Nephrotic Syndrome

A disorder of kidney function in which a large amount of protein is lost in the urine from damaged glomeruli.

Causes: Various abnormalities of glomeruli due to systemic disease (diabetes, systemic lupus erythematosus, amyloidosis); other forms: minimal change disease (lipoid nephrosis), focal glomerular sclerosis, membranous nephropathy, membranoproliferative glomerulonephritis.

History: Gradual onset of peripheral edema, with weight gain, dyspnea.

Physical Examination: Edema, ascites (excess fluid in abdominal cavity), anasarca (generalized edema); pulmonary edema, pleural effusion.

Diagnostic Tests: Marked increase in 24-hour urinary excretion of protein. Reduction of total protein and albumin in the serum. Increase in serum cholesterol level. There may be no cellular elements in the urine and no evidence of nitrogen retention. Renal biopsy provides histologic identification of the underlying disease process.

Treatment: Limitation of protein and salt intake; diuretics, cholesterol-lowering agents.

Diabetic Nephropathy

Progressive renal insufficiency with albuminuria and hypertension, occurring in persons with diabetes mellitus.

Cause: Thickening and degeneration of glomerular basement membrane and other pathologic changes that eventually occur in most patients with type 1 diabetes mellitus and in some patients with type 2. The incidence is higher in males, blacks, Hispanics, and Native Americans. Most patients also have hypertension, which hastens the advance of renal damage.

History: Symptoms, which do not occur until damage is far advanced, are those of nephrotic syndrome (see above), chronic renal failure, or both.

Physical Examination: Edema, ascites. Hypertension.

Diagnostic Tests: Periodic determination of 24-hour urinary protein excretion (part of the routine surveillance of patients with diabetes mellitus) can detect microalbuminuria, a reliable marker of renal damage, early in the course of disease. With further progression, larger amounts of albumin are excreted and measures of renal function show decline in glomerular filtration and in clearance of nitrogenous

wastes. Serum levels of BUN, creatinine, and potassium are elevated. Metabolic acidosis may occur as a result of renal tubular dysfunction.

Course: Continual deterioration of renal function is usual. Use of certain drugs and injection of radiographic contrast media can precipitate acute renal failure. Diabetic nephropathy is currently the chief cause of end-stage renal failure requiring renal dialysis.

Treatment: Rigorous control of diabetes, with maintenance of plasma glucose as near normal as possible, can delay onset or progression of disease, but no treatment has been shown to reverse renal damage. Limitation of dietary protein and aggressive treatment of hypertension with ACE inhibitors or angiotensin II receptor blockers can delay progression of nephropathy. Urinary tract infections are promptly treated, and radiographic contrast media and drugs known to be toxic to the kidney are avoided. End-stage renal failure is treated with kidney transplantation, hemodialysis, or peritoneal dialysis.

Urolithiasis (Kidney Stones)

Formation of stonelike concretions (calculi) in the urinary tract, which may obstruct a ureter at a site of natural narrowing such as the ureteropelvic junction (UPJ) and ureterovesical junction (UVJ).

Causes: Changes in the concentration of dissolved minerals or other substances in the urine: uric acid in gout; cystine in cystinuria; calcium in disorders of calcium metabolism. Local infection may play a part. Men are affected 4 times more often than women, and the disorder tends to run in families.

History: Passage of a stone into a ureter causes severe flank or abdominal pain radiating to the groin (ureteral colic), nausea, vomiting, restlessness, and often hematuria.

Physical Examination: There may be tenderness over the involved kidney in the flank or abdomen. Fever suggests infection resulting from urinary obstruction.

Diagnostic Tests: The urine shows microscopic or gross blood. X-ray or ultrasound examination identifies and localizes most stones, but about 15% are not radiopaque. Intravenous pyelography can be done to demonstrate obstruction of the tract. Examination of stones shows them to be aggregates of crystalline and organic materials. Chemical analysis of stones indicates which of five common types is present: calcium oxalate, calcium phosphate, ammoniomagnesium phosphate (struvite), uric acid, or cystine.

Course: Most stones pass spontaneously without treatment. Recurrences are common. Obstruction of a ureter can lead to renal failure (obstructive uropathy), infection, or both.

Treatment: Strong analgesics are prescribed, and all urine is collected and strained to identify stones or fragments. If infection is present or renal function is compromised, obstruction may be relieved by passing a ureteral catheter endoscopically from the bladder, or by percutaneous nephrostomy (inserting a drain through the skin into the renal pelvis). Stones lying low in a ureter may be extracted from below. Extracorporeal shock wave lithotripsy can be used to break stones into fragments, which then pass with the urine. A stone lodged in the renal pelvis or proximal ureter may be removed by percutaneous nephrolithotomy.

Acute Pyelonephritis

Acute inflammation of kidney tissue and the renal pelvis due to infection.

Cause: Bacterial infection with *Escherichia coli*, *Proteus*, *Pseudomonas*, *Klebsiella*, *Enterobacter*, or *Staphylococcus aureus*. Infection usually ascends from the lower urinary tract (bladder and urethra), but may be spread through the circulation from a remote focus. Obstruction to urine flow caused by prostatic enlargement, a ureteral stone, or pregnancy may be the underlying cause. Vesicoureteral reflux of urine or anomalies of the urinary tract (tortuous or duplicated ureter) are also risk factors.

History: Fever, chills, nausea, vomiting, flank pain, urinary urgency, pollakiuria, dysuria.

Physical Examination: The temperature and pulse are elevated. Tenderness at one or both costovertebral angles is usually noted on palpation.

Diagnostic Tests: The white blood cell count is elevated. Examination of the urine shows white blood cells, red blood cells, and bacteria. Urine culture identifies the infecting organism.

Course: Pyelonephritis resolves promptly with antibiotic treatment unless an underlying problem of septicemia or urinary obstruction remains unresolved.

Treatment: Antibiotics (trimethoprim-sulfamethoxazole, ciprofloxacin) are administered orally or intravenously. Urinary obstruction must be re-

lieved by catheterization, nephrostomy (draining urine from the renal pelvis), or other procedure.

DISORDERS OF THE BLADDER

Acute Cystitis

Acute inflammation of the bladder, usually due to bacterial infection.

Cause: Usually infection due to *Escherichia coli* or other organisms ascending from the urethra. Cystitis is much commoner in women, in whom the urethra is short and straight, with its orifice in the vaginal vestibule where it is exposed to fecal contamination and trauma from sexual intercourse. Less commonly, cystitis may be due to urethral obstruction (principally in males), viral infection, bladder trauma, or spread of infection from adjacent pelvic organs. Pregnancy, diabetes mellitus, presence of an indwelling catheter, and advanced age are risk factors.

History: Fairly sudden onset of pollakiuria, urgency, urinary burning, and bladder spasms after voiding. Hematuria may occur. Often there is suprapubic or low back discomfort.

Physical Examination: Essentially unremarkable. Fever is absent. There may be suprapubic tenderness.

Diagnostic Examination: Laboratory studies of urine show white blood cells (sometimes clumped), red blood cells or occult blood, and bacteria. Tests for leukocyte esterase and nitrites are often positive. Urine culture identifies the causative organism and sensitivity studies show which antibiotics are effective against it. However, culturing is not routinely performed except in atypical or recurrent disease. Cystitis is so uncommon in men that aggressive evaluation is usually undertaken in the male to identify any serious underlying cause such as obstruction or malignancy.

Course: The response to treatment is rapid, but many sexually active women experience frequent recurrences.

Treatment: Antibiotics (trimethoprim-sulfamethoxazole, cephalexin, ciprofloxacin) are often effective in courses of just 2-3 days. Urinary symptoms may be relieved by phenazopyridine (a bladder anesthetic taken orally) or antispasmodics. The frequency of recurrences in women can be reduced by regularly voiding just after intercourse. Long-term low-dose antibiotic prophylaxis also helps to prevent recurrences.

Interstitial Cystitis

A chronic disorder characterized by urinary frequency and pelvic pain.

Cause: Unknown. Possibly an autoimmune disorder due to defects in bladder mucosal cells, superficial mucin layer, or mast cells in the bladder wall. There is a significant association with migraine, irritable bowel syndrome, and chronic fatigue syndrome. Onset usually occurs in the 30s or 40s; 90% of patients are women.

History: Recurrent episodes of urinary urgency and frequency (15-40 voidings a day), pain in the bladder and pelvis relieved temporarily by voiding, dyspareunia (pain with intercourse). Pain may be worse before onset of menses and after consumption of caffeine, alcohol, carbonated drinks, citrus fruits, tomatoes.

Physical Examination: Unremarkable.

Diagnostic Tests: Cultures of urine are negative. Cystoscopy during distention of the bladder with saline may show pinpoint hemorrhages (glomerulations) or shallow ulcers (Hunner ulcers) of the mucosa. Biopsy may be performed to rule out other diseases, such as malignancy.

Course: The condition tends to recur throughout life.

Treatment: Counseling, education, avoidance of aggravating factors. Bladder analgesics, nonsteroidal anti-inflammatory drugs, antihistamines, tricyclic antidepressants, pentosan polysulfate. Intermittent injection into bladder of dimethylsulfoxide, heparin, corticosteroid.

Urinary Incontinence

Four distinct types of involuntary leakage of urine from the bladder are recognized.

Urge incontinence, which occurs after a sudden, intense, irresistible urge to void, is the commonest type of incontinence in elderly persons. It is due to overactivity of the detrusor muscle of the bladder, and often responds to treatment with the antispasmodic oxybutynin or the muscarinic antagonist tolterodine.

Stress incontinence, which is seen almost exclusively in women, occurs when mechanical stress is placed on the bladder, as by coughing, laughing, or changing position. It may result from structural damage to the bladder as in childbirth. Treatment with pelvic muscle exercises (Kegel exercises) or estrogens may help. Surgical correction of anatomic abnormalities is often necessary, and is highly successful.

Overflow incontinence is leakage of urine from an over-distended bladder, occurring almost exclusively in men with urinary obstruction due to prostatic disease. Treatment is correction of the obstruction.

Total incontinence is complete lack of control over voiding, usually due to neurologic disease, spinal cord injury, or radical prostatectomy. Continuous or intermittent catheterization may be the only effective means of controlling this type of incontinence. Incontinence is primarily a disorder of the elderly; besides the causes mentioned above it may be due to dementia, urinary tract infection, diuresis, drugs, diminished mobility, and, in women, atrophic vaginitis.

DISORDERS OF THE MALE REPRODUCTIVE SYSTEM

The male reproductive system consists of the paired testes (testicles), each with its collecting system (the epididymis, a coiled tubular structure attached to the testicle; and the spermatic duct or vas deferens, a tube that conducts sperm to the prostate), the penis, the scrotum (a cutaneous sac containing the testicles), the prostate (a gland surrounding the urethra just below the bladder), and the seminal vesicles (small pouchlike glands adjacent to the vas deferens). (See Figure 13.)

The testicle produces spermatozoa (singular, spermatozoon), the male gametes (sex cells). Each spermatozoon is capable of fertilizing a female ovum and carries the paternal contribution to the genetic makeup of the offspring. In addition, the testicles produce male hormones that are responsible for the development and maintenance of secondary sexual characteristics (facial and body hair, male body build, deep voice). The prostate contains secretory cells that produce the fluid component of semen. It also contains smooth muscle, and under sexual stimulation it closes off the bladder from the urethra and brings about ejaculation of semen (prostatic fluid + spermatozoa) through the urethra.

Figure 13 Male Genitourinary System

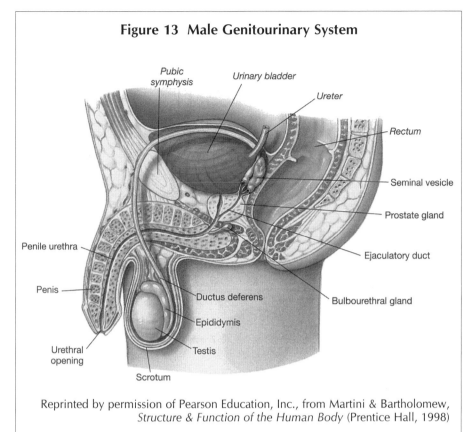

Reprinted by permission of Pearson Education, Inc., from Martini & Bartholomew, *Structure & Function of the Human Body* (Prentice Hall, 1998)

Epididymitis

Inflammation of the epididymis.

Causes: In younger men, typically due to sexually transmitted infection (gonorrhea or chlamydia); in older men, to spread of infection by gram-negative bacilli (*Escherichia coli*, *Proteus*, *Pseudomonas*, and others) from the urinary tract or prostate.

History: Pain and swelling in the scrotum adjacent to a testicle, urinary burning, fever.

Physical Examination: Fever, enlarged and tender epididymis, often enlargement of testicle and prostate as well.

Diagnostic Tests: Blood studies show leukocytosis. Stained urethral smear shows white blood cells and may show gonococci. The urine may show white blood cells, red blood cells, and bacteria.

Course: Complications include involvement of the testicle (epididymo-orchitis), abscess formation, and scarring of the epididymis with resultant infertility.

Treatment: An antibiotic, preferably selected on the basis of culture, and continued for 2-4 weeks. Scrotal support, ice, analgesics.

Testicular Torsion

Twisting of a spermatic cord. The condition runs in families, usually occurs before age 25, may follow strenuous activity, and may recur. Symptoms include pain, tenderness, and swelling in the affected cord. The affected testis lies higher than its fellow, because twisting shortens the cord. If spontaneous detorsion (untwisting) does not occur, the condition can lead to gangrene of the testicle within hours. Medical intervention is manual detorsion or, failing that, open surgery. Even when detorsion is accomplished without surgery, a procedure is eventually performed to anchor both testicles so as to prevent recurrence.

Prostatitis

Inflammation of the prostate, typically due to bacterial infection, which may be acute or chronic. In acute prostatitis the presenting complaints are fever, urinary frequency and burning, occasionally urinary retention, and pain in the perineum or back. On digital rectal examination the prostate is found to be enlarged, warm, and exquisitely tender. The white blood cell count is elevated, and the urine contains white blood cells, red blood cells, and bacteria. Treatment is with oral or intravenous antibiotics. In chronic prostatitis, symptoms are milder but of longer duration. Fever is absent and prostatic tenderness not so marked. The urinalysis is normal. Treatment is with antibiotics, and must often be continued for a long time.

Benign Prostatic Hyperplasia (BPH)

Enlargement of the prostate accompanying aging, with varying degrees of urinary obstruction.

Cause: Some prostatic enlargement due to overgrowth of androgen-sensitive glandular elements occurs naturally with aging. Causes of severely symptomatic enlargement are unknown.

History: Gradual onset of urinary symptoms, which may be obstructive (decreased force and caliber of urinary stream, hesitancy, intermittency) or irritative (frequency, urgency, nocturia).

Physical Examination: The prostate is symmetrically enlarged on digital rectal examination, firm but not hard. Abdominal examination may indicate distention of the bladder. Catheterization after voiding may indicate residual urine.

Diagnostic Tests: Urinalysis may indicate evidence of infection (white blood cells) or of bladder irritation (red blood cells). The blood urea nitrogen may be elevated if obstruction is advanced (obstructive uropathy). Intravenous pyelography may show bladder distention and bilateral ureteral dilatation. Urinary flowmetry gives an objective measure of the rate of flow from the bladder. Cystoscopy and urethroscopy may be of value in confirming the benign nature of the disorder.

Course: Symptoms may remain relatively mild for years, even decades. Obstruction may lead to infection and even to kidney failure. Benign prostatic hyperplasia does not evolve into carcinoma.

Treatment: Medical treatment with finasteride (an alpha-reductase inhibitor) or terazosin or doxazosin (alpha-adrenergic blocking agents) can reduce obstructive symptoms. In more severe cases, surgical excision of prostate tissue is indicated. Transurethral resection (TUR) is the usual procedure, but in some cases suprapubic (open) resection is preferred. Balloon dilatation of the prostate and transurethral laser excision are alternative procedures.

Adenocarcinoma of the prostate is discussed in Chapter 5.

Erectile Dysfunction (Impotence)

Failure of the penis to become erect after sexual stimulation, or to achieve and maintain sufficient rigidity for vaginal penetration in coitus. Possible causes include vascular disease (atherosclerosis), neurologic disease (multiple sclerosis, spinal cord injury), penile deformity including Peyronie disease (in which fibrotic plaques in the penis can block blood vessels), hormonal deficiency (hypothyroidism, testicular failure), side effects of drugs (tranquilizers, antihypertensives), and psychological factors (anxiety, depression). Risk factors are advancing age, diabetes mellitus, obesity, and cigarette smoking. The incidence of erectile dysfunction from all causes is about 20% at age 40 and 50% at age 70. About 50% of men with diabetes mellitus eventually develop erectile dysfunction. Treatment includes correcting underlying disorders if possible, counseling the patient and his sexual partner, and use of pharma-cologic or other measures to induce erection. Oral sildenafil is the preferred agent for most patients with organic erectile dysfunction, but in selected cases older methods may be used, including a vacuum device to induce erection mechanically, implantation of a penile prosthesis, and injection of a vasodilator into the penis with a fine-gauge needle.

SEXUALLY TRANSMITTED DISEASES

Diseases in this category are distinguished by being transmitted often, or almost exclusively, through sexual contact. Otherwise they have little in common: some are bacterial, some viral, some parasitic; some are trivial, some life-threatening or even uniformly lethal; some are easily cured, others are virtually unresponsive to treatment. The list of sexually transmitted diseases includes as many as 40 infections; only the more common and important are discussed in this book. Some sexually transmitted diseases are discussed in other chapters: AIDS in Chapter 4; genital warts, genital herpes, and pubic pediculosis in Chapter 7; hepatitis B in Chapter 11; and trichomoniasis in Chapter 13.

Syphilis (Lues)

A sexually transmitted spirochetal infection with widespread and life-threatening consequences.

Cause: *Treponema pallidum*, a spirochete that can enter the body through abraded skin or intact mucous membrane. Infection is usually transmitted sexually, but can also be spread by sharing needles. In addition, a woman infected with syphilis during the earlier months of pregnancy usually passes the infection along to her child, unless she is treated.

History: Primary stage: Appearance of a firm, painless papule or nodule (chancre), up to 2 cm in diameter, on the genitals or other site, 2-12 weeks after inoculation. The chancre eventually ulcerates and forms a crust, taking several weeks to heal and sometimes leaving a scar. Inguinal lymph nodes become swollen and tender. Second stage: Several weeks later, a generalized, nonspecific cutaneous rash may appear. Soft, moist plaques (condylomata lata) may occur on the skin of the genitals, perineum, perianal region, or groin, and ulcerations may also develop on oral or genital mucous membranes. There may be patchy hair loss. Symptoms of this stage may persist or recur over several weeks.

Tertiary (late) stage: Years after the first two stages, damage to cardiovascular and nervous tissue may result in cardiac symptoms, congestive heart failure, dementia, ataxia (tabes dorsalis), or paralysis. (Latent syphilis refers to a condition in which spirochetes remain alive in the body, but no signs or symptoms of infection occur after the secondary stage.)

Physical Examination: Findings are highly variable. Primary stage: The chancre and enlargement of inguinal nodes have already been described. Secondary stage: Nonspecific localized or generalized maculopapular rash, which often involves the palms and soles. Irregular zones of hair loss give the head a moth-eaten appearance. Condylomata lata and mucosal ulcers have already been described. Enlargement of spleen and lymph nodes may occur. Tertiary stage: Signs of aortic valvular insufficiency or aneurysm of the thoracic aorta, ataxia (incoordination), paresis (muscle weakness), dementia. Formation of gummata (rubbery fibrotic masses) in skin, bones, and liver.

Diagnostic Tests: Examination of material from a chancre or mucocutaneous ulcer by darkfield microscopy or fluorescent antibody testing confirms presence of *Treponema pallidum*. Serologic tests (VDRL, RPR) react to treponemal antigens, but may be falsely positive in autoimmune disorders. More specific tests for treponemal antibody (fluorescent treponemal antibody absorption test, FTA-ABS) yield reliable confirmation of the presence or absence of *T. pallidum* infection.

Course: The usual history of the disease has already been outlined. About 75% of persons with syphilis proceed to the latent stage and have no late manifestations. Treatment at any time before the late stage ordinarily yields complete cure. Without treatment, the late stage culminates in cardiovascular or neurologic death.

Treatment: A single intramuscular dose of benzathine penicillin G is usually curative. Alternative treatments are oral erythromycin or tetracycline.

Gonorrhea

Infection of the genital tract by the gonococcus.

Cause: *Neisseria gonorrhoeae* (gonococcus), a gram-negative diplococcus that is transmitted almost exclusively by sexual contact. It attacks genitourinary mucous membranes, producing a purulent inflammation that may spread to adjacent organs or the peritoneum, and may progress to scarring.

Infection of the pharynx or rectum can be acquired through oral or anal sex.

History: Men: After an incubation period of 3-5 days, severe pain on urination and a thick yellow or green urethral discharge. Women: Similar symptoms sometimes occur, along with vaginal or vulvar inflammation. Often, however, there are no symptoms unless pelvic inflammatory disease (PID) (spread of infection to the uterus and uterine tubes) occurs. PID causes pelvic pain and fever, with variable other symptoms.

Physical Examination: In men, evident purulent urethral discharge, with inflammation of the meatus. In women, acute disease may be manifested by urethritis, cervicitis, vaginitis, inflammation of Bartholin glands (secretory glands lateral to the vaginal vestibule), or proctitis (inflammation of the rectum). If PID ensues: fever, abdominal tenderness, extreme tenderness on manipulation of cervix.

Diagnostic Tests: DNA amplification tests performed on material obtained by cervical or urethral smear and on urine are valuable for diagnosis as well as for screening asymptomatic persons of either sex. Stained smear of pus or secretions shows gram-negative diplococci inside white blood cells. Culture on an appropriate medium grows gonococci. Oral and anal specimens are positive when infection is in those areas.

Course: Acute urethral infection may resolve spontaneously, but in men it often spreads to the epididymis or prostate, or progresses to a stage of scarring, with resultant infertility. In women, spread to the vagina, cervix, uterus, tubes, and rectum often occurs. Tubal infection (salpingitis, PID) with scarring causes infertility and a heightened risk of ectopic pregnancy. In either sex, infection occasionally involves the skin, conjunctivae, joints, tendon sheaths, cardiac valves, or meninges. Spread of infection from mother to newborn can cause conjunctivitis with ensuing blindness.

Treatment: Antibiotic treatment with a single dose of intramuscular ceftriaxone or oral ciprofloxacin is usually curative. It is standard practice to administer treatment for chlamydial infection at the same time since the infections so often occur together.

Chlamydial Infection

Urogenital infection with *Chlamydia trachomatis*.

Cause: Sexually transmitted infection of genital mucous membranes and related tissues with

Chlamydia trachomatis, an intracellular organism similar to gram-negative bacteria. Genital chlamydial infection (urethritis and cervicitis) is the commonest bacterial STD. Screening tests are positive in 10% of asymptomatic, sexually active women.

History: Men: Urethral itching or burning, dysuria, thin serous discharge beginning 1-4 weeks after exposure. Anorectal pain and bleeding with rectal infection, common in gay men. Women: Dysuria and pollakiuria due to acute urethral syndrome; dyspareunia (pain with intercourse), vaginal bleeding, and vaginal discharge due to cervicitis; abdominal pain and fever due to pelvic inflammatory disease. Most women with chlamydial infection are asymptomatic.

Physical Examination: May be unremarkable. Thin, watery urethral discharge may be noted in males. In women, cervical erythema with mucopurulent discharge indicates cervicitis. With development of PID, fever, abdominal pain, and cervical tenderness become evident.

Diagnostic Tests: DNA amplification testing of urine is used for both diagnosis and for screening of asymptomatic persons. A urethral or cervical smear may show organisms with direct fluorescence antibody examination, enzyme-linked immunosorbent assay, or DNA probe.

Course: Spontaneous resolution often occurs, but in many patients chlamydial infection has long-term consequences. In men, infection can spread to the epididymis, produce urethral stricture with resulting urinary obstruction or infertility, or trigger an autoimmune disorder called Reiter syndrome (arthritis, conjunctivitis, mucocutaneous lesions). In about one-fifth of infected women, infection spreads to the uterus and tubes (salpingitis, PID). Complications of PID include tubo-ovarian abscess, Fitz-Hugh–Curtis syndrome (localized peritonitis in the region of the liver), and tubal scarring with infertility or sterility and heightened risk of ectopic pregnancy. A child born to an infected mother is at risk of chlamydial conjunctivitis, with the danger of blindness.

Treatment: Oral antibiotic therapy with tetracycline, erythromycin, or a single dose of azithromycin is ordinarily curative. Treatment is often instituted on suspicion (urethritis or cervicitis with negative cultures of urine and discharge) because of the high probability of chlamydial infection in such cases. Persons treated for gonorrhea are also routinely treated for chlamydial infection.

QUESTIONS FOR STUDY AND REVIEW

1. List five causes of urinary obstruction:

   a. _____

   b. _____

   c. _____

   d. _____

   e. _____

2. List five conditions that predispose to urinary tract infection:

   a. _____

   b. _____

   c. _____

   d. _____

   e. _____

3. Give four sites of pain in urinary tract disease and indicate the probable origin of each type of pain:

   a. _____

   b. _____

   c. _____

   d. _____

4. Define or explain these terms:

   a. anuria _____
   _____

   b. chancre _____
   _____

   c. IVP _____
   _____

   d. microscopic hematuria _____
   _____

   e. overflow incontinence _____
   _____

   f. Peyronie disease _____
   _____

   g. pollakiuria _____
   _____

h. Reiter syndrome _____

_____

i. urolithiasis_____

_____

5. Distinguish between *pollakiuria* and *polyuria*, and for each symptom mention possible causes.

_____

_____

_____

_____

_____

_____

_____

_____

_____

_____

6. List three important similarities and three important differences between *chlamydial urethritis* and *gonorrhea*.

_____

_____

_____

_____

_____

_____

_____

_____

_____

_____

_____

CASE STUDY: YOU'RE THE DOCTOR

Eugene Vandenhall is a 77-year-old retired electrician who consults you, a urologist, about increasing urinary symptoms. He is accompanied to the office by his daughter and son-in-law, with whom he lives. His wife lives in a nursing home. Because Mr. Vandenhall is hard of hearing and has mild dementia, his son-in-law supplies part of the history. The patient has noted urinary frequency, diminished urine flow, hesitancy, nocturia, and occasional urinary burning for the past 10 years. For about 3 years he has been taking prazosin prescribed for prostatic hyperplasia by his primary care physician. In spite of that, his symptoms have become increasingly bothersome. He now has problems with leakage of urine when he is on the way to the bathroom and with dribbling after voiding, and he has to get up "at least once an hour" during the night to void. He has had no fever, chills, flank or perineal pain, hematuria, or urinary retention, but on some occasions he has to wait 2 or 3 minutes for urine flow to begin.

1. What diagnostic possibilities are raised by this history?

_____

_____

_____

_____

Mr. Vandenhall is in generally poor health. He had a stoke about 4 years ago which left him with mild weakness in the right arm and hand, gait disturbances, and balance problems. He has been hospitalized twice during the past year for congestive heart failure. He also has diminished renal function.

2. How might this background alter your way of assessing and treating this patient?

_____

_____

_____

_____

The patient is a thin, pale, feeble-appearing elderly male, who walks with difficulty and appears depressed and confused. Abdominal examination is negative. The patient's underwear is damp with urine. On rectal examination the prostate is 3+ enlarged and asymmetric, with a stony-hard nontender nodule measuring 2-3 cm occupying most of the right lateral lobe. Catheterization after voiding confirms the presence of about 80 mL of residual urine.

3. Give a reason in support of or against each of the following courses of action:

    a. Emergency testing of prostate specific antigen to rule out prostatic adenocarcinoma_____

    _____

    b. Ultrasound-directed prostatic biopsy _____

    _____

    c. Hospitalization for transurethral prostatectomy_____

    _____

    d. Instruct the patient in intermittent self-catheterization_____

    _____

    e. Prescription for tolterodine to control urge incontinence_____

    _____

    f. Discuss nursing home care with the family_____

    _____

    g. Arrange for primary care physician to review all medicines and consider antidepressant therapy __

    _____

    h. Suggest indwelling catheter with leg bag_____

    _____

SUGGESTIONS FOR ADDITIONAL LEARNING ACTIVITIES

1. Find out everything you can about dialysis. Start by determining possible research sources. Consider the sources mentioned in previous learning activities as well as any dialysis facilities in your local area. Use your research to prepare a report that answers these questions: What are the historical origins of dialysis? How is dialysis performed? What equipment is used? How often is it done and for how long? Who needs dialysis and why? What are the risks and complications associated with dialysis? What are the latest breakthroughs in this field? What will the future bring?

2. Visit your county health department and obtain literature and information on sexually transmitted diseases. Obtain statistics on the incidence of STDs in your area. Learn about the reporting procedures required by your county. Find out what community education programs are in place and what the results of these programs have been, i.e., has there been an increase or decrease in the rate of STDs over time?

3. Make a Reverse Crossword puzzle. Use graph paper or make your own gridwork, and write in as many terms from this chapter, across and down, as will fit within the grid. Take advantage of opportunities to overlap terms, so long as adjoining letters form legitimate words. When the grid is filled in, number each square that begins a word (up or down), numbering from left to right and top to bottom. Don't number a square that doesn't begin a word. On a separate sheet of paper, make a list of all the numbers for the "Across" entries and another for the list of all the "Down" entries. Solve this Reverse Crossword by filling in the definitions.

Disorders of the Female Reproductive System

LEARNING OBJECTIVES

Upon completion of this chapter, you should be able to

- describe the basic anatomy and physiology of the female reproductive system, including the breast;

- explain diagnostic procedures used in assessing disorders of the female reproductive system and breast;

- classify common diseases of the female reproductive system and breast by their signs, symptoms, and treatment.

DISORDERS OF THE FEMALE REPRODUCTIVE SYSTEM

ANATOMY AND PHYSIOLOGY OF THE FEMALE REPRODUCTIVE SYSTEM

The female reproductive system is concerned exclusively with procreation; unlike that of the male, it does not share structures with the urinary tract to any significant extent. The system consists of the internal genitalia (the ovaries, uterus, and vagina) and the external genitalia (the vulva, consisting of labia majora, labia minora, clitoris, and vaginal vestibule). The uterus is divided into the cervix (the lowermost portion, protruding into the vaginal vault) and the body (the remainder of the uterus, which lies in the pelvic cavity between bladder and rectum). (See Figures 14 and 15.) The system also includes the breasts, which provide nourishment to the newborn child.

GYNECOLOGIC SYMPTOMS AND SIGNS

Gynecology is the branch of medicine that is concerned with diseases peculiar to women, chiefly diseases of the reproductive system. The following are the principal indications of gynecologic disease.

Pain, local or generalized: Constant, intermittent, or related to menstruation. Various types of gynecologic pain can be distinguished:

Dysmenorrhea: Pain occurring with menstruation, typically felt low in the pelvis and in the low back, and often severe. The lay term for dysmenorrhea is "[menstrual] cramps."

Dyspareunia: Pain in the vulva, vagina, or pelvis with sexual intercourse.

Dysuria: Pain in the urethra or vulva with urination.

Ovulatory pain: Sharp pain, usually on one side of the pelvis, occurring midway between menstrual cycles (hence the common German term *mittelschmerz*

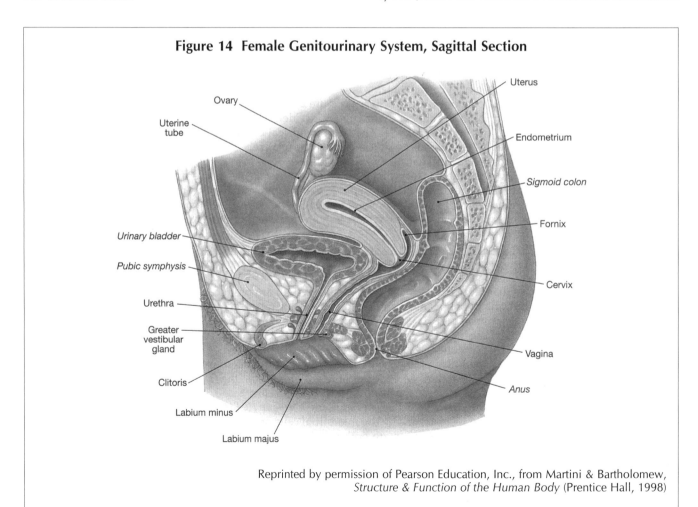

Figure 14 Female Genitourinary System, Sagittal Section

Reprinted by permission of Pearson Education, Inc., from Martini & Bartholomew, *Structure & Function of the Human Body* (Prentice Hall, 1998)

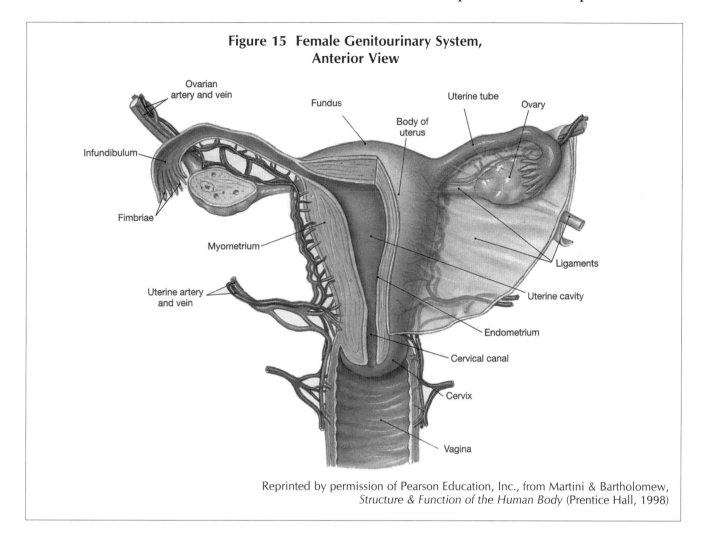

Figure 15 Female Genitourinary System, Anterior View

Reprinted by permission of Pearson Education, Inc., from Martini & Bartholomew, *Structure & Function of the Human Body* (Prentice Hall, 1998)

'middle pain') and due to peritoneal irritation by a small volume of blood escaping from the ovary at the time of ovulation.

Menstrual Abnormalities

Amenorrhea: Absence of menstruation.

Primary amenorrhea: Failure of menses to start at puberty (by age 14-16).

Secondary amenorrhea: Cessation of menses that have been normal in the past.

Anovulation: Failure of ovulation to occur at the expected times.

Dysfunctional uterine bleeding: Irregular, unpredictable menstrual flow (too frequent or too infrequent, too heavy or too light), or amenorrhea, occurring in the absence of pregnancy, infection, or neoplasm.

Hypermenorrhea: Abnormally high volume of menstrual discharge.

Hypomenorrhea: Abnormally low volume of menstrual discharge.

Menometrorrhagia: Excessive menstrual bleeding occurring both during menses and at irregular intervals.

Menorrhagia: Regularly occurring menstrual flow that is excessive in volume and lasts longer than a normal menstrual period.

Metrorrhagia: Menstrual bleeding occurring at irregular but frequent intervals.

Oligomenorrhea: Infrequent or scanty menstrual bleeding.

Polymenorrhea: Menstrual bleeding that occurs with abnormal frequency.

Abnormal vaginal discharge: Any discharge from the vagina that is abnormal in color, odor, or volume. Normal vaginal mucus discharge, originating from cervical glands, is nearly colorless, nearly odorless, and not heavy enough to stain underclothing except perhaps around the time of ovulation and just before onset of menses.

Vulvar burning, rawness, stinging, or itching.

A **lump, swelling, or ulcer** of the external genitalia, perineum, perianal region, pubes, or groin.

Breast symptoms: Pain, local or generalized swelling, palpable lump, discharge or bleeding from nipple.

DIAGNOSTIC PROCEDURES IN GYNECOLOGY

History: Age at menarche, menstrual history, sexual history, obstetric history, pelvic pain, bleeding, discharge, or other symptoms of gynecologic disease, general medical and surgical history.

Physical examination: General medical examination with attention to the abdomen and pelvis and to the breasts.

A standard **pelvic examination** consists of the following elements:

Inspection and palpation of the external genitalia and perineum, with particular attention to the urethral orifice and adjacent Skene glands, the vaginal vestibule and adjacent Bartholin glands, the integrity of the pelvic floor, and any redness, swelling, ulceration, scarring, or other abnormal lesions.

Examination of the vaginal vault and the uterine cervix with the help of a vaginal speculum, which has adjustable anterior and posterior leaves that distend the vagina. Acetic acid or Lugol solution may be applied to the cervix to highlight zones of abnormal (possibly malignant) tissue.

Palpation of pelvic organs: Cervix and body of uterus, adnexa (organs adjacent to the uterus—ovaries and tubes), bladder, pelvic walls and floor, rectum. Bimanual examination is performed with one or two fingers in the vagina and the palm of the other hand on the lower abdomen. Rectovaginal examination is performed with the index finger of one hand in the vagina and the middle finger of the same hand in the rectum.

A standard **breast examination** consists of the following elements:

Inspection of the breasts with the subject in the upright position, first with arms at sides, then with arms raised, and finally with hands pressed against hips to render underlying muscles taut.

Palpation of each breast in both the upright and supine positions, with attention to the axillae and assessment of nipples for inflammation, bleeding, or discharge.

Examination of cervical mucus for spinnbarkeit: When the estrogen level is high but the progesterone level is low (the conditions existing just before and just after ovulation), a specimen of cervical mucus can be drawn out into strings or strands several centimeters in length. This property is called *spinnbarkeit* (German, 'ability to be drawn out into a string'). When both estrogen and progesterone are present in large amounts, cervical mucus loses this property, and attempts to draw it out into a string fail. The physiology of the menstrual cycle is discussed fully below.

Basal body temperature: Daily determination of oral temperature on arising is useful in confirming and dating ovulation. Daily graphing of basal body temperature will show a rise of 0.75-1.0°F (0.2-0.5°C) approximately one day after ovulation.

Colposcopy: Examination of the cervix with an illuminated low-power microscope, which facilitates identification of suspicious cervical lesions requiring biopsy.

Pap (Papanicolaou) smear: Removal of superficial cells from the vagina and cervix for cytologic examination, to judge hormonal effect and to identify abnormal cell changes due to inflammation, infection, dysplasia (cell abnormalities heralding eventual development of malignancy), or actual malignancy. Specimens are taken from three areas: (1) the vaginal vault, with a flat wooden spatula; (2) the squamocolumnar junction (transition line between the squamous epithelium of the vagina and the columnar epithelium of the endocervical canal), with a specially shaped wooden spatula (Ayre spatula); (3) the endocervical canal, with a bristle brush to ensure sampling of columnar epithelial cells. Interpretation of the Pap smear, reported according to the Bethesda system, includes assessment of the adequacy of the specimen (presence of columnar cells from the endocervical canal); detection of hormonal effect (estrogen, progesterone); identification of inflammatory or degenerative changes in cells; and identification of dysplastic or malignant changes in cells. Cellular atypia without clear-cut evidence of premalignant change is reported as abnormal squamous cells of undetermined significance (ASC-US). Squamous cell changes formerly designated as mild dysplasia (including cellular atypia characteristic of HPV infection) are called low-grade squamous intraepithelial lesion (LGSIL). Moderate to severe dysplasia is called high-grade squamous intraepithelial lesion (HGSIL). Examination of a Pap smear can often also detect certain infections (candida, trichomonas, herpes simplex, human papillomavirus).

Smear and culture: Microbiologic study of secretions or other materials from the cervix, vagina, urethra, rectum, or from superficial lesions, to identify causes of infection.

Urine studies: Culture, colony count, and sensitivity to identify urinary tract infection.

Imaging: Plain x-ray studies, pelvic ultrasound, transvaginal ultrasound (TVUS), CT, MRI.

Pregnancy testing, usually by identification and measurement of the beta fraction of human chorionic gonadotropin (beta hCG) in serum.

Determination of blood levels of various hormones: Estrogens, TSH (thyroid stimulating hormone), T_4 (thyroxine), FSH (follicle-stimulating hormone), LH (luteinizing hormone), prolactin.

Biopsy: Removal of tissue from the cervix, the endometrium, or another part of the reproductive system for histologic examination to identify infection, neoplasm, or other abnormality. Cervical biopsy is performed under colposcopic view, and may involve removal of plugs of tissue with a punch-type instrument or removal of a cone of tissue including the entire squamocolumnar junction.

Dilatation and curettage (D&C): Scraping of the endometrium, after stretching of the cervix with graded dilators, to obtain specimen material for the diagnosis of endometrial disease. This procedure, performed under anesthesia (general, spinal, or intravenous), is also used therapeutically for various endometrial disorders.

Hysteroscopy: Endoscopic inspection of the uterine cavity; the instrument is passed through the cervix under local or general anesthesia.

Culdoscopy: Endoscopic inspection of the cul-de-sac (pouch of Douglas), the lowermost part of the peritoneal cavity, which lies between the uterus and the rectum. The instrument is introduced vaginally under anesthesia.

Laparoscopy: Inspection of pelvic viscera through a laparoscope, a tubular instrument with illumination and magnification, inserted through a small incision in the abdominal wall. Minor surgical procedures can be performed through the instrument.

MENSTRUATION AND ITS DISORDERS

Menstruation is the normal monthly discharge of blood and tissue from the uterus that results when ovulation is not followed by conception (see box). Menarche, the first onset of menstruation, occurs at puberty, between the ages of 11 and 15. Menopause, the final cessation of menstruation, occurs ordinarily

The English words *menses, menstrual,* and *menstruation,* and the Greek words *dysmenorrhea, menopause,* and many related terms, are all derived from the same Indo-European root meaning 'moon' and, by extension, 'month'. From earliest antiquity, women noticed that their menstrual cycles (interval from beginning of one menstrual period to the beginning of the next one) were normally the same number of days as the cycles of the moon (from one full moon to the next). Naturally the superstition followed that the two are related as cause and effect.

Mensis, the Latin word for 'month', is widely used in medicine (always in the plural) to refer to menstruation. Note that *menses* can have either of two meanings: 1. 'a single menstrual period' ("Menses began on April 14"), or 2. 'menstruation in general' ("Menses began at age 12").

Men, the cognate Greek word for 'month', appears in medical terms as the combining form *men(o)-: menarche, menorrhagia, polymenorrhea.* The same Greek word appears in *meniscus* (Greek *meniskos,* 'little moon', hence 'crescent moon') referring to the semilunar shape of the fibrocartilaginous menisci of the knee joint.

The notion of a connection between lunar cycles and menstrual cycles is deeply entrenched and ineradicable. Numerous women relate their menses to the calendar month ("My period always starts on the seventh"). In March, primary care physicians see many women who think their periods are late because February, having only 28 days, has foiled expectations based erroneously on the day of the month.

during the late 40s or early 50s. The normal menstrual cycle (interval from the first day of one menstrual period to the first day of the next menstrual period) is 21-35 days; the average is about 28 days. The normal menstrual period (time of menstrual flow) is 3-7 days; the average is 5 days. In lay and even professional parlance, the terms menstruation, menses, menstrual flow, and menstrual period are often used of any vaginal bleeding, even when it is evident that the bleeding in question is not normal menstrual flow. Similarly, the terms cycle and period are often applied to vaginal bleeding that is wholly irregular ("anovulatory cycle," "irregular periods").

The normal menstrual cycle depends on an intricate and interrelated series of chemical and biologic events. At puberty the hypothalamus secretes a neurohormone, gonadotropin-releasing hormone (GnRH), which stimulates the pituitary to release its gonadotropic hormones, follicle-stimulating hormone (FSH) and luteinizing hormone (LH).

FSH causes the ovary to begin producing estrogen, which is responsible for the development of secondary sexual characteristics (pubic and axillary hair, nipple and breast development, broadening of hips, feminine distribution of body fat). FSH also stimulates the monthly development or maturation of an ovarian (graafian) follicle, one of hundreds of immature microscopic units, each of which contains an ovum or female sex cell (gamete).

Under the influence of estrogen, the endometrium (lining of the uterus) undergoes changes concurrently with ripening of the follicle, to prepare it for implantation of the fertilized ovum should conception occur. This proliferative phase of endometrial development lasts 10-15 days, from the end of the last menstrual period to the time of ovulation.

Ovulation is the release of a mature ovum from its ovarian follicle into the pelvic cavity, from which it ordinarily passes into the uterine tube on the same side as the ovary from which it emerged, and so to the uterus. If sexual intercourse takes place around the time of ovulation, spermatozoa advancing through the female genital tract typically encounter the ovum during its passage through the uterine tube, and fertilization takes place in the tube. The fertilized ovum then migrates into the uterine cavity and implants on the endometrium. The physiology of pregnancy is discussed fully in the next chapter.

At ovulation, the pituitary release of LH greatly increases. This hormone stimulates the follicle from which the ovum was released to evolve into a *corpus luteum* (Latin, 'yellow body'), a small but powerful secretory organ that produces the hormone progesterone. The function of progesterone is to make further preparations for the development of the fetus should fertilization occur. The most striking early effect is a more lush development of the endometrium (secretory phase), with marked thickening, and formation of microscopic coiled glandular structures. (See Figure 16.)

If conception and implantation of a fertilized ovum do not occur, then the corpus luteum degenerates and ceases to produce progesterone. The endometrium, deprived of its stimulation, becomes ischemic and sloughs, with resultant menstrual flow. Menses predictably begin 14 days after ovulation if fertilization has not occurred.

The menstrual cycle is delicately regulated by various feedback mechanisms. For example, falling levels of either FSH or LH stimulate hypothalamic production of GnRH, and rising levels suppress GnRH.

Dysfunctional Uterine Bleeding

Unusually heavy or light bleeding from the uterus, typically unpredictable, or amenorrhea, in the absence of pregnancy or any demonstrable abnormality (neoplasm, infection) of the uterus.

Causes: Most cases are due to anovulation (failure to ovulate). This is a common occurrence and can result from physical or emotional stress, marked weight loss (as in anorexia nervosa or stringent dieting), strenuous exercise (running, gymnastics), excess or deficiency of thyroid hormone, polycystic ovary disease, recent discontinuance of oral contraceptives, lactation, and other causes. About one-third of patients with amenorrhea have elevated levels of prolactin; in rare cases, this is due to overproduction of prolactin by a pituitary tumor.

History: Unusually heavy or light bleeding, typically irregular; often, amenorrhea lasting for three or more cycles. Symptoms of underlying disease may also be present.

Physical Examination: Generally unremarkable. May show obesity or emaciation, stigmata of thyroid or ovarian disease (goiter, exophthalmos, hirsutism), or other evidence of an underlying disorder. Cysts may be palpable in the ovaries. Presence of normal breast development and axillary and pubic hair confirms normal estrogen effect. A palpable, nontender uterus of normal size and shape rules out congenital absence of the uterus (a diagnostic possibility in primary amenorrhea) and helps to exclude uterine tumors or infection.

Diagnostic Tests: A pregnancy test is always done to rule out normal or ectopic pregnancy or recent miscarriage or abortion. Determination of blood levels of estrogen, LH, FSH, T_4, TSH, and prolactin is standard. In amenorrhea in which pregnancy has been ruled out, oral administration of a progesterone (medroxyprogesterone acetate) for 5 days is normally followed within 10 days by a discharge of blood from the uterus if the endometrium is healthy and the estrogen level adequate. Absence of a response suggests a severe uterine disorder (endometrial scarring) or estrogen deficiency due to pituitary or ovarian disease. Pelvic ultrasound may help to confirm the presence or absence of uterine or ovarian disease. Laparoscopy may be needed for definitive diagnosis. CT or MRI of the head may be performed if a pituitary tumor is suspected.

Course: Depends on the underlying condition. Extremely heavy bleeding can lead to shock or anemia. Female athletes who remain amenorrheic for extended periods of time as a result of vigorous

training are at risk of developing osteoporosis, which may be irreversible.

Treatment: Depends on the underlying condition. For many patients, a course of oral contraceptive provides cyclical hormone levels sufficient to induce what seem like normal menstrual cycles and flow. Clomiphene may be given to an anovulatory woman who wants to conceive. Hyperprolactinemia (abnormal elevation of prolactin) in the absence of a pituitary neoplasm is treated with bromocriptine. Thyroid, ovarian, or pituitary disease, or abnormalities of pelvic anatomy and physiology, may require other specific treatment.

Dysmenorrhea

Pelvic pain occurring with menstruation.

Causes: Primary: "Normal" menstrual cramps, occurring in 50-75% of all women, are due to uterine vasoconstriction and spasm resulting from withdrawal of progesterone effect. Secondary: Endometriosis, PID, use of an IUD (intrauterine contraceptive device), tumor of the uterus, cervical stenosis (due, for example, to scarring after induced abortion).

History: Cramping pain felt low in the pelvis, often radiating to the back or inner thighs, often accompanied by nausea, diarrhea, headache, or prostration. Pain begins usually on the first day of

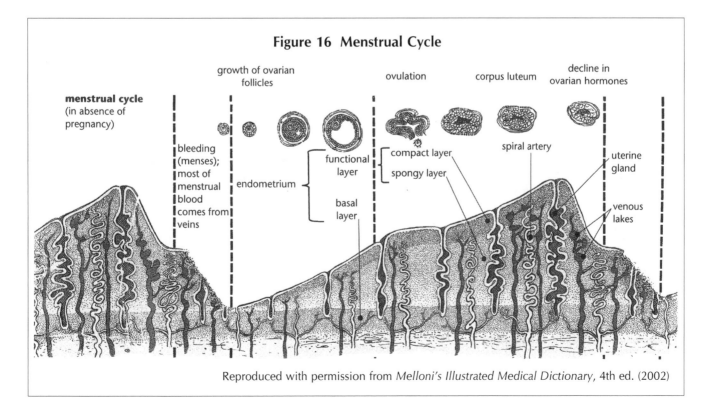

Figure 16 Menstrual Cycle

Reproduced with permission from *Melloni's Illustrated Medical Dictionary*, 4th ed. (2002)

the menstrual period and lasts 1-2 days. In secondary dysmenorrhea, symptoms are more variable.

Physical Examination: Generally unremarkable in primary dysmenorrhea. Endometriosis, salpingitis, or uterine neoplasm may be detected as a cause of secondary dysmenorrhea.

Diagnostic Tests: In secondary dysmenorrhea, pelvic ultrasound or MRI may identify the underlying cause. Diagnostic D&C may disclose a cause within the uterine cavity. Laparoscopy identifies endometriosis or PID.

Course: Primary dysmenorrhea tends to diminish in severity after age 25, and particularly after childbirth. Without treatment, secondary dysmenorrhea may continue throughout the reproductive years.

Treatment: Nonsteroidal anti-inflammatory drugs (ibuprofen, naproxen, mefenamic acid) usually provide good symptomatic relief. Oral contraceptives may be prescribed for more sustained control. Endometriosis is treated with drugs or surgery.

Endometriosis

Growth of endometrial tissue outside of the uterus, particularly in the ovaries and on the pelvic walls.

Cause: Unknown. The problem affects about 2% of American women. Implants of endometrial tissue can occur in a wide variety of locations, including any peritoneal surface, the rectal mucosa, and the ovaries (causing endometrial or "chocolate" cysts, so-called because of their color).

History: Onset is usually during the middle to late 20s. Severe dysmenorrhea, often beginning days before the onset of menstruation and continuing for a week or more. Pain is constant and may be diffuse, with rectal pain and dyspareunia. Many patients are infertile (unable to conceive). Rectal bleeding may occur from implants in the rectum.

Physical Examination: Tender nodules of endometrial tissue may be palpated in the pelvis, particularly the cul-de-sac (lowermost part of pelvic cavity, between uterus and rectum), the ovaries, or the rectum.

Diagnostic Tests: Ultrasound, MRI, or barium enema may identify endometrial implants. Often laparoscopy is required to arrive at a definitive diagnosis. At laparoscopy, endometrial implants often appear as hemorrhagic cysts or "powder burn" lesions on peritoneal surfaces.

Course: Pain (including dyspareunia) and infertility tend to persist throughout the reproductive years. Medical or surgical treatment may diminish pain, but most treatment methods may further impair fertility.

Treatment: Analgesics and various hormone analogues (leuprolide, nafarelin, oral contraceptives) or hormone inhibitors (danazol) may help. Focal endometriosis may be ablated laparoscopically with a laser. For severe or generalized disease, hysterectomy (removal of uterus), oophorectomy (removal of ovaries), or both may be indicated.

Premenstrual Syndrome (PMS, Premenstrual Tension, Late Luteal Phase Dysphoria)

A group of distressing physical and psychologic symptoms experienced in varying degrees and proportions by many women during the week preceding onset of menstruation: swelling of breasts, waist, and ankles, breast soreness, weight gain, irritability, drowsiness, depression, changes in appetite and libido. The cause is unknown, but hormonal and possibly psychological or psychosocial factors are thought to play a part. Cyclical treatment with fluoxetine is often effective. Other measures that may help are counseling, a regular program of exercise, and restriction of sodium, caffeine, alcohol, and sugar.

INFECTIONS OF THE FEMALE REPRODUCTIVE SYSTEM

Pelvic Inflammatory Disease (PID), Salpingitis, Endometritis

Acute or chronic bacterial infection of the uterus and tubes.

Causes: Sexually transmitted infection with *Neisseria gonorrhoeae* or *Chlamydia trachomatis* ascending from the lower genital tract; infection with other organisms (streptococci, *Haemophilus influenzae*) may be bloodborne. Risk factors include nulliparity (never having borne a viable child), nonwhite race, smoking, and sexual contact with many partners.

History: Pelvic pain, chills, fever, menstrual irregularities, purulent vaginal discharge, dyspareunia. Acute symptoms are more likely to occur during menses. With Fitz-Hugh–Curtis syndrome, right upper quadrant pain.

Physical Examination: Fever, abdominal tenderness; marked tenderness on manipulation of cervix and palpation of adnexa. Right upper quadrant tenderness in Fitz-Hugh–Curtis syndrome.

Diagnostic Tests: The white blood cell count is variably elevated. Smear and culture of material obtained from the cervix (or from the cul-de-sac by culdoscopy) may identify the infecting organism. Pelvic ultrasound and laparoscopy are used to refine the diagnosis.

Course: In about 25% of patients, the condition becomes recurrent or chronic even after treatment, with pelvic pain, infertility, and increased risk of ectopic pregnancy. Complications of PID include tubo-ovarian abscess with danger of rupture into the peritoneal cavity, and Fitz-Hugh–Curtis syndrome, a localized peritonitis in the right upper quadrant.

Treatment: Hospitalization, intravenous antibiotics (cefoxitin, clindamycin). For milder disease, outpatient treatment with oral antibiotics may suffice. Surgical drainage of abscesses; for severe disease, hysterectomy with bilateral salpingo-oophorectomy.

Vaginitis, Vulvovaginitis

Inflammation of the vagina and vulva, generally due to infection and manifested by vaginal discharge and vulvar itching or pain. The following three types account for nearly all cases.

Vaginal candidosis: *Candida albicans*, a yeastlike fungus, frequently causes vulvar pruritus and a thick white curdy discharge. Infection is more common in diabetes mellitus and pregnancy and in women taking oral contraceptives or broad-spectrum antibiotics. Examination shows intense erythema of the vulva and curdy white material in the vaginal vault. A wet preparation of this material in potassium hydroxide examined microscopically identifies the causative organism. Culture may also be performed. Treatment is with topical antifungal medicines (miconazole, terconazole, clotrimazole) in vaginal suppositories, creams, or ointments, or with oral fluconazole in a single dose. Recurrences are common.

Trichomonal vaginitis: *Trichomonas vaginalis* is a sexually transmitted protozoan parasite that causes vulvar itching and vaginal discharge. Vaginal examination shows erythema, particularly of the cervix ("strawberry cervix"), and a watery, frothy, malodorous, yellowish-brown discharge. Wet preparation of vaginal discharge shows motile protozoa. Treatment is with oral metronidazole for the patient and all sexual partners. (Symptoms in men are usually absent; dysuria and urethral discharge may occur.)

Bacterial vaginosis: *Gardnerella vaginalis* is at least one of the organisms involved in bacterial vaginosis, a mixed vaginal infection that causes a thin grayish discharge with a foul fishy odor but not much vulvar irritation or itching. Microscopic examination of discharge material shows clue cells (epithelial cells heavily studded with bacteria). This condition is associated with increased risk of premature labor and preterm birth. Treatment is with oral or vaginal metronidazole or clindamycin.

PELVIC NEOPLASMS

Uterine Myoma (Fibromyoma, Fibroid)

A common benign neoplasm of uterine muscle.
Cause: Unknown.

History: There may be no symptoms. Abdominal or pelvic pain or pressure, heavy vaginal bleeding, dysmenorrhea, urinary frequency, infertility.

Physical Examination: Pelvic examination shows one or more discrete, firm masses in the uterine wall. With heavy bleeding there may be tachycardia, pallor, or even shock.

Diagnostic Tests: With heavy bleeding the hemoglobin level may be low. Ultrasound or MRI studies can clearly delineate the nature of the problem.

Course: Uterine myomas tend to grow larger and more numerous with time. With significant bleeding there is a risk of chronic anemia or sudden onset of shock. Myomas in the pregnant uterus can lead to fetal loss, premature or difficult labor, or severe postpartum hemorrhage.

Treatment: Small or solitary myomas can be removed surgically (myomectomy). If tumors are large or numerous, hysterectomy (removal of the uterus) may be indicated. Before surgery, leuprolide or nafarelin is administered to reduce the size and vascularity of tumors.

Carcinoma of the Cervix

A slowly growing, invasive carcinoma of the uterine cervix, predominantly of squamous-cell origin.

Causes: Squamous cell carcinoma of the cervix develops as a consequence of cervical dysplasia, which in turn is caused in a majority of cases by cervical infection with human papillomavirus (genital wart virus), particularly types 16, 18, and 31. The progression from dysplasia to invasive carcinoma typically takes 5-10 years. Peak incidence of cervical carcinoma occurs in the late 30s. Risk factors for cervical carcinoma are smoking, prolonged use of oral contraceptives, sexual contact with many partners, and HIV infection.

History: Irregular vaginal bleeding or spotting, particularly after intercourse; abnormal vaginal discharge; bowel or bladder pain or dysfunction.

Physical Examination: Cervical ulceration. With advanced disease, evidence of pelvic invasion or metastasis; a fistula (abnormal passage or communication) between the vagina and the bladder or rectum may occur.

Diagnostic Tests: Premalignant cellular changes can be detected early by routine Pap smear. About 20% of women with ASC-US (abnormal squamous cells of undetermined significance) eventually develop squamous intraepithelial lesions or invasive carcinoma. Detection of cellular dysplasia (LGSIL, HGSIL) calls for follow-up in the form of colposcopy, cervical biopsy, and possibly surgical or laser excision of a cone of cervical tissue including the entire squamocolumnar junction. These provide precise information about the type and stage of disease.

Course: Severe bleeding may occur from ulceration and erosion of the cervix and surrounding tissues. Extension can lead to bilateral ureteral obstruction, with resultant kidney failure, or to rectovaginal or vesicovaginal fistula. The 5-year survival rate after treatment is about 60%.

Treatment: Early removal of localized disease by conization or, preferably, hysterectomy. In advanced disease, radiation is an alternative to radical surgery.

Endometrial Carcinoma

Adenocarcinoma of the uterine lining.

Causes: Unknown. Most patients are over 50. The risk is increased in childless women, those with obesity, diabetes mellitus, or polycystic ovary disease, and those who have taken postmenopausal estrogen replacement therapy without progesterone, or have been treated for breast cancer with tamoxifen.

History: Abnormal vaginal bleeding, particularly postmenopausal bleeding; pelvic pressure or pain.

Physical Examination: Often unremarkable. There may be uterine enlargement or pelvic tenderness.

Diagnostic Tests: Endometrial biopsy (occasionally, Pap smear) shows malignant cells. Ultrasound examination helps to assess the nature and extent of the problem.

Course: Extension and metastasis occur eventually. With prompt treatment, the 5-year survival rate is about 80%.

Treatment: Removal of uterus, tubes, and ovaries (bilateral salpingo-oophorectomy), with supplemental radiation. Progesterone may be given to palliate metastatic disease.

Hydatidiform mole and choriocarcinoma are discussed in the next chapter.

DISORDERS OF THE BREAST

The breasts consist of glandular elements (dormant except during pregnancy and lactation) and their duct system (discharging at the nipple), interspersed with variable amounts of fat.

Fibrocystic Disease (or Condition) of the Breast (Cystic Mastitis, Mammary Dysplasia)

Formation of benign but painful cysts in the breasts.

Cause: Probably inappropriate response of breast tissue to ovarian hormones. The condition affects as many as one-third of all women between the ages of 25 and 50. The theory that caffeine (from coffee, tea, and chocolate) exacerbates symptoms remains unproven.

History: One or more lumps in the breast, typically painful and tender, and more so just before the onset of menses. Lumps are frequently multiple and may change markedly in size within a period of 2-3 days. Lumps typically disappear eventually, but meanwhile others often develop.

Physical Examination: One or more fluctuant, usually tender masses in one or both breasts. Occasionally nipple discharge is noted.

Diagnostic Tests: Needle aspiration of a cyst usually leads to its disappearance. Biopsy material obtained by fine-needle aspiration or other method from a solid or cystic mass helps to rule out malignant change. Biopsy may show hyperplasia of epithelial tissues, associated with an increased risk of malignant tumor of the breast. Mammography and ultrasound examinations may help to distinguish cysts from solid tumors.

Course: Fibrocystic disease tends to persist, with remissions and exacerbations, until menopause, and then to resolve completely and permanently. Forms of fibrocystic disease associated with proliferation of epithelial elements carry a slightly higher risk of progression to carcinoma of the breast.

Treatment: Analgesics, education, close observation for persisting or dominant lump, which may prove to be a solid tumor requiring further observation. For severe disease, danazol and, rarely, mastectomy may be advised.

Fibroadenoma of the Breast

A benign solid tumor of the breast, occurring typically in younger women. The mass is not usually tender and may be discovered accidentally. It is firm, discrete, spherical, and about 1-5 cm in diameter. Occasionally more than one tumor may be found. Aspiration does not yield fluid and does not collapse the lesion. The principal concern is in distinguishing fibroadenoma from adenocarcinoma, and in the small risk of progression of this lesion to cystosarcoma phyllodes, a rapidly growing tumor that is not histologically malignant but tends to recur after excision. Treatment of fibroadenoma is simple excision under local anesthesia.

Carcinoma of the breast is discussed in Chapter 5.

QUESTIONS FOR STUDY AND REVIEW

1. Name two effects of GnRH (gonadotropin releasing hormone):

   a. _____

   b. _____

2. Name two effects of FSH (follicle stimulating hormone):

   a. _____

   b. _____

3. Briefly describe how a Pap (Papanicolaou) test is done and what it shows:

   _____

   _____

   _____

   _____

   _____

   _____

   _____

4. Define or explain these terms:

   a. anovulation _____

   _____

   b. clue cell_____

   _____

   c. dyspareunia_____

   _____

   d. menarche _____

   _____

   e. mittelschmerz _____

   _____

   f. spinnbarkeit _____

   _____

   g. *Trichomonas vaginalis*_____

   _____

5. Compare and contrast *breast* and *cervical carcinoma* as to incidence, mortality rate, risk factors, and measures for early detection.

_____

_____

_____

_____

_____

_____

6. Name five conditions that can cause amenorrhea or irregular vaginal bleeding:

    a. _____

    b. _____

    c. _____

    d. _____

    e. _____

7. Name two conditions that can cause heavy uterine bleeding:

    a. _____

    b. _____

CASE STUDY: YOU'RE THE DOCTOR

Beverlee Taylor is a 51-year-old African-American woman who is seen by you, her family physician, for a routine checkup. She is employed as a secretary at an elementary school and volunteers on weekends at a senior citizens' center. Her health history is essentially negative except for mild hypertension, well-controlled with medicine. She has had no menstrual periods for the past 3 years and no postmenopausal bleeding. She has a family history of arteriosclerotic heart disease and type 2 diabetes mellitus, but no family history of breast cancer. A Pap smear 2 years ago was normal. She offers no complaints today except vaginal dryness during coitus and occasional hot flashes. Your examination discloses no abnormalities except mild atrophic vaginitis and about 25 pounds of overweight. She would like to start estrogen replacement therapy because, after considering all the pros and cons, she believes the expected relief from menopausal symptoms and the protection against osteoporosis outweigh the risks of cardiovascular disease, breast cancer, thrombophlebitis, and gallbladder disease.

1. What specific health risks might you consider for this patient?

_____

_____

_____

_____

_____

Most authorities currently recommend a baseline mammogram by age 40 (earlier in women with a family history of early-onset breast cancer), but Ms. Taylor has never had a mammogram because her insurance won't pay for one until she is 55 unless she has abnormal findings on physical examination. Since laboratory screening for diabetes mellitus and hypercholesterolemia yielded normal results one year ago, Ms. Taylor's insurance won't pay for another screening until next year. In addition, her insurance won't pay for estrogen replacement therapy in a postmenopausal woman unless there are documented medical indications for it.

2. Which of the following courses will you adopt?

   ___ a. Omit mammography and diabetic screening and withhold estrogen replacement therapy.

   ___ b. Try to persuade Ms. Taylor to pay for these out of her own pocket.

   ___ c. Order the testing and the medicine and invent or exaggerate indications for them in completing insurance claim forms.

3. Explain the reasons for your choice:

   _____

   _____

   _____

   _____

   _____

   _____

   _____

SUGGESTIONS FOR ADDITIONAL LEARNING ACTIVITIES

1. Draw a "Wanted" poster for a disorder discussed in this chapter. Be sure to include all the relevant features of the disorder in the description of this "outlaw" disorder, including symptoms, lab tests, treatment, and so on. Use poster board or cardboard, and make your poster standard poster size or a minimum of 2 feet in height. Use marking pens, crayons, paint, or pictures from magazines to illustrate your poster. Display it in the classroom or at home.

2. This chapter contains eight major sections. For each section, write a summary paragraph containing five sentences. Summarize each of the eight paragraphs you've written in a single sentence per paragraph, so that you have reduced the chapter to just eight sentences. Now distill these eight sentences into a single comprehensive summary sentence. Compare your results with those of other students. How is your work similar to or different from their work?

3. Play Definition Bingo by compiling terms and definitions from this chapter. Use at least 75 terms. Write the definitions on slips of paper and put them in a large bowl. Make Bingo cards from card stock, construction paper, or plain paper. Draw a grid five squares across and five down. Put a star in the center square as the "free space." Write terms in the squares at random. Each Bingo card will hold 24 terms. Play begins by having someone pull a definition slip from the bowl and read it aloud. If the definition matches a term on your card, mark it. Call out "Bingo!" when you complete a row up, down, or diagonally. Then continue play until you or someone else can call out "Blackout" with every space on the card filled in. For a more enjoyable learning game, use M&Ms or other small edibles as markers.

Pregnancy and Childbirth

LEARNING OBJECTIVES

Upon completion of this chapter, you should be able to

- outline the process of conception, fetal development, and normal childbirth;

- explain routine prenatal care and the conduct of labor and delivery;

- describe common disorders of pregnancy and complications of labor and delivery.

PREGNANCY AND CHILDBIRTH

Although pregnancy is scarcely a disease in the usual sense of the word, all phases of childbearing from conception to delivery and the events immediately following it are subject to variations and complications that can endanger the life or well-being of the mother, the infant, or both. The medical supervision of pregnancy and childbirth is the province of the specialty of obstetrics (see box).

For most of human history, **pregnancy** and **childbirth** have been outside the realm of medical practice. Although some ancient medical authors wrote treatises on these topics, women in labor were nearly always attended, from ancient times until the early modern era, by one or more midwives, mature women who were experienced in assisting at childbirth. In sixteenth-century Europe, barber-surgeons began to encroach on the turf of the midwives, and by the eighteenth century obstetrics had become a medical specialty.

Midwife means '[one who is] with [that is, in attendance on] a woman'. Similarly, the Latin noun *obstetrix* 'midwife', from which English *obstetrics* is derived, means literally, 'she who stands by'. At present in many parts of the United States, midwives are legally authorized to attend uncomplicated births and to provide limited obstetrical intervention as necessary.

ANATOMY AND PHYSIOLOGY OF PREGNANCY

The anatomy and physiology of the female reproductive system and the formation and fertilization of the ovum (oocyte) have been described in the preceding chapter.

As mentioned there, FSH (follicle stimulating hormone) produced by the pituitary gland stimulates the maturation each month of an ovum or female sex cell in one ovary. Simultaneously, estrogen causes changes in the the endometrium (lining of the uterus) that begin preparation for implantation of a fertilized ovum if conception occurs.

After ovulation (the release of a mature ovum from its follicle into the pelvic cavity), the production of LH (luteinizing hormone) by the pituitary

gland rises sharply. This hormone causes the ovarian follicle from which the ovum was released to develop into a corpus luteum. Progesterone secreted by the corpus luteum stimulates more complex development of the endometrium, further preparing it for implantation of a fertilized ovum.

The released ovum enters the adjacent uterine tube and migrates toward the uterus. If intercourse takes place around the time of ovulation, spermatozoa advancing through the female genital tract typically encounter the ovum during its passage through the uterine tube, and fertilization takes place in the tube. The fertilized ovum then migrates into the uterine cavity and implants on the endometrium.

At the site of implantation, the fertilized ovum (now called an embryo) forms a specialized plate of tissue, the chorion, through which it draws nourishment from the underlying endometrium by way of fingerlike projections (villi). During the third week after conception, the embryo differentiates into three primitive cell layers: ectoderm, from which epidermis, the nervous system, the eye, the ear, and dental enamel develop; mesoderm, the source of muscle, bone, connective tissue, the circulatory system, and the genitourinary system; and endoderm, which gives rise to the liver, the pancreas, and the epithelial linings of the respiratory, digestive, and genitourinary systems.

Further development consists of a complex series of divisions, foldings, and fusions as the basic framework of the body is laid down and the formation of organ systems (organogenesis) proceeds. By the end of the eighth week, organogenesis is largely complete. After the ninth week of gestation, the embryo is called a fetus. Its further development is largely a matter of growth and maturation.

The chorion evolves into the placenta, a round flat disk of tissue to which the blood vessels in the umbilical cord are attached. (See Figure 17.) Although interchange of oxygen, carbon dioxide, nutrients, and wastes takes place in the placenta by diffusion between maternal and fetal circulations, the circulations do not mix. The placenta produces progesterone and gradually takes over this function from the corpus luteum (which may, however, persist through at least the first half of pregnancy). The placenta also produces (human) chorionic gonadotropin (hCG), the basis of virtually all current pregnancy tests.

Figure 17 Placental and Fetal Circulation

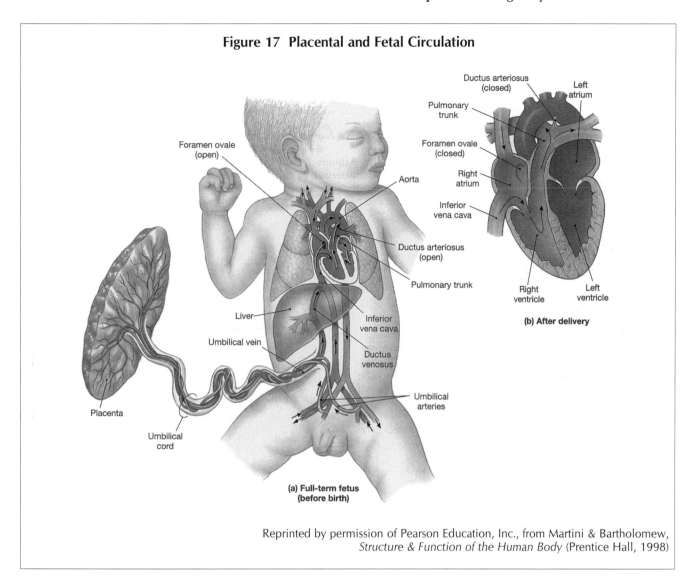

(a) Full-term fetus
(before birth)

(b) After delivery

Reprinted by permission of Pearson Education, Inc., from Martini & Bartholomew,
Structure & Function of the Human Body (Prentice Hall, 1998)

The fetus develops within a fluid-filled membranous sac, the amnion. Amnionic fluid serves as a shock-absorber and also participates in nutrient and excretory functions. During pregnancy the lining of the uterus undergoes structural change and is called the decidua. Chorion, amnion, and decidua are known collectively as fetal membranes. (See Figure 18.)

Multiple pregnancy (twins, triplets) can occur as a result of either fertilization of a single ovum by more than one spermatozoon (identical twins) or fertilization of more than one ovum, each by a different spermatozoon (fraternal twins). The average duration of a normal pregnancy from conception to delivery is 280 days (40 weeks). This period is divided into three trimesters of three months each.

Note the following terms:

Nulligravida: A woman who has never been pregnant.

Nullipara: A woman who has never given birth.

Primigravida: A woman who is pregnant for the first time.

Primipara: A woman who has given birth once.

Multigravida: A woman who has been pregnant more than once.

Multipara: A woman who has given birth more than once.

Parturition: Childbirth.

Parturient: A woman in labor.

Antepartum: Before childbirth.

Postpartum: After childbirth.

Puerperium: The period between the birth of the child and the return of the uterus to its normal size, with regeneration of endometrium.

Puerperal: Pertaining to the puerperium.

Figure 18 Fetal Membranes

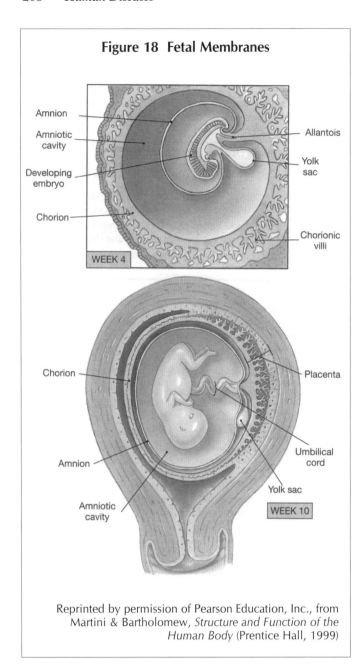

Reprinted by permission of Pearson Education, Inc., from Martini & Bartholomew, *Structure and Function of the Human Body* (Prentice Hall, 1999)

SYMPTOMS AND SIGNS OF PREGNANCY

Amenorrhea (cessation of menses).

Nausea and vomiting. Typically confined to the earlier part of the day, or worse then ("morning sickness"), and often aggravated by the smell, sight, or even the thought of food. About 50% of pregnant women experience some nausea between the sixth and the sixteenth weeks of pregnancy.

Swelling and soreness of the breasts due to edema (milk secretion does not occur until after childbirth).

Enlargement of the uterus. Enlargement can be detected on pelvic examination by about the sixth week of pregnancy. After the twelfth week, the fundus (curved upper surface or dome) of the uterus rises above the pubic bone and the uterus becomes an abdominal organ. Uterine enlargement may be responsible for symptoms occurring at various stages of pregnancy such as urinary frequency, varicosities of the vulva and lower limbs, constipation, hemorrhoids, and heartburn.

Weak and irregular contractions of the uterus (Braxton Hicks contractions) begin early in pregnancy.

Purplish discoloration of the cervix and vagina (Chadwick sign) is due to increased vascularity.

Softening of the cervix (Hegar sign) can sometimes be observed on palpation during pelvic examination.

Presence of a fetus can be detected by ultrasound examination at and after six weeks' gestation. X-ray examination (avoided during early pregnancy because of the risk of fetal damage) shows fetal development somewhat later.

Fetal heart action can be detected by echocardiography by the sixth week and by Doppler ultrasonography by the eighth week. Fetal heartbeat can be heard with a special stethoscope (fetoscope) by about 18 weeks' gestation. The rate is normally 120-160 beats per minute, and the heart tones sound like the ticking of a watch.

Other circulatory sounds that can occasionally be heard are a **funic souffle** (a whistling sound synchronous with fetal heartbeat, due to flow of blood in the umbilical cord) and a **uterine souffle** (a softer rushing sound synchronous with maternal heartbeat, due to increased flow of blood in uterine arteries).

Fetal movement (quickening) is first appreciable around 16-20 weeks' gestation.

Skin changes: Increased pigmentation of areolae (darker zones around nipples); chloasma (brownish patches on the face and elsewhere).

Positive pregnancy test: Chemical tests for the beta fraction of human chorionic gonadotropin in blood or urine become positive between 6 and 10 days after implantation.

PRENATAL CARE

At the first prenatal visit, pregnancy is confirmed and the probable date of delivery is estimated. According to the time-honored Naegele Rule, the EDC (expected date of confinement; "confinement" is an old euphemism for childbirth) is found by going back three months and then forward seven days from the first day of the last menstrual period (LMP). Thus, if the LMP began on August 8 the EDC would be May 15.

The mother's history is carefully reviewed, with particular attention to prior reproductive history (stillbirths, miscarriages, abortions, premature labor or other complications of pregnancy, previous cesarean delivery). The salient points of the reproductive history are customarily noted according to one of two formulas. In one of these, pregnancies, term deliveries, and miscarriages are recorded respectively as gravida, para, and abortus (or G, P, and Ab) with a numeral. Thus, G 3, P 2, Ab 1 refers to a woman who has been pregnant three times, has delivered two children at term, and has had one miscarriage. The other formula consists of a set of four numerals (for example, 2-0-1-2) representing respectively deliveries at term, premature deliveries, miscarriages, and children currently living. Either of these systems can prove ambiguous with respect to multiple pregnancies and their outcome.

Other elements of the history that may have an impact on the course and outcome of pregnancy are the mother's use of tobacco, alcohol, coffee, prescription and nonprescription medicines, or drugs of abuse; history of sexually transmitted diseases such as chlamydia, genital herpes, or AIDS; personal or family history of genetically transmitted disorders; presence of systemic disease such as diabetes mellitus, hypertension, thyroid disease, or heart disease; and occupational exposures, such as lead or radiation, that could cause fetal harm.

The initial prenatal examination includes determination of maternal height, weight, and blood pressure; assessment of general health and nutritional status; and a search for significant disorders. Naturally the examination focuses on the reproductive system and the developing fetus. Pelvimetry refers to certain standard measurements of the bones of the pelvis to assure an adequate birth passage for the fetus.

Laboratory studies carried out as part of routine prenatal care include a complete blood count, urinalysis, blood type, Rh antibody screen, rubella titer (to confirm maternal immunity to rubella, a potential cause of fetal damage), serologic test for syphilis, and Pap smear. Other tests that may be performed depending on risk factors include screening for sexually transmitted diseases (chlamydia, gonorrhea, HIV, syphilis) and for genetic diseases (sickle cell anemia).

Attention to maternal nutrition includes assuring adequate intake of protein, iron, calcium, and vitamins including folic acid. A weight gain of 20-30 pounds is considered most compatible with good maternal and fetal health. The patient is advised to avoid alcohol and tobacco and to limit caffeine intake. Maternal use of alcohol, caffeine, or nicotine is associated with lower birth weight, a sensitive indicator of suboptimal fetal development. Maternal alcoholism can induce a syndrome of facial dysmorphism (short palpebral fissures, broad flat nose, hypoplastic upper lip) and cardiac and spinal defects. Maternal cocaine abuse can lead to genitourinary anomalies and central nervous system infarcts in the fetus.

Prescription and nonprescription medicines are avoided if possible, and taken only when the expected benefit outweighs the risk of fetal harm. Nearly any drug administered to a pregnant woman will reach the fetal circulation in some concentration. Drugs that are capable of causing developmental anomalies are called teratogens. The risk of teratogenesis is limited almost exclusively to the period from the third through the eighth week of development, but a few drugs (ACE inhibitors, sulfonamides, tetracyclines) can cause fetal harm later in pregnancy.

Fetal malformations that can result from administration of drugs during early pregnancy include cleft lip and palate, heart valve abnormalities, optic atrophy, malformation of the brain with mental retardation, and neural tube defects such as meningomyelocele and spina bifida. Drugs that are absolutely contraindicated during pregnancy because of unacceptably high risk include sex hormones (estrogens, androgens, progesterones), certain antibiotics (fluoroquinolones, tetracyclines, vancomycin), isotretinoin, radionuclides, valproic acid, and warfarin.

Certain maternal infections are also associated with a risk of fetal malformation. These include rubella in the first trimester and toxoplasmosis, cytomegalovirus, and herpes simplex later in pregnancy.

Standard prenatal care consists of regular visits every four weeks through the seventh month of gestation. During the eighth month visits are every two weeks, and after the 36th week they are weekly. At each visit the patient's weight and blood pressure are recorded, the urine is tested for protein and sugar, and the height of the uterine fundus above the pubic symphysis is measured. The examiner palpates the uterus and listens for fetal heart tones. As pregnancy progresses, more and more information about the fetus can be gained by palpation.

Fetal ultrasound is routinely performed at 18-20 weeks to confirm fetal size and assess development. The examination may be repeated later to resolve any doubts. Repetition at four-week intervals is standard in multiple pregnancy. If needed for prenatal diagnosis of suspected anomalies, chorionic villus sampling is done at 10-12 weeks, amniocentesis at 12-18 weeks.

At 26-28 weeks the patient is screened for gestational diabetes (discussed later in this chapter) by determination of plasma glucose one hour after a standard oral glucose load. An Rh-negative mother is given a prophylactic dose of an immune globulin to suppress possible immune response to blood from an Rh-positive fetus.

NORMAL LABOR AND DELIVERY

Childbirth is a natural process that only occasionally requires skilled medical or surgical intervention. The role of the obstetrician or midwife is to observe the progress of labor while attending to the comfort of the mother and monitoring fetal and maternal well-being, prepared to render assistance as needed but generally allowing events to proceed naturally.

The **stages of labor** (Figure 19) are as follows:

- 1st stage: from the onset of labor to full dilatation of the cervix.
- 2nd stage: from full dilatation of the cervix to delivery of the fetus.
- 3rd stage: from delivery of the fetus to delivery of the placenta.

The onset of labor is usually signaled by intermittent pelvic and back pains due to uterine contractions, at first mild and random but eventually growing stronger and coming at shorter and more regular intervals. Once labor has begun, the parturient may experience a bloody show—passage of a small amount of bloody material from the vagina, representing a plug of mucus that has been expelled from the cervix by uterine contractions. Eventually the amnionic sac ruptures, releasing a gush of fluid ("breaking of the waters") from the vagina.

The following terms are used in describing the relation between the fetal and maternal bodies:

Lie: The relation of the long axis of the fetus to that of the mother. Generally the lie is longitudinal (fetal axis parallel to mother's); in 1% of pregnancies it is transverse (fetal axis at right angle to mother's).

Presenting part: The part of the fetus that is nearest to, or has entered, the birth canal. With a longitudinal lie this is either the head or the breech (buttocks).

Presentation: Cephalic when the head is the presenting part, breech when the breech is the presenting part. May be more precisely distinguished: occiput presentation (back of head nearest birth canal, or starting into it), brow presentation, face presentation.

Position: The relation of the presenting part to the right or left side of the birth canal. For example, right occiput anterior (ROA): the fetal occiput is anterior and directed toward the right side of the mother.

The birth canal consists of two concentric passages—an inner soft-tissue tube made up of the cervix, vagina, and vulva and an outer rigid channel formed by the pelvic bones—through which the fetus must pass. The force that propels the fetus through this canal is supplied chiefly by uterine contractions, augmented by voluntary or involuntary contractions of the abdominal muscles including the diaphragm ("bearing down").

The principal soft-tissue obstacle to the advance of the fetus is the cervix. Near the end of pregnancy the cervix undergoes a process of softening ("ripening") so that when labor begins it can stretch to accommodate the presenting part. Cervical stretching consists of two more or less simultaneous processes. **Effacement** is the flattening of the cervix from a tubular structure to a ring, and **dilatation** is

Figure 19 Stages of Labor

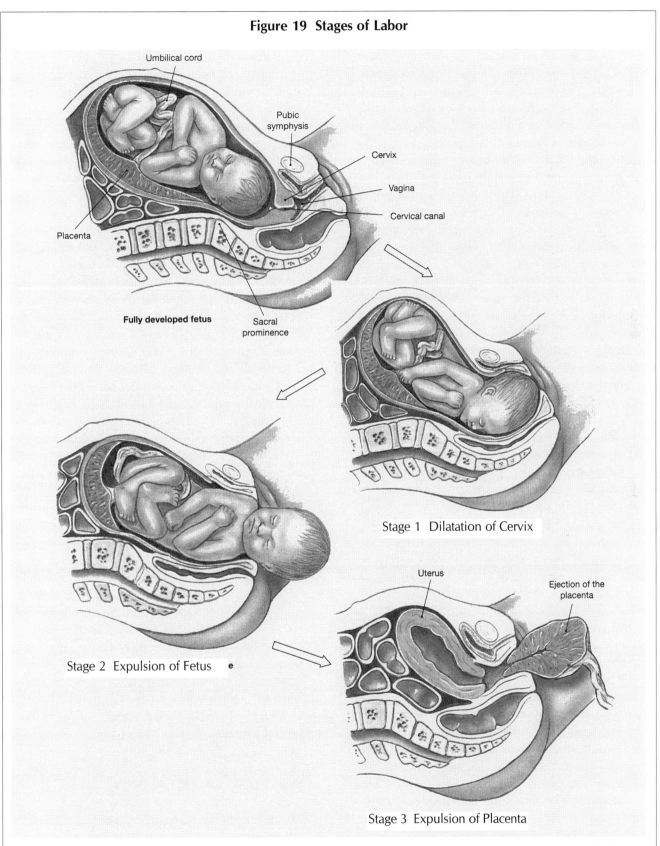

Umbilical cord

Pubic symphysis

Cervix

Vagina

Cervical canal

Placenta

Fully developed fetus

Sacral prominence

Stage 1   Dilatation of Cervix

Stage 2   Expulsion of Fetus   e

Uterus

Ejection of the placenta

Stage 3 Expulsion of Placenta

the expansion of that ring to a size (about 10 cm) through which the fetal head can pass.

A lesser soft-tissue obstacle to delivery is the vulva. Encirclement of the largest diameter of the fetal head by the vulva is called **crowning**. Delivery typically ensues shortly after crowning has occurred, unless the passage of the fetus through the bony pelvis is delayed or arrested.

The bony birth canal is not only rigid and barely large enough to accommodate passage of the fetal head, but also tortuous. The pelvic inlet, or superior pelvic strait, is formed by the pubic bones, the ilia, and the promontory of the sacrum. In entering the pelvic inlet, the greatest diameter of the presenting part (the anteroposterior diameter of the fetal head) must rotate into an oblique position. The pelvic outlet, or inferior pelvic strait, is formed by the inferior rami of the ischia and pubic bones and the sacrotuberous and sacrospinous ligaments. In passing through the pelvic outlet the presenting part must rotate back to an anteroposterior orientation.

The mechanism of normal labor is classically described as consisting of seven sequential movements. These will be described here only for a fetus in the left occiput anterior (LOA) position.

Engagement: The presenting head moves downward into the pelvic inlet, assuming an oblique position with the occiput directed anteriorly and inclined toward the mother's left side.

Descent: The presenting part descends further into the pelvic inlet, with the result that the uterine fundus drops down somewhat from its former height in the upper abdomen. This is known as "lightening." These first two steps may occur days or weeks before the onset of labor, or only after it.

Flexion: As uterine contractions push the presenting part more deeply into the bony pelvis, the shape of birth canal forces the fetal head into flexion (chin closer to chest).

Internal Rotation: With further descent, the head rotates about one-eighth of a circle from the oblique position it occupied in the pelvic inlet to an anterior-posterior orientation imposed by the pelvic outlet. The fetal shoulders are still held in an oblique orientation by the bones of the pelvic inlet.

Extension: The fetal head extends again (chin further away from chest) as it moves through the lower pelvic strait and is born.

External Rotation: Freed of the constraints of the pelvic bones, the head moves back one-eighth of a circle into a normal position with respect to the shoulders just before they are delivered in turn.

Expulsion: The entire fetus is delivered.

The obstetrician follows the progress of the first stage of labor by performing periodic rectal examinations to note the extent of cervical effacement and dilatation and the **station** of the presenting part, that is, its position with respect to the ischial spines. ("Station minus two" means that the presenting part is 2 cm above the spines.) When the cervix is fully dilated ("complete") the parturient is positioned on a delivery table or birthing bed, obstetrical anesthesia (if any) is administered, continuous fetal monitoring is begun (usually by electronic pulse detector applied to the maternal abdomen), and the attendant dons sterile gown and gloves.

Failure of the second stage of labor to progress at the expected rate, evidence of fetal distress, inability of the mother to assist or cooperate (heart disease, mental illness), or certain complications (maternal hemorrhage, prolapse of the umbilical cord) may dictate one or more forms of obstetrical intervention: **episiotomy** (an incision in the posterior midline to enlarge the soft tissue passage), application of forceps or a vacuum cup extractor to the fetal head, or **cesarean section** (delivery of the fetus through a surgical incision into the uterus through the abdominal wall).

During and immediately after the birth process the upper respiratory passages of the newborn are cleared of mucus and amnionic fluid, resuscitation measures are undertaken if spontaneous respirations do not begin immediately, and the umbilical cord is clamped and cut. The placenta is spontaneously expelled from the uterus within the next few minutes by further uterine contractions. The birth canal is carefully inspected for injuries or unexpected bleeding. Any laceration found (or an episiotomy, if one was performed) is surgically repaired. Hormones are administered by injection to hasten contraction of the uterus so as to arrest postpartum bleeding.

DISORDERS OF PREGNANCY

Miscarriage (Spontaneous Abortion)

Spontaneous termination of pregnancy before the fetus is sufficiently developed to survive. The dividing line between abortion and premature delivery (with at least the possibility of survival of the infant) is arbitrarily placed at 20 weeks' gestation or a birth weight of 500 g.

At least 10% of pregnancies are believed to end in miscarriage, usually during the first trimester. More than 60% of these early miscarriages occur after embryonic or fetal death due to developmental abnormality. Inherited genetic disorders account for very few of these abnormalities. Miscarriage can also be due to a variety of maternal factors: severe illness or malnutrition, endocrine deficiency, uterine infection or trauma, cervical incompetence, and alcohol or nicotine use.

Threatened abortion: Any vaginal bleeding, with or without uterine cramping, during the first half of pregnancy.

Inevitable abortion: Rupture of membranes before the period of fetal viability.

Incomplete abortion: Expulsion of a nonviable fetus with retention of part or all of the placenta in the uterus.

Missed abortion: Retention of a dead fetus in the uterus for an extended period (often several weeks) before diagnosis is made.

Habitual abortion: A history of three or more consecutive spontaneous abortions.

Threatened abortion is treated with rest, careful observation, and attention to blood loss. Inevitable, incomplete, and missed abortion are treated by cervical dilatation and curettage of the uterus to remove all products of conception.

Ectopic Pregnancy

Implantation of a fertilized ovum at a site other then the endometrium, usually (95%) in a uterine tube (tubal pregnancy).

Cause: Often unknown. The risk of tubal implantation is increased by any factor that delays migration of the fertilized ovum from the tube to the uterine cavity (developmental anomaly, neoplasm, scarring due to infection or surgery). Development of a fetus in a uterine tube eventually leads to rupture of the tube and life-threatening maternal hemorrhage.

History: Highly variable. The classical triad of amenorrhea followed by scanty vaginal bleeding and severe abdominal pain occurs often but not always.

Physical Examination: Pallor, tachycardia, and hypotension reflect severe hemorrhage. An adnexal mass representing a tubal pregnancy may be felt on pelvic examination.

Diagnostic Tests: Serum pregnancy test is positive but progesterone level is low. In tubal pregnancy, ultrasound shows an adnexal mass but no gestational sac in the uterus. Laparoscopy allows direct visualization of the dilated tube. Uncommonly, an ectopic pregnancy may implant on the abdominal or pelvic wall or on an ovary.

Treatment: Surgical control of hemorrhage, blood transfusion if necessary, and removal of the ectopic pregnancy with preservation of the tube if possible.

Abruptio Placentae

Separation of the placenta from the endometrium before onset of labor.

Cause: Unknown. Trauma is sometimes implicated. The risk is increased by advanced maternal age, multiparity, hypertension, and cigarette smoking.

History: Abdominal or pelvic pain coming on gradually or abruptly, due to stretching of placenta and dissection of leaking blood into uterine muscle. Premature labor often begins within a few hours, in which case abdominal pain persists between labor pains. Vaginal bleeding preceding or following onset of pain.

Physical Examination: Confirms that bleeding is from the external cervical os. The uterus is tender and may show asymmetric swelling.

Diagnostic Tests: Ultrasound may show placental separation but often fails to do so. Blood studies may show hemorrhagic anemia. In disseminated intravascular coagulation (discussed in Chapter 16), fibrinogen and platelets are depleted and fibrin degradation products appear in the blood.

Course: Without treatment, maternal hemorrhage often leads to shock and loss of both mother and child. Complications include disseminated intravascular coagulation and failure of the uterus to contract after delivery, both predisposing to postpartum hemorrhage.

Treatment: Intensive maternal and fetal monitoring. Fluid replacement or blood transfusion as necessary. With heavy bleeding or fetal distress, delivery by cesarean section to save the fetus and prevent life-threatening maternal hemorrhage.

Placenta Previa

Implantation of the placenta partially or entirely over the internal cervical os.

Cause: Unknown. The risk is increased by advanced maternal age, multiparity, and multiple pregnancy. Uterine anomalies or previous uterine surgery may be contributory. Significant placenta previa occurs in about 0.5% of all pregnancies.

History: Painless vaginal bleeding in the third trimester, resulting from separation of the malpositioned placenta from the endometrium as the fetus enlarges.

Physical Examination: Confirms flow of blood from cervix. The uterus is soft and nontender.

Diagnostic Tests: Ultrasound examination quickly and accurately confirms placental position. The finding of placenta previa on ultrasound in the second trimester is common (up to 40% of pregnancies), but most of these have resolved on repeat ultrasonography in the third trimester. MRI may be of use when the diagnosis is doubtful. Blood studies may show hemorrhagic anemia.

Course: Without treatment, maternal hemorrhage often leads to shock and loss of both mother and child. If labor begins, blockage of the internal cervical os by the placenta may interfere with the expulsion of the fetus.

Treatment: Intensive maternal and fetal monitoring. Fluid replacement or blood transfusion as necessary. Preterm delivery (usually by cesarean section) is often required to save the fetus and prevent life-threatening maternal hemorrhage.

Premature (Preterm) Labor

Premature labor is defined as onset of labor after attainment of fetal viability but before fetal maturity is reached, usually at 40 weeks' gestation. Premature labor is the most common complication of pregnancy occurring in the third trimester. Possible causes are numerous: premature rupture of membranes, cervical incompetence, multiple pregnancy, polyhydramnios (excessive volume of amnionic fluid), placenta previa, abruptio placentae, uterine anomalies, maternal trauma or surgery. Risk factors include low socioeconomic status, maternal age under 17 or over 40, previous pregnancy with preterm labor and term delivery, cigarette smoking, poor nutrition or anemia, inadequate prenatal care, and maternal illness (diabetes mellitus, hypertension, pyelonephritis, hyperthyroidism). The prognosis depends largely on the degree of fetal maturity and hence on the length of gestation. Management includes careful maternal and fetal monitoring,

maintenance of maternal hydration, and avoidance of analgesics and anesthetics as much as possible because of their possible adverse effects on the premature infant. Labor is permitted to continue if the cervix is dilated to 4 cm or more, if membranes are ruptured, if there is evidence of fetal distress, and especially in the presence of pre-eclampsia or other complication of pregnancy for which prompt delivery would be beneficial. Otherwise labor is arrested by administration of a tocolytic drug: a beta-adrenergic agonist (isoxsuprine, ritodrine, terbutaline), calcium channel blocker (nifedipine), or magnesium sulfate.

Gestational Diabetes

Carbohydrate intolerance that begins, or is first recognized, during pregnancy.

Cause: May be due to hormonal and physiologic alterations of pregnancy, and hence fully reversible. Although most cases of gestational diabetes resolve after delivery, at least half of women with this disorder eventually develop clinical diabetes mellitus. Gestational diabetes occurs in 3-6% of pregnancies.

History: Usually asymptomatic.

Physical Examination: Usually unremarkable.

Diagnostic Tests: Abnormal elevation of 1-hour postprandial glucose on routine testing at 24-28 weeks' gestation; abnormal result confirmed by 3-hour glucose tolerance test. Occasionally, incidental discovery earlier or later in pregnancy.

Course: May be associated with fetal macrosomia (excessive body size and weight), congenital anomalies, and polyhydramnios (excessive quantity of amniotic fluid); heightened risk of urinary tract infection (pyelonephritis) in the mother.

Treatment: Strict attention to diet, with avoidance of concentrated sugar and fats. Insulin may be required for adequate control of blood sugar level. Labor may be induced early if fetal size threatens to complicate delivery.

Urinary Tract Infection (UTI)

Bacterial infection of the bladder, ureter, or kidney.

Cause: Usually gram-negative bacilli (*E. coli*, *Klebsiella pneumoniae*, *Proteus*, *Pseudomonas*). A predisposing factor is compression of the ureters, especially the right one, by the enlarging uterus. Elevated progesterone level dilates ureters, leading to stagnation and predisposing to infection.

History: Often asymptomatic, or symptoms may be attributed to mechanical pressure of enlarged uterus on bladder. Dysuria, urinary frequency, chills, fever, flank pain.

Physical Examination: Fever, costovertebral angle tenderness if pyelonephritis is present.

Diagnostic Tests: Urinalysis shows white blood cells. Culture identifies the organism.

Course: Possible complications of UTI in pregnancy include impairment of renal function, perinephric abscess, septic shock, premature labor, pulmonary edema with respiratory insufficiency (2%) due to an endotoxin; may progress to adult respiratory distress syndrome.

Treatment: Aggressive treatment even of asymptomatic bacteriuria is the rule in pregnancy because of the risk of complications. Nitrofurantoin, amoxicillin, and cephalosporins are considered safe.

Toxemia of Pregnancy

A syndrome of hypertension and proteinuria (pre-eclampsia) occurring during the second half of pregnancy, which can progress to a stage characterized by seizures (eclampsia).

Cause: Widespread spasm of blood vessels. Metabolic or immunologic factors induced by the developing chorion appear to be involved. The risk is greater for very young mothers or those over 40, and for those with preexisting hypertension or vascular or renal disease. There also appears to be a genetic predisposition. In early pregnancy the syndrome may be induced by hydatidiform mole (discussed below).

History: Pre-eclampsia: Usually there are no symptoms. Headache, blurring of vision, or abdominal pain due to swelling of the liver indicate severe disease with likelihood of progression to eclampsia. Eclampsia: Tonic-clonic seizures.

Physical Examination: Diastolic hypertension. Excessive weight gain, swelling of face, fingers, ankles. Enlargement and tenderness of liver.

Diagnostic Tests: Protein in urine.

Treatment: Hospitalization, bed rest, close observation of maternal blood pressure, weight, and renal function. Fetal monitoring, early induction of labor. Severe elevation of blood pressure is controlled with intravenous hydralazine or labetalol. Eclamptic seizures are treated with intravenous magnesium sulfate.

Placental Neoplasms

Neoplasms occasionally develop from placental tissue. Hydatidiform mole is a benign tumor consisting of clusters of blisterlike vesicles arising from chorionic villi. A molar pregnancy may enlarge more rapidly than a normal pregnancy, but no fetus can be detected by palpation or ultrasound examination. The chorionic gonadotropin level is very high. The mother is at risk of hypertension developing before the 24th week of gestation (earlier than typical pre-eclampsia). A hydatidiform mole is a common cause of irregular second-trimester bleeding. Occasionally a molar pregnancy is expelled spontaneously, but usually it must be surgically removed.

Choriocarcinoma is a malignant tumor arising from the chorion of a normal or abnormal pregnancy. About 25% develop through malignant transformation of hydatidiform moles. The tumor grows rapidly and metastasizes early to lung, vagina, kidney, liver, and brain. Choriocarcinoma may cause vaginal bleeding during pregnancy or after miscarriage or abortion, but symptoms of metastatic disease may occur first. With prompt diagnosis, surgical excision, and chemotherapy, the prognosis in choriocarcinoma is favorable.

DISORDERS OF PARTURITION

Dystocia

Dystocia (literally "difficult childbirth") is any abnormal slowing or arrest of the progress of labor once it has begun. Dystocia can be due to maternal factors (uterine dysfunction, excessive anesthesia, pelvic deformity), fetal factors (large baby, hydrocephalus, breech presentation), or some combination of these. Cephalopelvic disproportion means that the fetal head is too large to pass through the maternal pelvis. Dystocia that cannot be readily corrected by pharmacologic measures or nonsurgical manipulation is a principal indication for cesarean delivery.

Nonreassuring Fetal Status (Fetal Distress)

Findings on fetal cardiac monitoring that suggest fetal hypoxemia (reduction in plasma oxygen tension).

Cause: Various. Often no cause is found and labor and delivery proceed normally. May be a consequence of maternal anesthesia or of administration of oxytocin to induce labor. Serious causes include developmental abnormality of the placenta, prolapse (premature descent through the cervix) or compression of the umbilical cord, and uterine rupture.

Diagnostic Tests: The fetal cardiac monitor shows prolonged or nonuniform deceleration of the pulse rate (bradycardia). Normally the fetal pulse slows during a uterine contraction because of compression of the fetal head, and returns to a normal rate (120-160/ minute) afterwards. Departures from this pattern, or fetal tachycardia, can indicate significant abnormality or threat to fetal welfare. The pH of fetal blood obtained by scalp incision (in a cephalic presentation) is 7.2 or lower in the presence of significant fetal hypoxemia.

Treatment: Administration of oxygen to the mother. Search for and correction of any mechanical cause (umbilical cord prolapse). Depending on cause and the progress of labor, prompt delivery or cesarean section may be indicated.

QUESTIONS FOR STUDY AND REVIEW

1. List three symptoms of pregnancy:

   a. _____

   b. _____

   c. _____

2. List three signs of pregnancy:

   a. _____

   b. _____

   c. _____

3. Which signs and symptoms of pregnancy are most reliable? How early in a pregnancy do they occur or can they be detected?

   _____

   _____

   _____

   _____

   _____

   _____

4. How does the obstetrician follow the progress of labor?

   _____

   _____

   _____

   _____

   _____

5. Define or explain these terms:

   a. chorion_____

   _____

   b. crowning _____

   _____

   c. eclampsia _____

   _____

   d. effacement_____

   _____

e. multipara _____

_____

f. presenting part _____

_____

g. puerperium _____

_____

6. Distinguish the three stages of labor:

a. _____

_____

b. _____

_____

c. _____

_____

7. List three serious complications or disorders of the second stage of labor:

a. _____

_____

b. _____

_____

c. _____

_____

8. List three maternal factors that can contribute to dystocia:

a. _____

b. _____

c. _____

9. List three fetal factors that can contribute to dystocia:

a. _____

b. _____

c. _____

CASE STUDY: YOU'RE THE DOCTOR

Veska Troy is a 19-year-old gravida 2, para 1 who has been seeing you for maternity care since the fourth month of her current pregnancy. She is now in her seventh month (35 weeks by ultrasound dating). Her previous pregnancy, at age 15, ended at term with a cesarean delivery because of cephalopelvic disproportion and non-reassuring fetal status. Her first child is thriving. Ms. Troy and her husband have expressed a wish for a trial of labor with vaginal delivery and for natural childbirth (no general anesthetic).

1. Give at least one reason for and one against each of the following courses of action:

   a. Allow only a brief trial of labor and then go ahead with a repeat cesarean delivery.

      For: _____

      _____

      Against: _____

      _____

   b. Deliver the baby vaginally if possible but insist on general anesthesia.

      For: _____

      _____

      Against: _____

      _____

   c. Accede to the wishes of the parents as fully as possible while remaining attentive to professional standards and the safety of mother and child.

      For: _____

      _____

      Against: _____

      _____

Ms. Troy is Rh positive. Screening for gestational diabetes yielded normal results. Her weight gain since conception has been approximately 22 pounds She is taking prenatal vitamins. She does not drink alcohol or take prescription medicines. She had been smoking about one-half pack a day before beginning prenatal care, but has now reduced her smoking to one cigarette after each meal. She drinks two to four caffeine-containing beverages a day. She is doing well, with no complaints of headaches, ankle swelling, nausea, heartburn, abdominal cramping, backache, vaginal discharge, or bleeding. She does notice that the baby is increasingly active and also complains of bladder pressure and urinary frequency, without burning or hematuria.

2. What tests and observations will you make today?

_____

_____

_____

_____

Ms. Troy's blood pressure is normal at 116/75. Her urine is negative for sugar, protein, occult blood, and leukocyte esterase. Fundal height is appropriate for developmental age and fetal heart tones are strong and regular at 144. Palpation of the abdomen confirms a cephalic presentation. The fetal head is not yet engaged. You advise Mrs. Troy to continue her prenatal vitamins and urge her to curtail nicotine and caffeine intake as much as possible. You also enjoin increasing caution about falls as her center of gravity continues to shift. You ask her to return in 2 weeks for her next routine prenatal visit.

3. Based on the history and course thus far, what is your prediction for the remaining course and ultimate outcome of this pregnancy?

_____

_____

_____

Eleven days later Mrs. Troy's husband calls you at 3:15 a.m. to report that for about 4 hours she has been experiencing pelvic cramping and has now noted light vaginal bleeding.

4. What is your tentative diagnosis?

____ a. normal onset of labor

____ b. premature onset of labor

____ c. miscarriage

____ d. abruptio placentae

____ e. placenta previa

5. Formulate a treatment plan from the options below:

____ a. bed rest for 24 hours

____ b. ibuprofen for cramps

____ c. heating pad to the abdomen

____ d. nothing by mouth

____ e. transport to hospital by ambulance

The patient is taken to the hospital maternity unit by rescue squad, and you meet her there. On arrival she has a pulse of 93, blood pressure 138/59. She is in no acute distress but is experiencing irregularly spaced uterine contractions lasting 20-30 seconds. The amniotic sac has not yet ruptured. A perineal pad is about half saturated with bright red blood. Abdominal examination shows moderate uterine tenderness and intermittent contractions. The fetal head is not fully engaged. Fetal heart tones are strong at 140.

6. Which of the following options do you recommend? Rank your choices in order:

____ a. Prepare the patient at once for cesarean delivery.

____ b. Perform speculum and digital pelvic examination immediately.

____ c. Order pelvic ultrasound examination.

____ d. Type and crossmatch 4 units of whole blood.

____ e. Order emergency hemoglobin and hematocrit.

Explain your rationale: _____

_____

_____

_____

Laboratory studies show low normal hemoglobin and hematocrit. Ultrasound examination rules out placenta previa but is otherwise inconclusive. When blood is ready for transfusion you perform a speculum and digital examination, which confirms brisk bleeding from the cervical os. The os is not effaced or dilated. Fetal monitor does not suggest fetal distress. Ms. Troy's pulse is now 108, blood pressure 121/54. You explain to the Troys that this looks more like abruptio placentae, an obstetrical emergency, than premature labor. Because bleeding is brisk and the cervix has not begun to dilate, observation could be perilous. You advise immediate cesarean delivery.

7. What are the risks to delaying the cesarean delivery at this point?

_____

_____

_____

_____

Mr. Troy now expresses extreme dissatisfaction with your handling of his wife's condition. He feels you have betrayed their trust by proceeding with a repeat cesarean delivery even though you had assured them that you endorsed their wish for a trial of vaginal birth. Ms. Troy, who is apprehensive and in considerable pain, becomes tearful and upset and shouts at you and her husband that while you are carrying on your debate she may be bleeding to death.

8. Choose a course of action from among the following:

___ a. Put off the cesarean delivery for 24 hours.

___ b. Advise the Troys to get another obstetrician.

___ c. Prescribe a tranquilizer for Ms. Troy.

___ d. Continue patiently explaining the current situation and the basis for your decision regarding its management.

Justify your decision: _____

_____

_____

_____

_____

SUGGESTIONS FOR ADDITIONAL LEARNING ACTIVITIES

1. Make arrangements to tour a community birthing center or hospital labor and delivery department. Make note of the names of equipment or procedures discussed during your tour. Find out what information is available to prospective parents. Take home any literature that is available from this facility. Make a brief oral presentation on your experience.

2. Make a mind map or concept map for each of the disorders of pregnancy listed in this chapter. Write the name of the disorder in a circle in the center of your map. Draw five short lines extending from the center circle, each connected to another circle. Label this ring of secondary circles as Cause, History, Physical Exam, Diagnostic Tests, and Treatment. Extend short lines from each of the secondary circles and attach new circles filled in with the data related to that topic. For example, on a mind map for UTI, the circles attached to the History circle might be filled in with these terms: dysuria, urinary frequency, chills, fever, flank pain, pressure, asymptomatic.

3. View a video of a cesarean birth. If one is not available through your school or scheduled for television broadcast on one of the cable networks, contact your local hospital or a Lamaze group for suggestions on where to borrow one. As you watch the video, make notes of terminology you hear that is used in this chapter. Look up any terms you don't recognize. Watch the video with another student or a family member and compare your notes.

15

Disorders of Metabolism, Nutrition, and Endocrine Function

Chapter Outline

DISORDERS OF METABOLISM, NUTRITION, AND ENDOCRINE FUNCTION

METABOLISM AND NUTRITION
    Obesity
    Disorders of Lipid Metabolism

DISORDERS OF ENDOCRINE FUNCTION

DISEASES OF THE PITUITARY GLAND
    Hypopituitarism
    Acromegaly, Gigantism
    Diabetes Insipidus

DISEASES OF THE THYROID GLAND
    Hypothyroidism
    Hyperthyroidism (Thyrotoxicosis)
    Thyroiditis
    Hashimoto Disease (Chronic Lymphocytic
        Thyroiditis

DISEASES OF THE PARATHYROID GLANDS
    Hypoparathyroidism
    Hyperparathyroidism

(Outline continued on next page)

LEARNING OBJECTIVES

Upon completion of this chapter, you should be able to

- discuss the physiology of metabolism and nutrition;

- describe the functions of the principal endocrine glands;

- classify common metabolic disorders by their signs, symptoms, and treatment.

DISORDERS OF METABOLISM, NUTRITION, AND ENDOCRINE FUNCTION
(continued)

DISEASES OF THE ADRENAL GLANDS
Adrenal Insufficiency (Addison Disease)
Cushing Syndrome (Hyperadrenocorticism)
Congenital Adrenal Hyperplasia

DISORDERS OF PANCREATIC ENDOCRINE FUNCTION
Diabetes Mellitus (DM)
Type 1 Diabetes Mellitus
Type 2 Diabetes Mellitus

DISORDERS AFFECTING MORE THAN ONE ENDOCRINE GLAND
Multiple Endocrine Neoplasia
(Multiple Endocrine Adenomatosis)
Polyglandular Deficiency Syndrome
(Polyglandular Autoimmune Syndrome)

QUESTIONS FOR STUDY AND REVIEW

DISORDERS OF METABOLISM, NUTRITION, AND ENDOCRINE FUNCTION

METABOLISM AND NUTRITION

Metabolism is a general term for the sum of all the chemical and electrical processes that occur in the living body. A principal part of metabolism is the oxidation of foods so as to release energy in tiny amounts that are usable at the cellular level. Most metabolic processes are at least partially under the control of hormones.

A hormone is a chemical messenger or mediator produced by a cell, tissue, or gland. Hormones are released into the circulation, and perform their functions at sites remote from their origins. Some hormones stimulate cellular functions, while others inhibit them. A tropic hormone stimulates the cells of a remote gland to produce its secretion, and a releasing hormone (relin) promotes release of a specific hormone into the circulation.

Many of the important hormones are produced by endocrine ("internal secretion") glands (also called ductless glands because their secretions pass directly into the circulation)—pituitary, thyroid, adrenal, and others. Some of these endocrine glands (for example, the pancreas and the gonads), perform nonhormonal functions as well.

Nutrition refers to the intake and use of foods by the body. Each of the three main types of food (protein, fat, carbohydrate) has its own function in human nutrition.

A normal adult requires one gram of protein per kilogram of body weight per day to supply sufficient materials for maintenance and repair of tissues and organs and for production of intracellular enzymes, hormones, and other substances. Proteins are built up of long strands of amino acids, which are relatively simple nitrogen-containing organic compounds. Only 20 different amino acids have been found in all the complex proteins of the human organism. About half of these can be synthesized in the body; the rest, called essential amino acids, must be obtained from the diet.

Carbohydrate (consumed in the form of starches and sweets) is the most important source of energy in most diets. Carbohydrate foods are chemically degraded in the digestive system to simple sugars, especially glucose, a six-carbon sugar that is the most plentiful in the blood and the principal fuel of cellular energy metabolism.

Fats (lipids) are oily or greasy substances built up of fatty acids (long, straight-chain organic acids). Fats in the diet come mainly from animal foods, but the term fat is often extended to include oils of plant origin.

All three basic types of food can be and are burned in the body as fuel. The amount of energy that a foodstuff can supply can be determined by burning the food outside the body in a calorimeter (a small furnace equipped with a sensitive means of measuring heat production). The energy released by food is measured in calories per gram (cal/g). The large calorie or kilocalorie (kcal, 1000 calories) is a more convenient unit of measure in nutrition; in modern parlance, kilocalories are usually called simply calories.

Whereas proteins and carbohydrates both supply about 4 calories (kcal) per gram, fats supply about 9. The active adult requires 2500-4000 kcal/day: 1200-1800 kcal to meet the energy demands of basic life processes, plus those needed for physical exertion. In the average middle-class American diet, 50% of calories come from carbohydrate, 35% from fat, and 15% from protein.

By convention, the subject of nutrition also includes materials usually not thought of as foods: water, minerals, and vitamins. Water is the most abundant substance in the body and the principal constituent of blood. Intracellular fluid accounts for about 40% of total body weight, interstitial fluid (in tissue spaces, outside of cells) another 15%, and plasma (the fluid part of blood) about 5%. The water content of plasma, and indirectly that of the intracellular and interstitial compartments, is regulated within narrow limits by a complex system of checks and balances involving the sensation of thirst, perspiration, gastrointestinal fluid losses, renal excretion and reabsorption of water and electrolytes, and other chemical processes.

Essential dietary minerals include iron (needed for the production of red blood cells and as a catalyst in many metabolic processes), calcium (a principal constituent of bones and teeth), sodium, potassium, zinc, magnesium, and many more.

Vitamins are organic compounds, normally present in many foods, that the human body needs in trace amounts, usually to serve as boosters or catalysts in essential metabolic processes.

Disorders of nutrition are relatively common, and have many causes, among them overeating, alcoholism, stringent dieting, anorexia nervosa, malabsorption due to inherited abnormalities or to gastrointestinal disease or surgery, and any severe chronic disease including metastatic carcinoma. Specific vitamin deficiencies occur but are rare in our culture. Most nutritional deficiencies are complex and occur as part of a more general pattern of illness.

Obesity

The most common nutritional disorder, except among the extremely poor, is not undernutrition but obesity, an excess of subcutaneous fat in proportion to lean body mass.

Body mass index (BMI), the weight in kilograms divided by the body surface in square meters, is a useful measure of the proportion of fat to lean body mass. The National Institutes of Health (NIH) has defined obesity as a BMI of 30 or more, and overweight as a BMI between 25 and 30. By these criteria, 55% of adults in the United States are either overweight or obese, and the prevalence of obesity is increasing in both children and adults.

The cause of obesity is unknown, but in most cases it appears to be genetically determined. Most obese persons do not have faulty eating habits or endocrine disease.

Obesity is an independent risk factor for hypertension, hypercholesterolemia, type 2 diabetes mellitus, myocardial infarction, some cancers, osteoarthritis, gastroesophageal reflux disease, and a number of other conditions.

Weight reduction leads to reduction in many of these risks, but cannot repair damaged arteries or joints. Most safe and effective weight-reduction programs include a diet low in fat and in total calories and 30 minutes of strenuous physical exercise on most or all days of the week. Other methods include the use of behavior modification therapy, hypnosis, or drugs to suppress appetite, and gastrointestinal surgery to reduce the size of the stomach or diminish intestinal absorption of food.

Disorders of Lipid Metabolism

Fats (triglycerides) and cholesterol are not soluble in the watery medium of plasma. They are therefore transported in the blood in loose chemical combination with carrier substances called lipoproteins. Produced by the liver and by cells of the intestinal mucosa, lipoproteins occur in several forms, which are distinguished according to molecular weight and density. Each lipoprotein has a specific function. Chylomicrons transport dietary cholesterol and triglycerides from the intestine to the liver and other tissues. Very low density lipoproteins (VLDL) transport triglycerides from the intestine and the liver to muscle and fatty tissue. Low density lipoproteins (LDL) transport cholesterol to tissues other than the liver, such as the walls of arteries. High density lipoproteins (HDL) transport cholesterol to the liver for excretion in bile.

Persons with any of several inherited abnormalities in the synthesis and metabolism of lipoproteins are at increased risk of atherosclerosis (deposition of cholesterol crystals in the walls of arteries, discussed in Chapter 8). A total cholesterol above 220 mg/dL, an LDL cholesterol above 160 mg/dL, a fasting triglyceride level above 250 mg/dL, or HDL cholesterol below 35 mg/dL all increase the risk of coronary artery disease.

Factors besides heredity that can elevate LDL cholesterol include diabetes mellitus, hypothyroidism, nephrotic syndrome, and some drugs. Dietary saturated fat can raise LDL cholesterol more than any other dietary component, but excess dietary intake of fats and cholesterol is seldom solely responsible for dangerous elevation of cholesterol.

Reducing elevated LDL cholesterol is important in reducing the risk of coronary artery disease, stroke, and peripheral arterial disease, and in the treatment of these conditions when they are present. About 75% of persons with elevated LDL cholesterol can achieve normal levels with diet, exercise, and correction of overweight. Most of the remainder can gain satisfactory control of lipid levels with niacin, bile acid sequestrants (cholestyramine, colesevelam, colestipol), HMG-CoA reductase inhibitors or "statins" (atorvastatin, fluvastatin, pravastatin, simvastatin) and other drugs (fenofibrate, gemfibrozil).

DISORDERS OF ENDOCRINE FUNCTION

Diseases of the pituitary, thyroid, adrenal, and parathyroid glands, and diabetes mellitus, are discussed in this section.

DISEASES OF THE PITUITARY GLAND

The pituitary gland or hypophysis, situated on the undersurface of the brain, consists of two distinct masses of endocrine tissue. The anterior pituitary (adenohypophysis) produces hormones that regulate the development and function of other endocrine glands: thyroid stimulating hormone (TSH), adrenocorticotropic hormone (ACTH), which stimulates the adrenal cortex, and the gonadotropins: follicle-stimulating hormone (FSH) and luteinizing hormone (LH), which stimulate gonadal functions. The anterior pituitary is also the source of growth hormone (somatotropin, which regulates the natural growth process) and prolactin (required for lactation after pregnancy).

The posterior pituitary (neurohypophysis) is in direct continuity with the part of the brain called the hypothalamus. It produces two hormones: oxytocin, which stimulates uterine contractions in labor; and vasopressin (antidiuretic hormone, ADH), which helps to control water balance by promoting reabsorption of water by the kidneys.

Hypopituitarism

Deficiency of pituitary hormones, with resultant structural and functional disturbances.

Causes: Benign or malignant neoplasms of the pituitary gland or surrounding tissues, cerebral vascular disease, infection, trauma, shock, autoimmune disease.

History: Weakness, fatigue, weight loss, diminished libido, amenorrhea.

Physical Examination: Wasting, loss of axillary and pubic hair, hypotension. Visual field defects may be noted if a causative tumor affects the optic chiasm (crossing of optic nerve fibers close to the pituitary gland).

Diagnostic Tests: The levels of pituitary hormones (ACTH, TSH) in the serum are diminished, as well as the levels of hormones produced by organs stimulated by these hormones (thyroxine, cortisol). Fasting blood sugar and sodium are depressed, lipids increased.

Course: Any stressing illness can precipitate shock, vascular collapse, and death.

Treatment: Surgical excision of a tumor, if present. Endocrine replacement therapy as needed (cortisol, thyroid hormone, gonadal hormones).

Acromegaly, Gigantism

Overgrowth of body structures in adulthood (acromegaly) or in childhood (gigantism) due to excessive somatotropin (growth hormone).

Cause: Benign pituitary adenoma producing abnormal amounts of somatotropin. May occur as part of multiple endocrine adenomatosis.

History: Excessive long-bone growth (when onset is before puberty); excessive growth of hands, feet, jaw. Weakness, amenorrhea, headache, hoarseness, obstructive sleep apnea, sweating.

Physical Examination: Coarse facial features, hypertension, visual field defects, cardiomegaly.

Diagnostic Tests: Serum level of growth hormone is elevated, and is not suppressed by administration of oral glucose. The blood sugar is elevated. X-ray of the skull may show an enlarged sella turcica (the saddle-shaped bony depression in which the pituitary rests). MRI may show a pituitary tumor.

Course: Premature cardiovascular disease. Other complications include pituitary failure, hypertension, diabetes mellitus, cardiac enlargement and failure, carpal tunnel syndrome, and visual field defects.

Treatment: Surgical excision of the tumor is usually successful. Radiation may also be used. Bromocriptine is administered to reduce the level of growth hormone. Octreotide, a synthetic analog of somatostatin (a hormone that inhibits production and release of growth hormone) is also effective.

Diabetes Insipidus

A disorder in which deficiency of antidiuretic hormone (ADH, vasopressin) leads to excessive output of urine containing no sugar.

Cause: Failure of the posterior lobe of the pituitary to produce ADH because of trauma, infection, neoplasm, or inherited pituitary disease.

History: Polyuria (increased urine output), polydipsia (excessive thirst).

Physical Examination: There may be signs of dehydration. The pulse may be rapid and the blood pressure low.

Diagnostic Tests: The serum sodium is elevated. The specific gravity of urine is low, and urine contains no sugar. Administration of vasopressin corrects polyuria.

Course: Complications include dehydration (if the patient is unable to replace renal losses with oral fluid intake) and hypertonic encephalopathy (brain injury, causing lethargy or coma, due to elevation of serum sodium).

Treatment: Desmopressin, a synthetic analog of vasopressin administered intranasally or intramuscularly, controls polyuria and polydipsia. Intravenous fluid replacement may be necessary if severe dehydration or encephalopathy occurs.

DISEASES OF THE THYROID GLAND

The thyroid gland, whose name means "shield-shaped," is situated in the front of the neck overlying the junction of the larynx and trachea. The thyroid gland produces two iodine-containing hormones, thyroxine (T_4) and triiodothyronine (T_3), which circulate in the blood bound to a plasma protein (thyroid binding globulin, TBG). These hormones influence general metabolism, chiefly by regulating gene transcription of body proteins (including growth hormone).

The term goiter refers to a palpable and often visible enlargement of the thyroid gland. Goiter can occur with elevated, normal, or decreased levels of thyroid hormone, depending on its cause.

Hypothyroidism

A syndrome resulting from deficiency of circulating thyroid hormone. When the disorder appears at birth or in early infancy it is called cretinism; hypothyroidism occurring after early childhood is called myxedema.

Causes: Congenital absence or hypoplasia of the thyroid gland; intrinsic thyroid disease (Hashimoto thyroiditis), deficiency of dietary iodine, goitrogenic foods or medicines, deficiency of pituitary thyroid stimulating hormone.

History: Weakness, lethargy, myalgia, constipation, depression, intolerance to cold, polymenorrhea, weight gain, hoarseness.

Physical Examination: Dry, sallow skin, brittle hair and nails, thinning of scalp hair and outer thirds of eyebrows, puffy face, sluggish speech, bradycardia, nonpitting edema. A goiter may be present when disease is due to iodine deficiency, antithyroid agents, or thyroiditis.

Diagnostic Tests: The T_4 and other measures of thyroid hormone are depressed, the TSH level elevated (except when disease is due to pituitary TSH deficiency). There may be reduction of red blood cells, blood sugar, and sodium, and elevation of cholesterol. Antibody to thyroid may be found in Hashimoto thyroiditis.

Course: With treatment the prognosis is excellent. Complications of untreated disease include coronary artery disease, congestive heart failure, heightened susceptibility to infection, psychosis, and coma.

Treatment: Deficiency of thyroid hormone can be corrected by administration of levothyroxine. Maintenance treatment must be continued indefinitely unless a treatable cause of hypothyroidism can be found and eliminated.

Hyperthyroidism (Thyrotoxicosis)

A syndrome resulting from excessive thyroid hormone in the circulation.

Causes: The principal cause is autoimmune disease of the thyroid gland, with production of thyroid-stimulating immunoglobulin by the immune system. This condition (Graves disease) is eight times more common in women and usually comes on between ages 20 and 40. Graves disease may be accompanied by other autoimmune disorders (pernicious anemia, myasthenia gravis, diabetes mellitus). Less common causes of hyperthyroidism are acute thyroiditis and inappropriate administration of thyroid hormone.

History: Restlessness, nervousness, fatigue, intolerance to heat, sweating, cardiac palpitation, weight loss, frequent bowel movements, menstrual irregularities, enlargement of thyroid gland (goiter). In Graves disease, bulging of eyes, conjunctival drying or irritation.

Physical Examination: Tachycardia, warmth and moistness of skin, resting tremor of hands, hyperactive deep tendon reflexes, loosening of nails. In Graves disease, diffuse or nodular enlargement of thyroid, sometimes with arterial bruit (a vascular hum synchronous with heartbeat, heard with a stethoscope); exophthalmos (undue prominence of eyes due to edema of orbital contents), staring gaze, lid lag (slowness of upper eyelids to move with eye movements).

Diagnostic Tests: The levels of T_3 and T_4 are elevated, and TSH is depressed. The radioactive iodine uptake is increased. Thyroid-stimulating immunoglobulin is present in the serum. Antinuclear antibody may also be present. There may be mild anemia and hypercalcemia.

Course: Complications include atrial fibrillation, paralysis, and hypercalcemia.

Treatment: End-organ effects of thyroid hormone (tachycardia, tremor, restlessness) can be reduced by beta-blocker treatment. Glandular hyperactivity can be reduced by antithyroid medicines (propylthiouracil, methimazole), radioactive iodine, or thyroidectomy.

Thyroiditis

Thyroiditis is a general term for inflammation of the thyroid gland. Several types are recognized, differing in their causes, symptoms, and effects on thyroid function. Two of the more common types are discussed below.

Hashimoto Disease (Chronic Lymphocytic Thyroiditis)

A relatively common disorder, often asymptomatic. It occurs more frequently in women, and tends to run in families.

Cause: Development of antibody to one's own thyroid tissue.

History: Gradual painless enlargement of the thyroid gland, with symptoms of mild hypothyroidism. Often there are no symptoms at all.

Physical Examination: The thyroid gland is enlarged, symmetric, firm, and nontender.

Diagnostic Tests: The erythrocyte sedimentation rate is elevated. Testing of serum may disclose presence of autoantibody to thyroid tissue. Thyroid function tests give variable results.

Course: Tendency to resolve spontaneously, but may lead to progressive decline of thyroid function.

Treatment: Thyroid hormone supplementation and long-term observation for progression of hypothyroidism.

de Quervain Disease (Subacute Thyroiditis, Granulomatous Thyroiditis, Giant Cell Thyroiditis)

Cause: Probably viral infection of the thyroid gland.

History: Acute, painful enlargement of the thyroid gland, with dysphagia. There may also be malaise and symptoms of thyrotoxicosis.

Physical Examination: The thyroid gland is enlarged and tender. Signs of hyperthyroidism may be present.

Diagnostic Tests: The sedimentation rate is markedly elevated and the radioactive iodine uptake is reduced. Antibody to thyroid tissue may be present in the serum.

Course: Self-limited.

Treatment: Aspirin. If hypothyroidism is present, thyroid hormone supplementation is given. Propranolol is used to control transitory thyrotoxicosis.

DISEASES OF THE PARATHYROID GLANDS

The four parathyroid glands are so called because they lie on or in the capsule of the thyroid gland. These glands produce parathyroid hormone (PTH), which regulates the serum calcium level within narrow limits. Calcium control is important for proper maintenance of bones and teeth; more critically, the level of calcium in the serum and in tissue fluids exerts a potent influence on nerve and muscle function. Parathyroid hormone maintains the level of calcium in serum by moving calcium ions out of the bones, reducing the renal clearance of calcium, and increasing the rate of intestinal absorption of calcium. Calcitonin, a hormone produced by the thyroid gland, is also involved in regulation of serum calcium.

Hypoparathyroidism

Causes: The most common cause is accidental removal of the parathyroid glands during thyroidectomy. Rarely the parathyroid glands may be damaged by trauma, infection, neoplasm, or chemical poisons, or by autoantibodies, which may be formed in the polyglandular autoimmune syndrome, discussed later in the chapter.

History: With acute onset, tetany, tingling of face, hands, and feet, muscle cramps, carpopedal spasm (painful cramps of wrists and ankles), laryngospasm with respiratory obstruction, seizures. With more chronic onset, mental retardation, abnormalities of bones and teeth, cataract, parkinsonlike disorder due to calcification of basal ganglia.

Physical Examination: The skin may be dry and coarse. Deep tendon reflexes are hyperactive, and the Chvostek sign (twitching of face after percussion over facial nerve in front of ear) and Trousseau sign (spastic contraction of the hand after application of a constricting cuff to the arm) are present.

Diagnostic Tests: The serum calcium is low and the serum phosphorus is high. Excretion of phosphorus in the urine is reduced. The level of parathyroid hormone in the serum is low.

Treatment: Calcium replacement, intravenously in acute tetany, and vitamin D. Treatment must be continued indefinitely.

Hyperparathyroidism

Causes: Hyperplasia, adenoma, or carcinoma of a parathyroid gland. Adenoma may occur as part of multiple endocrine adenomatosis, discussed later in this chapter.

History: Bone pain; weakness, fatigue, polyuria, polydipsia, urolithiasis.

Physical Examination: Unremarkable.

Diagnostic Tests: The serum calcium is elevated, the phosphorus depressed. Urinary calcium and phosphorus are both elevated. X-ray may show osseous or dental abnormalities, or cysts or pathologic calcification of the kidneys.

Course: Complications include peptic ulcer, pancreatitis, renal damage.

Treatment: Surgical removal of neoplasm. Reduction of serum calcium by administration of furosemide or other agents.

DISEASES OF THE ADRENAL GLANDS

The adrenal glands are two crescent-shaped caps of endocrine tissue, one situated on top of each kidney. Each adrenal gland consists of two essentially different bodies of endocrine tissue: the outer cortex, and the inner medulla.

The adrenal cortex produces three classes of hormones, two of which play crucial roles in the control of sugar, protein, and mineral metabolism.

The glucocorticoids (principally cortisol) increase glucose production by the liver, affect protein and fat metabolism, help to regulate blood pressure, mediate many of the responses of the body to stress, and tend to suppress immune and inflammatory responses.

The mineralocorticoids (principally aldosterone) regulate electrolyte and water balance by promoting renal retention of sodium ions and renal excretion of potassium, hydrogen, and ammonium ions.

Adrenal androgens play a minor role in reproductive physiology in both men and women. They are chiefly of interest as a cause of hirsutism and virilization in certain adrenal diseases.

The adrenal medulla is part of the sympathetic nervous system (see Chapter 19). Cells of the adrenal medulla are stimulated directly by sympathetic nerve endings to produce epinephrine, norepinephrine, and dopamine, which (although not essential to life) play a critical part in the body's response to severe stress. These hormones affect many tissues, increasing the rate and force of cardiac contractions, relaxing the smooth muscle of the bronchi, constricting some blood vessels and dilating others, stimulating liver and muscle tissue to produce and release glucose, and controlling fat breakdown and insulin production.

Adrenal Insufficiency (Addison Disease)

An acute or chronic deficiency of cortisol and related hormones from the adrenal cortex.

Causes: Degeneration of the adrenal cortices, usually as an autoimmune phenomenon sometimes involving other endocrine glands as well. Other diseases (infection, malignant tumors) may account for destruction of the adrenal glands in rare cases. Deficiency of pituitary ACTH also causes some adrenal insufficiency, but not the full-blown clinical picture of Addison disease. Adrenal crisis may be precipitated by severe physical stress (surgery) or systemic disease (meningococcemia) or by sudden withdrawal of steroid therapy.

History: Weakness, easy fatigability, anorexia, nausea, vomiting, diarrhea, abdominal pain, amenorrhea, emotional lability. In addisonian crisis, fever, confusion, collapse, coma.

Physical Examination: Weight loss, wasting, hypotension, sparseness of axillary hair; increased pigmentation of skin, especially over pressure points, skin creases, and nipples. In crisis, severe hypotension and evidence of dehydration.

Diagnostic Tests: The eosinophil count is elevated. The serum sodium is low, the potassium and BUN (blood urea nitrogen) elevated. Serum cortisol is abnormally low and does not rise in response to administration of ACTH. Chest x-ray shows a small, vertical heart.

Course: Without treatment, steady progression is likely. Addisonian crisis can be rapidly fatal. Fluid and electrolyte depletion, wasting, cardiovascular collapse.

Treatment: The basic treatment is replacement of missing corticosteroids. Supportive treatment and elimination of any identifiable underlying or precipitating cause are important. In crisis, intravenous fluid and electrolyte replacement may be lifesaving.

Cushing Syndrome (Hyperadrenocorticism)

A syndrome due to prolonged elevation of adrenal cortical hormones in the circulation.

Causes: The most frequent cause of Cushing syndrome today is medicinal administration of adrenocortical hormones. The condition can also result from production of excessive adrenocortical hormones by a neoplasm of the adrenal cortex, from medicinal administration of ACTH, or from production of ACTH-like substances by other neoplasms (such as bronchogenic carcinoma). When excessive adrenal cortical activity results from an elevated level of adrenocorticotropic hormone (ACTH) from a tumor (basophil adenoma) of the pituitary, the condition is called Cushing disease.

History: Increasing obesity, stretch marks especially on trunk and thighs, acne, easy bruising, impaired wound healing, weakness, thirst, headache, amenorrhea or impotence, increased body hair, personality change.

Physical Examination: Truncal obesity, moon face, buffalo hump (soft tissue prominence over upper back), protuberant abdomen with purple striae (stretch marks), hirsutism, acne, hypertension.

Diagnostic Tests: Blood glucose is elevated and potassium is low. The serum level of cortisol is high and does not fall after administration of dexamethasone, a synthetic corticosteroid. Urinary excretion of cortisol is also increased. In Cushing disease and other disorders due to excessive ACTH, the blood level of ACTH is elevated. Otherwise the ACTH level is subnormal, its production by the pituitary having been suppressed by high circulating levels of corticosteroid. An adrenal tumor may be shown by abdominal CT scan. Tumor of the pituitary is identified by cranial MRI.

Course: Depends on the origin of the problem. Untreated Cushing syndrome can be complicated by osteoporosis, nephrolithiasis, psychosis, heightened susceptibility to infection, and consequences of hypertension and diabetes mellitus; it is generally fatal within a few years.

Treatment: Discontinuance of corticosteroid treatment, or reduction of dose. Surgical removal of a causative pituitary or adrenal neoplasm. Ketoconazole or metyrapone can be used to suppress cortisol levels when surgery is not feasible.

Congenital Adrenal Hyperplasia

A genetically determined deficiency of the enzymes normally involved in the formation of cortisol. The resulting deficiency of cortisol leads to overproduction of ACTH by the pituitary, which in turn stimulates excessive androgen production by the adrenal glands. Signs of abnormality due to excessive androgen levels are evident at birth or shortly after: virilization of female children, precocious genital development of males. Signs of adrenal insufficiency include electrolyte and water imbalances, which may be evident within the first few days of life. Laboratory studies show elevation of androgen (dehydroepiandrosterone) in serum and urine. Serum ACTH levels are increased and cortisol levels are diminished. Treatment is lifelong replacement of missing adrenal cortical secretion with dexamethasone or prednisone.

DISORDERS OF PANCREATIC ENDOCRINE FUNCTION

The digestive function of the pancreas is discussed in Chapter 11. As mentioned earlier, the pancreas is an endocrine gland as well as an exocrine one (one that produces a secretion released through a duct). The endocrine function of the pancreas is performed by the islets of Langerhans, tiny aggregations of endocrine cells interspersed among the exocrine secretory elements.

The B or beta cells of the islets of Langerhans produce insulin, which increases glucose utilization and exerts other complex influences on the metabolism of carbohydrates, proteins, and fats. The A or alpha cells produce glucagon, an inhibitor of glucose activity, and the D or delta cells produce somatostatin, which inhibits secretion of growth hormone by the anterior pituitary.

Diabetes Mellitus (DM)

A disorder of metabolism in which body cells are unable to use glucose as fuel because of a deficiency of insulin. Two major types of diabetes are recognized.

Type 1 Diabetes Mellitus

Cause: A lack of insulin in the circulation due to failure of pancreatic B cells to respond to normal stimuli to insulin production. This type of diabetes shows a familial tendency. Failure of insulin production may be due to toxic, infectious, or autoimmune damage to B cells in genetically predisposed persons.

History: Polyuria (increased output of urine), polydipsia (excessive thirst), polyphagia (excessive appetite), weakness, and weight loss, coming on gradually or suddenly, usually in a person under 40 years of age. With fulminant onset, type 1 diabetes mellitus may present as ketoacidosis with dyspnea, drowsiness, collapse, and coma.

Physical Examination: Unremarkable in uncomplicated diabetes. In ketoacidosis: tachypnea, tachycardia, hypotension, flushing, fruity breath, and stupor or coma. Symptoms of cardiovascular, neurologic, or ocular complications may be evident in long-established or neglected disease.

Diagnostic Tests: Fasting blood sugar is over 140 mg/dL and 2-hour postprandial blood sugar is over 200 mg/dL. Sugar is present in the urine. Serum cholesterol is often elevated. In ketoacidosis, ketones are found in the serum and the urine, and there is chemical evidence of metabolic acidosis (low blood pH, low blood HCO_3^-). Glycosylated hemoglobin (Hb_{Alc}) reflects the average of blood sugar levels during the preceding 4-6 weeks and is used to monitor control. Laboratory studies may also show evidence of systemic complications (infection, renal disease).

Course: Type 1 diabetes is a lifelong derangement of carbohydrate metabolism. In most patients, careful attention to diet and general health and proper use of insulin permit good control of blood sugar and fair protection against complications. Diabetes predisposes to numerous other conditions, including hypercholesterolemia, atherosclerosis, ocular cataracts and retinopathy, renal disease, infections of the urinary tract, skin, and other tissues, neuropathy, and microvascular disease in the extremities.

Treatment: Type 1 diabetes mellitus is by definition a disease that must be treated with insulin as a condition of the patient's survival. The mainstay of treatment, however, is diet, with limitation of total calories and restriction of carbohydrate and cholesterol. Increased fiber helps to stabilize carbohydrate

metabolism, and artificial sweeteners are substituted for sugar. Injections of insulin are given one to four times a day. The patient monitors plasma glucose level by self-testing of fingerstick blood with a portable electronic meter. A variety of insulin products, including synthetic variants such as lispro and glargine insulins, are available with different patterns of absorption and peak activity. The proper management of diabetes requires scrupulous attention to general health, care of the skin and the feet, and vigorous treatment of complications. Regular eye examinations and periodic testing for microalbuminuria provide early detection of retinopathy and nephropathy respectively. Diabetic ketoacidosis is treated with intravenous fluids, insulin, and general supportive measures.

Type 2 Diabetes Mellitus

Cause: A relative deficiency of circulating insulin accompanied by insensitivity or resistance of tissues, particularly liver and muscle cells, to insulin effect. There is a genetic predisposition to this form of diabetes, but the mechanism of transmission is unknown. Type 2 diabetes accounts for 90% of all cases of diabetes mellitus. Most patients are over 40 and obese.

History: The condition may remain asymptomatic for months or years. Polyuria, polydipsia, and sometimes weakness or fatigue occur as in insulin-dependent disease, but weight loss and ketoacidosis do not occur.

Physical Examination: Unremarkable except for obesity, unless complications have developed. Hypertension is often present.

Diagnostic Tests: Fasting blood sugar over 140 mg/dL; 2-hour postprandial blood sugar over 180 mg/dL. There is sugar in the urine. Ketones are not found in serum. The cholesterol is often elevated. With advanced disease there may be chemical or electrocardiographic evidence of complications.

Course: Mild type 2 diabetes mellitus may cause few symptoms, particularly with treatment. Complications are the same as those for type 1 diabetes, with the exception of ketoacidosis. Complications typically do not develop as rapidly or become as severe as in type 1 diabetes.

Treatment: Dietary restriction of carbohydrate alone may suffice to control blood sugar levels and abolish symptoms of polyuria and fatigue. Cholesterol restriction is also advised. When diet does not control hyperglycemia, oral drugs (sulfonylureas, biguanides, other classes) are prescribed. Drugs such as pioglitazone and rosiglitazone help to overcome insulin resistance. Alpha-glucosidase inhibitors (acarbose, miglitol) impede absorption of dietary carbohydrate. To achieve optimal control, the use of insulin may be required. Care of general health and avoidance of skin injury and infection are important in the management of all forms of diabetes.

DISORDERS AFFECTING MORE THAN ONE ENDOCRINE GLAND

Multiple Endocrine Neoplasia (Multiple Endocrine Adenomatosis)

At least three genetically determined disorders have been identified in which benign or malignant neoplasms occur in two or more endocrine glands, particularly the parathyroid glands and pancreatic islets. Pancreatic tumors may produce insulin, gastrin, VIP (vasoactive intestinal polypeptide), or other hormonelike substances.

Polyglandular Deficiency Syndrome (Polyglandular Autoimmune Syndrome)

Any of several familial autoimmune disorders in which deficiencies in the hormonal products of two or more endocrine glands result from autoantibodies directed against the glands.

QUESTIONS FOR STUDY AND REVIEW

1. Give three examples of diseases caused by endocrine deficiency:

   a. _____

   b. _____

   c. _____

2. Give three examples of diseases caused by excessive hormone production:

   a. _____

   b. _____

   c. _____

3. Give two examples of endocrine disorders present (but not necessarily evident) at birth:

   a. _____

   b. _____

4. List five general types of substances that are essential in the human diet:

   a. _____

   b. _____

   c. _____

   d. _____

   e. _____

5. Define or explain these terms:

   a. Addison disease _____

   _____

   b. carbohydrate_____

   _____

   c. glucose_____

   _____

   d. goiter_____

   _____

   e. hormone_____

   _____

   f. insulin_____

   _____

g. metabolism_____

_____

h. thyrotoxicosis_____

_____

i. thyroxine _____

_____

j. vasopressin _____

_____

6. The pituitary gland is called the master gland because it controls other glands. List four endocrine glands whose function is regulated by the pituitary:

a. _____

b. _____

c. _____

d. _____

7. List four types of endocrine disorder that can result from pituitary disease:

a. _____

b. _____

c. _____

d. _____

8. Give some examples of feedback control between two hormones or the glands that produce them:

_____

_____

_____

_____

_____

_____

_____

CASE STUDY: YOU'RE THE DOCTOR

> Orpha Roudebush is a 44-year-old married white woman with type 2 diabetes mellitus who is referred to you by her family physician because of poor response to treatment.

1. What kind of background information would you like to have about Ms. Roudebush?

   _____

   _____

   _____

   _____

> She teaches music and art at an elementary school. Her past health history is generally unremarkable. She has a family history of overweight, diabetes mellitus, hypertension, and heart disease. She has never been pregnant. She quit smoking about 5 years ago. She admits to being a "foodaholic." For the past 5 months she has been following an 1800-calorie ADA diet and taking metformin, 500 mg twice daily. She is also taking pravastatin for moderately elevated cholesterol and triglycerides and lisinopril for moderate diastolic hypertension. She tests her blood sugar at least once on most days and finds it is "usually below 200 [mg/dL]." Her most recent glycated hemoglobin was 9.1%. Recent repeat lipid studies have shown some improvement, and liver and renal function tests and electrolytes have been normal. Ocular assessment by an ophthalmologist yielded normal findings. At the urging of her family physician she has tried to lose weight, but with little success.

2. What risk factors does Ms. Roudebush have for premature death due to cardiovascular disease?

   _____

   _____

   _____

   _____

3. Check all of the factors that may be contributing to her metabolic problems:

   ___ a. overeating

   ___ b. sedentary occupation

   ___ c. lack of will power

   ___ d. excess fat in diet

   ___ e. hypothyroidism

   ___ f. insulin resistance

   ___ g. failure of the pancreas to make insulin

   ___ h. occupational stress

4. Which of these factors do you think is at the root of most of her metabolic problems? Why?

_____

_____

_____

_____

> Ms. Roudebush is a pleasant, voluble, overweight woman appearing younger than her stated age. Her blood pressure is 140/88. Skin is warm, moist, and free of lesions. Head and body hair is of normal texture and distribution. Head, eyes, ears, nose, and throat are normal on examination. No cervical masses, thyromegaly, or carotid bruits are noted. The heart tones are regular at 78, with no murmurs, clicks, rubs, S3, or S4, and the lungs are clear to auscultation. No breast masses or tenderness is noted. No axillary lymph nodes are palpable. The abdomen is somewhat protuberant and some striae are noted over the iliac crests. No abdominal tenderness, guarding, organomegaly, masses, tympanites, or fluid wave is noted. Pelvic and rectal examinations and Pap smear have been performed within the past 8 months by her gynecologist and yielded normal results. The extremities show no tremor, edema, or cyanosis. Neurologic examination shows no abnormality of cranial nerves II through XII. Motor strength and sensation are normal and symmetrical in all extremities and no pathologic reflexes are noted.

5. What measures might you take to improve Ms. Roudebush's blood sugar control and general health?

_____

_____

_____

_____

> You counsel her about strict adherence to her diet and urge her to adopt a regular exercise program to help bring down her weight and improve blood pressure control. You remind her that rigorous control of blood pressure has been shown to reduce complications and mortality arising from diabetes mellitus. You increase her dose of metformin and add rosiglitazone to her regimen in order to improve tissue sensitivity to endogenous insulin.

6. Considering what you know so far about this patient, what do you think is the likelihood that she will comply with your treatment plan?

_____

_____

_____

_____

At her next visit 6 weeks later, Ms. Roudebush has lost 4 pounds and her blood pressure is 130/84. A fasting blood sugar is 124 mg/dL and glycated hemoglobin is 8.4%. She looks well. You encourage her to continue her regimen and ask her to return in another 6 to 8 weeks for re-examination and repeat glycated hemoglobin, lipid studies, and (because she is taking pravastatin and rosiglitazone) liver function studies.

7. Has your opinion of her chances for successful compliance changed? Why or why not?

_____

_____

_____

_____

She postpones her next visit twice because of vacations and a death in the family. When you next see her, she has gained 9 lb., her blood pressure is 151/93, a random blood sugar is 210 mg/dL, and glycated hemoglobin is 10.1% Lipid studies are also abnormal, but liver function is normal. She reports that she omitted her medicines for about 4 days because she forgot to take them with her when she went out of town for her husband's aunt's funeral about a month ago. She says she has been checking blood sugar regularly but has forgotten to bring in the record she has kept. As on her first visit, she says her sugar levels have been below 200 mg/dL.

8. What do you think has happened to Ms. Roudebush's diabetic control?

_____

_____

_____

_____

She says she finds it hard to exercise regularly because of lack of free time from occupational, family, and household obligations. But she insists that she has been following her diet conscientiously. As you discuss her condition further and suggest that she may need to take injections of insulin to enhance the effectiveness of her oral medicine, she becomes upset and tearful. Eventually she reveals that she has not been following her diet during recent weeks. A door-to-door salesman for a food club was so eager to sign her up for membership that he persuaded her that she could eat whatever she wanted and still maintain a normal blood sugar. All she had to do was visit a licensed reflexologist and zone therapist, who would correct her pancreatic physiology by massaging the soles of her feet for 20 minutes twice a week.

9. What do you do now?

_____

_____

_____

_____

SUGGESTIONS FOR ADDITIONAL LEARNING ACTIVITIES

1. Track everything you eat for a week and calculate daily totals for major nutrients, including protein, carbohydrates, fat, fiber, vitamins, and minerals, relying on the nutritional information required on food packaging and paying particular attention to _portions_ of foods. How well did you meet your needs? What changes do you need to make?

2. Play a learning game based on the old television show, "What's My Line?" A player chooses a disease or disorder described in this chapter and relies on this information to answer questions posed by a panel of contestants. Contestants take turns asking the player a single "yes" or "no" question in order to compile enough information to make a correct diagnosis and win the game. Example questions might include "Do you cause weight loss?" or "Could you lead to premature cardiovascular disease?" or "Would a T_4 level be elevated in your presence?"

3. Interview a registered dietitian or nutritionist. Ask questions about the training and/or credentialing necessary for this field, the kinds of nutritional or metabolic disorders encountered on the job, and the results this healthcare worker feels are achieved through his or her efforts. Prepare your questions in advance and, if your interview is conducted in person, make an audio recording to refer to later. Write a one page summary of this interview.

16

Disorders of Blood Cells, Blood-Forming Tissues, and Blood Coagulation

(Outline continued on next page)

LEARNING OBJECTIVES

Upon completion of this chapter, you should be able to

- describe the basic anatomy and physiology of the blood cells and lymphatic system;

- explain diagnostic procedures and treatments used in diseases of hemolymphatic disorders;

- classify common diseases of the blood cells and lymphatic system by their signs, symptoms, and treatment.

DISORDERS OF BLOOD CELLS, BLOOD-FORMING TISSUES, AND BLOOD COAGULATION

(continued)

DISEASES OF WHITE BLOOD CELLS

LEUKEMIA
Acute Lymphocytic Leukemia
(Acute Lymphoblastic Leukemia, ALL)
Chronic Myelogenous Leukemia (CML)
Chronic Lymphocytic Leukemia

LYMPHOMA
Hodgkin Disease
Non-Hodgkin Lymphoma
Multiple Myeloma

COAGULATION DISORDERS
Thrombocytopenia
Idiopathic Thrombocytopenic Purpura (ITP,
Immune Thrombocytic Purpura)
Glanzmann Disease (Thrombasthenia)
Hemophilia
Disseminated Intravascular Coagulation (DIC)

QUESTIONS FOR STUDY AND REVIEW

DISORDERS OF BLOOD CELLS, BLOOD-FORMING TISSUES, AND BLOOD COAGULATION

ANATOMY AND PHYSIOLOGY

The blood is an opaque, viscous fluid that can be classed as a tissue because of its complex structure and cellular components. Nearly half of the volume of the blood is made up of formed or cellular elements: red blood cells, white blood cells, and platelets. These are suspended in a fluid medium called plasma, whose chief component is water. Plasma carries electrolytes, proteins, nutrients, wastes, and dissolved gases. Among the proteins is fibrinogen, which under certain conditions is converted to fibrin, the insoluble material that is responsible for blood clotting. Plasma from which the fibrin has been removed is called serum.

Red blood cells (RBCs, erythrocytes) contain hemoglobin, a complex iron-containing protein that transports oxygen from the lungs to tissues and carbon dioxide from tissues to the lungs. On microscopic examination, red blood cells appear as flat, round, faintly pink disks with both faces concave. When seen on edge they thus have a dumbbell appearance.

Red blood cells are formed in bone marrow and released into the circulation as needed to maintain the normal red blood cell count. The process of red cell production is called erythropoiesis. It depends on adequate supplies of iron, protein, certain vitamins (especially folic acid and vitamin B_{12}), and a hormone produced in the kidney (erythropoietin). After about three months, a red blood cell disintegrates and is removed from the circulation in the spleen; the iron is recycled.

Mature red blood cells have no nuclei. The presence of many nucleated red blood cells in the circulation indicates increased production and release of red blood cells. The presence of reticulocytes (red blood cells containing fragments of nuclear material that can be detected by staining) has the same significance.

White blood cells (WBCs, leukocytes) differ from red blood cells in being somewhat larger and far less numerous, having nuclei, and lacking a reddish tinge. In addition, white blood cells are subdivided into several distinct categories on the basis of origin, form, and function.

White blood cells that arise and mature in bone marrow are called myeloid cells. They fall into two major groups: granulocytes (so called because they have stainable granules in their cytoplasm) and monocytes (so called because each has a solitary, non-lobed nucleus). Monocytes are phagocytes (cells that engulf and destroy dead tissue, bacteria, and other foreign material). Similar cells called histiocytes appear in various tissues and organs of the body (spleen, liver).

Granulocytes are also called polymorphonuclear leukocytes because their nuclei are characteristically divided into two to five lobes. These are further classified on the basis of the appearance of their granules after staining by a standard method (Wright or Giemsa stain) as eosinophils, with coarse reddish-orange granules; basophils, with dark blue to black granules; and neutrophils, with fainter granules that take up equal amounts of blue (basic) and red (acidic) stains. (See Figure 20.)

Eosinophils are phagocytes and function in allergic and other immune responses. Basophils contain histamine, heparin, and other active biochemical agents, which they release as appropriate. Neutrophils, the most numerous polymorphonuclear leukocytes and in fact the most numerous white blood cells, function primarily as phagocytes. Their numbers in the circulation rise soon after any injury or inflammatory process occurs, and they are transported by the blood to the site of trouble. Here they leave the circulation (squeezing through capillary walls by a process known as diapedesis) and enter the tissues to surround, engulf, and destroy devitalized tissue or invading microorganisms. Less mature neutrophils, whose nuclei are not divided into lobes, are called band cells or simply bands.

The only white blood cells not produced in the bone marrow are lymphocytes. These arise from precursor cells in the marrow but develop to maturity in lymphoid tissue (spleen, thymus gland, tonsils, lymph nodes). Their classification and functions are discussed in Chapter 4.

Platelets are not cells and have no nuclei. They are small round or oval bodies formed in bone marrow by cells called megakaryocytes. They function in blood coagulation. Coagulation is a complex process, in which, as a final stage of various possible reaction chains, soluble fibrinogen is converted by thrombin into insoluble fibrin. Thrombin also causes formation of plasmin, which breaks down fibrin. An intact coagulation mechanism depends

Figure 20 Composition of Blood

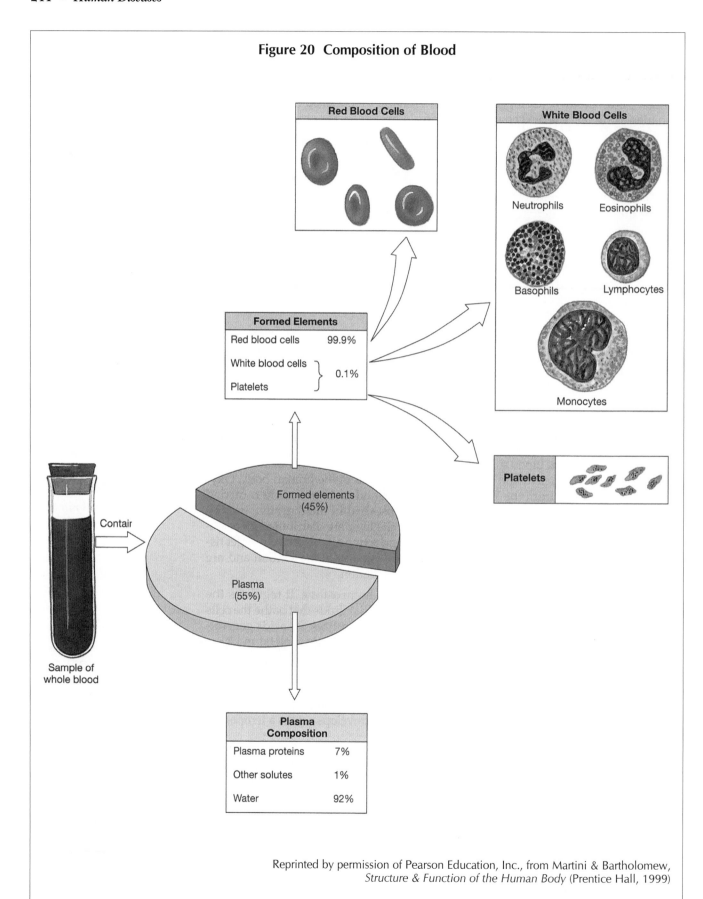

Reprinted by permission of Pearson Education, Inc., from Martini & Bartholomew,
Structure & Function of the Human Body (Prentice Hall, 1999)

on sufficient numbers of normally functioning platelets and on the presence in the plasma of adequate levels of a number of proteins, any of which can be congenitally deficient.

DIAGNOSTIC PROCEDURES IN HEMATOLOGIC DISEASE

Complete blood count (CBC): Enumeration and classification of formed elements in the blood, generally with electronic instruments rather than by visual inspection. The components of the complete blood count are as follows.

Red blood cell count (RBC): Enumeration of red blood cells in a standard volume of blood (reported as cells/mm^3 or cells/L).

Hemoglobin (Hb, Hgb): Measurement of concentration of hemoglobin in whole blood (reported in g/dL or mmol/L).

Hematocrit (Hct): Proportion of mass of cellular elements in blood to total blood volume, after centrifugation, reported as a decimal (if cell mass is 44% of total blood volume, the hematocrit is reported as 0.44); reflects chiefly red blood cell volume.

From these three values (RBC, Hb, Hct), three **red cell indices** are calculated as follows:

• Mean corpuscular hemoglobin (MCH): Hgb ÷ RBC; average weight of hemoglobin per red blood cell (reported as pg/cell).

• Mean corpuscular hemoglobin concentration (MCHC): Hgb ÷ Hct; average concentration of hemoglobin in red blood cells (reported as g/dL or g/L).

• Mean corpuscular volume (MCV): Hct ÷ RBC; average size of red blood cells (reported in μm^3 or fL).

White blood cell count (WBC): Enumeration of white blood cells in a standard volume of blood (reported as cells/mm^3 or cells/L). A count of 7000/mm^3 would be reported in SI units as 7 x 10^9/L.

Platelet count (Plt): Enumeration of platelets in a standard volume of blood (reported as platelets/ mm^3 or /L).

Stained smear of peripheral blood: This examination allows a detailed inspection of all formed elements, with an estimate of their size, shape, staining properties, maturity, and other structural features, and identification of abnormal cells or immature forms not normally found in peripheral blood.

Differential count of white blood cells: Determination of the relative proportions of the six principal white blood cells (mature neutrophils, band neutrophils, eosinophils, basophils, lymphocytes, and monocytes). This examination can be performed either by visually inspecting a stained smear of blood and counting 100 cells, or by sophisticated electronic equipment. Proportions are reported as percents (lymphocytes 30%) but may also be given as integers without units (lymphocytes 30). Multiplying the relative count of a particular cell type by the total number of white blood cells in the specimen yields the absolute count of that cell type. If lymphocytes make up 30% of all white blood cells, and the total white blood cell count is 7000/mm^3 (7 x 10^9/L), then the absolute lymphocyte count is 2100 x 10^6/L.

Bone marrow biopsy: An examination of bone marrow removed by aspiration from the sternum or iliac crest. The marrow may be smeared and stained like whole blood, or it may be compacted, embedded in wax, and sectioned before staining like a specimen of solid tissue.

Erythrocyte sedimentation rate (ESR) (sed rate): Determination of the rate at which erythrocytes settle in a specimen of anticoagulated blood standing in a glass column of standard dimensions. Principally an index of inflammation, which accelerates sedimentation of cells by leading to production of acute phase reactants (serum proteins generated as part of the inflammatory process).

Reticulocyte count: Enumeration of reticulocytes (immature red blood cells) as an estimate of red blood cell production.

Serum iron, serum iron-binding capacity, serum ferritin: These are all measures of the iron available for erythropoiesis. Ferritin is the plasma protein that carries iron in bound form.

Osmotic fragility test: Determination of the osmotic concentration of a solution of saline that will cause hemolysis of red blood cells; altered in conditions affecting the chemical or physical structure of cells.

Hemoglobin electrophoresis: Analysis of the various hemoglobins, normal and abnormal, found in the patient's blood.

Sickling test: Application of chemicals that cause sickling of red blood cells from persons with sickle cell anemia or sickle cell trait.

Carboxyhemoglobin: A measure of the percent of hemoglobin that has formed carboxyhemoglobin with inhaled carbon monoxide.

Assays of serum B$_{12}$ and folate: To determine adequacy of these vitamins for RBC production.

Serum indirect-reacting bilirubin: A measure of the formation of bilirubin by breakdown of RBCs.

Clotting time: The time in which a specimen of blood clots under standard conditions.

Prothrombin time: A measure of prothrombin activity; the standard test to monitor therapy with the oral anticoagulant warfarin.

Activated partial thromboplastin time: A specialized coagulation test to identify deficient clotting factors; the standard test to monitor therapy with the intravenous or intramuscular anticoagulant heparin.

Coagulation factor assay: Chemical or immunologic tests to measure concentrations of various coagulation factors in the blood.

DISORDERS OF RED BLOOD CELLS

ANEMIA

Anemia, a reduction in the number of red blood cells in the circulation, can be due to deficient production of red blood cells, their destruction within the body (hemolysis), or their loss through hemorrhage.

ANEMIA DUE TO DEFICIENT OR ABNORMAL PRODUCTION OF RED BLOOD CELLS

Iron Deficiency Anemia

Anemia due to deficient iron stores; the most common type of anemia.

Cause: Depletion of iron stores usually results from chronic or recurring blood loss (gastrointestinal hemorrhage, menstruation, repeated blood donation). It can also occur in certain metabolic states (pregnancy, chronic infection) and, rarely, because of inadequate iron intake (vegetarians, dieters).

History: Fatigue, poor exercise tolerance, cardiac palpitation, shortness of breath. Dysphagia occurs in Plummer-Vinson syndrome (due to formation of esophageal webs). Pica (eating non-food materials such as clay).

Physical Examination: Pallor, tachycardia, smooth tongue, brittle nails, cheilosis (chapping and fissuring of lips).

Diagnostic Tests: The red blood cell count is abnormally low. With advanced disease, cells become microcytic (smaller than normal; MCV reduced) and hypochromic (containing less hemoglobin than normal; MCH reduced). Abnormal cells, including target cells (cells so thin that the central portions of opposite sides touch, causing a bull's-eye appearance), may occur. The serum iron and serum ferritin are abnormally low. Administration of iron produces a prompt improvement in the red blood cell count, with elevated reticulocyte count. Diagnostic evaluation may include an aggressive search for a site of blood loss.

Treatment: Oral iron replacement continued for several months restores the red blood cell values and serum iron and ferritin to normal.

Pernicious Anemia

A chronic anemia due to deficiency of vitamin B$_{12}$ absorption.

Cause: Pernicious anemia is an inherited autoimmune disorder that typically does not cause symptoms until after the age of 35. The biochemical cause is lack of secretion of intrinsic factor by glands in the gastric mucosa, with resultant failure to absorb vitamin B$_{12}$. All patients have gastric achlorhydria (lack of hydrochloric acid in gastric juice). Neurologic symptoms (ataxia, confusion, dementia) eventually occur.

History: Gradual onset of weakness, paresthesia in the fingers and toes, dysequilibrium, anorexia, sore tongue, and diarrhea.

Physical Examination: Pallor, icterus. The tongue appears red and smooth. Ataxic gait, diminished sense of vibration and position in extremities; later, loss of perception of light touch and pinprick.

Diagnostic Tests: The red blood cell count is low. Red blood cells are large (macrocytosis; increased MCV) and variable in size (anisocytosis). The reticulocyte count is low. Polymorphonuclear leukocytes have multilobulated nuclei. Bone marrow smear shows large precursors of red blood cells with abnormal morphology. The serum indirect bilirubin is elevated. The serum vitamin B_{12} is abnormally low. The Schilling test (administration of radioactively tagged B_{12} orally before and after administration of intrinsic factor) shows an increase in the urinary excretion of B_{12}. Endoscopy shows atrophic gastritis, and chemical studies indicate achlorhydria.

Course: This is an irreversible condition requiring lifelong treatment, without which neurologic damage may become irreversible. There is a heightened risk of gastric carcinoma in persons with achlorhydria.

Treatment: Administration of vitamin B_{12} regularly throughout life.

Aplastic Anemia

Failure of marrow production of red blood cells (also white blood cells and platelets).

Cause: Damage to bone marrow by chemicals (benzene), drugs (chloramphenicol), radiation, neoplastic infiltration, or autoantibodies.

History: Gradual onset of weakness, fatigue, dyspnea, headache.

Physical Examination: Pallor, purpura or petechiae, tachycardia, oral or pharyngeal infection or ulceration.

Diagnostic Tests: The red blood cell, white blood cell, and platelet counts are abnormally low. Marrow smear shows hypoplastic or acellular marrow.

Treatment: Blood transfusion to correct anemia. Oxygen and control of hemorrhage as needed. Antibiotics for infection. Corticosteroids, immunosuppressive agents, colony stimulating factors. Marrow transplantation if possible.

HEMOLYTIC ANEMIA

Anemia due to abnormal destruction of red blood cells. Hereditary hemolytic anemias are due to genetically induced abnormalities in the structure of the red blood cell (spherocytosis, elliptocytosis, sickle cell disease) or sensitivity to certain biochemical challenges (glucose-6-phosphate dehydrogenase deficiency).

Sickle Cell Anemia

A congenital abnormality of red blood cells causing hemolytic anemia and other adverse effects.

Cause: An autosomal recessive gene, present in 8% of African-Americans, results in formation of variable amounts of an abnormal hemoglobin (hemoglobin S). Persons with the homozygous form (abnormal gene inherited from both parents) have significant numbers of abnormal red blood cells, which are subject to sickling (assumption of a sickle-shaped distortion), with a tendency to hemolysis and formation of arterial obstructions, in the presence of reduced arterial oxygen, acidosis, or other biochemical alterations in blood. Persons with the heterozygous form are said to have sickle cell trait; they rarely or never have symptoms.

History: Weakness, poor exercise tolerance, jaundice, ulcers of the shins, susceptibility to infections, hemolytic crises (acute episodes of bone pain in extremities and back).

Physical Examination: Jaundice, hepatomegaly, splenomegaly, cardiomegaly.

Diagnostic Tests: The red blood cell count is abnormally low and the bilirubin is elevated. The blood smear shows reticulocytes, nucleated red blood cells, target cells, and sickled cells. Laboratory screening for sickling is positive, and hemoglobin electrophoresis shows the presence of hemoglobin S. Persons with sickle cell trait have smaller amounts of hemoglobin S on electrophoresis, and their blood counts and smears are normal. Prenatal diagnosis can be made by studying fetal DNA.

Course: Complications include ischemic necrosis of bone, osteomyelitis due to *Staphylococcus* or *Salmonella*, splenic and renal infarction, increased risk of infection, retinopathy with visual loss, formation of bilirubin gallstones.

Treatment: Largely supportive, with avoidance of precipitating factors. For hemolytic crisis, oxygen inhalation and blood transfusion.

Glucose-6-Phosphate Dehydrogenase (G-6-PD) Deficiency

An inherited deficiency of the enzyme glucose-6-phosphate dehydrogenase, which causes episodes of hemolytic anemia in response to infection or on exposure to certain drugs or foods.

Cause: Absence of glucose-6-phosphate dehydrogenase from red blood cells. An X-linked recessive disorder seen primarily in males of African, Mediterranean, or Asian ancestry. Occurs in 10-15% of African-American men.

History: Jaundice at birth. In later life, susceptibility to episodes of hemolysis (manifested by weakness, jaundice, and dark urine) during infections or after eating fava beans or taking certain drugs (quinidine, quinine, nitrofurantoin, sulfonamides, phenazopyridine, and others).

Physical Examination: During hemolytic episodes: pallor, jaundice, possibly evidence of congestive heart failure. At other times, no physical findings.

Diagnostic Tests: During hemolytic episodes: anemia, reticulocytosis, abnormally shaped red blood cells on smear. Elevation of indirect bilirubin. At other times: no hematologic abnormalities, but deficiency of G-6-PD in red blood cells.

Course: Hemolytic episodes occur during infections or after consumption of certain drugs and foods, and sometimes spontaneously. They are rarely severe or life-threatening.

Treatment: Avoidance of drugs known to induce hemolysis, and fava beans. Prompt treatment of severe or systemic infection.

Acquired Hemolytic Anemia

Causes: Acquired hemolytic anemias result from formation of antibody to one's own red blood cells in certain systemic diseases (lupus erythematosus, leukemia, lymphoma), in response to certain drugs (methyldopa, quinidine), or for unknown reasons (50%).

History: Gradual or abrupt onset of fatigue and dyspnea due to anemia. There may be a family history of hemolytic anemia.

Physical Examination: Pallor, jaundice, splenomegaly.

Diagnostic Tests: The red blood cell count is low, the reticulocyte count elevated. Indirect bilirubin is elevated in serum. The direct Coombs test is positive, indicating sensitization of the patient's red blood cells. The indirect Coombs test may also be positive, indicating presence of anti-RBC antibody in serum.

Treatment: If anemia is severe, blood transfusion may be indicated. Corticosteroid treatment may block hemolysis. In severe or refractory cases, splenectomy, immunosuppressive agents, and immune globulin are often beneficial.

Erythroblastosis Fetalis (Hemolytic Disease of the Newborn)

Hemolytic anemia affecting a newborn, due to destruction of fetal red blood cells by antibodies formed by the mother's immune system.

Cause: The child's red blood cells contain some antigen not found in the mother's red blood cells. If fetal and maternal blood become mixed (as in ante-

natal trauma, amniocentesis, or chorionic villus biopsy), the maternal immune system may form antibody to this antigen, which then enters the fetal circulation and causes hemolysis. Mixing of blood during delivery stimulates maternal antibody that cannot affect the child just born, but will affect any future fetuses having the same red cell antigen.

The usual cause of severe erythroblastosis is presence of the D antigen of the Rh system in the red blood cells of a fetus borne by an Rh-negative mother. Milder degrees of hemolysis occur with other red blood cell incompatibilities, including those in the ABO system. The mother is unaffected in hemolytic disease of the newborn. The incidence of the disorder has been much reduced by the administration to Rh-negative mothers of high-titer Rh_O (D) immune globulin during each pregnancy and immediately after delivery.

History: Jaundice becoming evident within hours of birth. Pallor, generalized swelling, lethargy, poor feeding, spasms.

Physical Examination: Jaundice, pallor (often masked by jaundice), anasarca (generalized edema), pleural effusion, ascites (fluid in the abdominal cavity), enlargement of liver and spleen, cardiac murmurs, lethargy, spasticity, hyperactive reflexes, cardiac or pulmonary failure.

Diagnostic Tests: The red blood cell count is low and the unconjugated (indirect-reacting) bilirubin is high. Blood glucose may be depressed. Increased numbers of nucleated red blood cells and reticulocytes are found in the circulation. The direct Coombs test shows the red blood cells of the newborn to be coated with hemolytic antibody. The indirect Coombs test on the mother's blood confirms that she has formed antibody to fetal red cell antigen.

Course: Very mild cases may resolve spontaneously, but even with treatment a child showing profound jaundice and lethargy in the first 24 hours may die. Stillbirths are not uncommon. Anemia may correct itself over a few days once further exposure to maternal antibody ceases. However, severe anemia may lead to cardiac failure or death. A more severe threat is marked elevation of bilirubin, which is toxic in the newborn to the basal ganglia of the brain. Deposition of unconjugated bilirubin in the nerve tissue of the basal ganglia, called kernicterus, produces spasticity and unless quickly treated and reversed may lead to a parkinson-like movement disorder and often mental retardation and deafness.

Treatment: Exchange transfusion (replacement of fetal blood, a little at a time, with donor blood lacking harmful antigen) may be needed if anemia is profound or hyperbilirubinemia very high. Respiratory and cardiac function may require support.

Polycythemia Vera

A myeloproliferative disorder in which the red blood cell count is abnormally high.

Cause: A clonal stem cell disorder leading to increase in all cellular elements of bone marrow and peripheral blood, most conspicuously erythrocytes but to a lesser degree granulocytic leukocytes and platelets. Onset is usually between 50 and 60 years of age.

History: Headaches, dizziness, tinnitus, visual blurring, fullness in the epigastrium, redness of skin, pruritus (worse after a hot bath).

Physical Examination: Reddish-purple skin and mucous membranes. Hypertension, splenomegaly, hepatomegaly.

Diagnostic Tests: Red blood cell count, hemoglobin, and hematocrit are increased, as well as white blood cell and platelet counts. Serum iron and ferritin are reduced. Marrow biopsy shows increased cellularity.

Course: Average survival time is 10-12 years. Arterial and venous thromboses, hemorrhage, and infection are common complications. As the disease progresses, the marrow cells become replaced by fibrous tissue, and zones of extramedullary hematopoiesis (formation of red blood cells elsewhere than in the marrow) develop in the spleen and liver. Secondary gout may develop as a result of rapid DNA turnover with excessive uric acid production. Many cases evolve into a terminal acute leukemia-like blast stage.

Treatment: Phlebotomy to reduce blood volume and red blood cell count. Radioactive phosphorus, busulfan, chlorambucil, hydroxyurea.

DISEASES OF WHITE BLOOD CELLS

LEUKEMIA

Any of several disorders characterized by increased white blood cell count and the appearance of immature and abnormal white blood cells in the circulation. Leukemias result from genetic abnor-

mality of stem cells in the bone marrow, due either to mutation of cells or to chromosomal aberrations occurring before conception. As a consequence, the body produces increased amounts of one or more types of blood cells (erythrocytes, granulocytes, monocytes, lymphocytes, platelets), which are abnormal in structure and function. Leukemias vary broadly in clinical features and course. Three common types are discussed here.

Acute Lymphocytic Leukemia (Acute Lymphoblastic Leukemia, ALL)

A rapidly progressive hematologic malignancy of children.

Cause: Mutation of lymphocyte precursor cells, possibly due to drugs, radiation, or genetic predisposition or chromosomal aberration. Onset is in childhood, usually before age 5.

History: Pallor, weakness, irritability, repeated infections, bleeding tendency, bone pain, headache, stiff neck, vomiting, cranial nerve palsies and other neurologic abnormalities.

Physical Examination: Pallor, lethargy, neurologic findings, evidence of opportunistic infections, hemorrhagic phenomena.

Diagnostic Tests: The white blood cell count may be low, elevated, or normal. Anemia and thrombocytopenia are often present. Serum levels of uric acid and creatinine may be elevated. Bone marrow examination shows replacement of normal elements by infiltrations of blast cells. Cerebrospinal fluid shows lymphoblasts (extremely immature lymphocytes) in central nervous system involvement. Imaging studies including radionuclide bone scans may show abnormalities due to infiltration of organs or tissues by malignant lymphoblastic cells.

Course: The disease is ordinarily fatal in less than six months. With vigorous treatment, many patients achieve long-term survival and apparent cure. Anemia, thrombocytopenia, susceptibility to infection, invasion of the central nervous system (50%), and infiltration and damage of the liver and other organs often prove lethal.

Treatment: Chemotherapy with vincristine, daunorubicin, or asparaginase, combined with corticosteroid. For central nervous system involvement, cranial irradiation and injection of methotrexate intrathecally (into the subarachnoid space). Control of anemia (transfusions if necessary), bleeding, and infection; personal and family counseling.

Chronic Myelogenous Leukemia (CML)

A malignancy of the marrow characterized by markedly elevated levels of circulating white blood cells formed there, with immature and abnormal cells.

Cause: The Philadelphia chromosome, the first oncogene to be associated with a specific malignancy; this is a reciprocal translocation of strands of genes between chromosomes 9 and 22. It results in malignant proliferation of myelogenous (marrow-produced) white blood cells (granulocytes and monocytes), which, however, retain their functions for years, until the disease reaches its terminal stage. Onset generally occurs in middle life (30s, 40s, and 50s).

History: Weakness, fatigue, fever, night sweats, bone pain.

Physical Examination: Low fever, enlargement of the spleen, tenderness over the sternum due to hyperactive marrow.

Laboratory Tests: Marked elevation of the white blood cell count (100,000-500,000/μL), with modest increases in immature forms. Other cells in the circulation are generally normal in number and form. The uric acid may be elevated. Marrow smear shows increased cellularity and increased immature white blood cells. Chromosomal studies identify the Philadelphia chromosome.

Course: Usual survival is less than 5 years. However, long-term survival, and apparent cure, occur in half of patients who undergo successful bone marrow transplantation. The disease typically ends in a phase of greatly accelerated production of wholly immature and undifferentiated stem cells (blastic crisis), in which marrow dysfunction can lead to marked anemia, bleeding disorders, and toxemia.

Treatment: Largely supportive and palliative. Chemical suppressants of marrow activity (hydroxyurea, interferon alfa) lower white blood cell counts and mitigate symptoms. In the blast stage, chemotherapy protocols including vincristine, daunorubicin, and prednisone provide brief remission. Allogeneic bone marrow transplant (from a sibling or unrelated donor matched with respect to critical antigens, particularly HLA) is apparently curative in about one-half of patients, and is more likely to be effective in younger patients.

Chronic Lymphocytic Leukemia

A malignancy of B lymphocytes.

Cause: Malignant change in a B-cell precursor, with formation of a clone of abnormal, immunologically incompetent cells. This results in infiltration of bone marrow and other tissues with abnormal lymphocytes and failure of immune response. Most cases occur in the middle-aged and elderly.

History: Gradual onset of weakness and fatigue, often with enlarged lymph nodes. In some asymptomatic patients the condition is discovered incidentally on routine blood testing.

Physical Examination: Enlargement of lymph nodes, liver, spleen, or all of these. Pallor or jaundice may be present.

Diagnostic Tests: Relative and absolute lymphocytosis (increase in the percentage of lymphocytes among white blood cells, and in their total number). The lymphocytes are small but normal in appearance. Bone marrow may show infiltrations of lymphocytes. Red blood cell or platelet count may be reduced. There may be a deficiency of IgG in serum.

Course: Typically chronic, with mild or absent symptoms. Most patients survive 5-10 years after diagnosis. Possible complications include autoimmune hemolytic anemia, thrombocytopenia, and lymphoma (development of a malignant solid neoplasm of lymphoid tissue).

Treatment: Largely supportive and palliative. Chlorambucil, fludarabine, and adrenal corticosteroids may be used in severe or terminal disease. Splenectomy may be needed to control hemolytic anemia.

LYMPHOMA

A malignant tumor consisting of lymphocytes. Several types are recognized.

Hodgkin Disease

Cause: Unknown. Genetic influences and viral infection have been implicated, but without conclusive proof.

History: Painless enlargement of one or more lymph nodes, fever, sweats, pruritus, abdominal pain (aggravated by alcohol).

Physical Examination: Enlargement of lymph nodes, possibly spleen; fever.

Diagnostic Tests: Lymph node biopsy shows Reed-Sternberg cells (characteristic large cells with two nuclei).

Prognosis: The overall survival rate is about 50%; with early diagnosis and treatment, about 80%.

Treatment: Radiation, chemotherapy.

Non-Hodgkin Lymphoma

A variegated group of lymphocyte malignancies. Oncogenes have been identified for some types.

History: Painless enlargement of lymph nodes, fever, sweats, weight loss, abdominal pain.

Physical Examination: Enlargement of lymph nodes, spleen.

Diagnostic Tests: The peripheral blood may be normal. Lymph node biopsy shows characteristic malignant changes, and bone marrow biopsy shows infiltration of abnormal lymphoid aggregates. The serum LDH is elevated. Chest x-ray and CT scan of the abdomen and pelvis may show hilar and abdominal or pelvic lymphadenopathy.

Treatment: Radiation, chemotherapy, bone marrow transplantation.

Multiple Myeloma

A malignant tumor of plasma cells.

History: Bone pain, usually in the back or ribs. Onset is usually in later life.

Physical Examination: Pallor, bone tenderness, neurologic abnormalities.

Diagnostic Tests: The red blood cell count is low, the erythrocyte sedimentation rate elevated. The serum calcium level is elevated. Serum protein electrophoresis shows abnormal proteins, and Bence Jones protein appears in urine. Marrow biopsy shows infiltration of abnormal plasma cells. X-rays show lytic lesions in ribs, spine, other bones.

Complications: Renal failure, amyloidosis, cardiomegaly, neurologic impairment.

Prognosis: Average survival is about 3 years.

Treatment: Radiation, chemotherapy, marrow transplant.

COAGULATION DISORDERS

Numerous disorders of blood coagulation have been identified, some acquired but the majority inherited. They fall into three categories: disorders of platelets, abnormalities of platelet function, and disorders of clotting factors. A major distinction among coagulation disorders is between platelet disorders and deficiencies of one or more plasma coagulation proteins.

Thrombocytopenia

Deficiency of platelets in the circulation, which can result from diminished production, accelerated destruction, or sequestration in the spleen.

Idiopathic Thrombocytopenic Purpura (ITP, Immune Thrombocytic Purpura)

An acquired hemorrhagic disorder due to autoimmune destruction of platelets.

Cause: Antiplatelet antibody formed in response to acute viral infection (acute ITP) or other factors (chronic ITP). Acute ITP occurs chiefly in children between 2 and 6 who are recovering from a viral illness such as varicella or infectious mononucleosis. Chronic ITP is a disease of adults affecting more women than men by a ratio of 4:1.

History: Acute: Sudden onset of easy bruising, nosebleeds, blood in urine or stool. Chronic: Insidious onset of bruising, heavy menstrual flow, and spontaneous bleeding from mucosal surfaces (epistaxis, hematemesis, hematochezia or melena, hematuria).

Physical Findings: Petechiae, purpura, ecchymoses; frank or occult blood in sputum, urine, stool. Blood blisters in the mouth.

Diagnostic Tests: Marked lowering of the platelet count in peripheral blood. Prolonged bleeding time and abnormal clot retraction. Bone marrow shows normal to hyperactive platelet production. Serologic studies show antibody bound to platelets.

Course: In acute ITP, spontaneous return of platelet count to normal usually occurs within 6 months. In chronic disease the course tends to be protracted. Severe hemorrhage and anemia due to chronic blood loss are unusual, but can occur. The most dangerous kind of hemorrhage is intracranial.

Treatment: Acute ITP requires mainly support, observation, and treatment of severe complications. In chronic ITP, splenectomy and therapy with corticosteroids or other immunosuppressive agents are usually required.

Glanzmann Disease (Thrombasthenia)

An inherited coagulation disorder (autosomal recessive) in which platelets occur in normal numbers, but do not function normally because of deficiency or absence of platelet membrane glycoprotein. The condition is more common in persons of Semitic or Indian origin. Symptoms are the same as for thrombocytopenia: bruising, epistaxis, menorrhagia, and other spontaneous mucosal bleeding. Laboratory studies show normal numbers of platelets in the circulation, but tests of platelet function (clot retraction, observation for adhesion and aggregation) yield abnormal results. Treatment is with platelet transfusions and oral iron supplementation. Allogeneic bone marrow transplant is sometimes successful.

Hemophilia

A hereditary clotting disorder leading to spontaneous hemorrhages.

Cause: Very low levels of coagulation factor VIII (antihemophilic globulin, AHG), due to an X-linked recessive genetic defect. Males are affected almost exclusively, but genetic transmission is by female carriers. Approximately one male in 10,000 is affected.

History: Abnormal bleeding in response to mild trauma, or even spontaneously: hemarthrosis (bleeding into joints), gastrointestinal bleeding, and excessive bleeding after surgery or dental extractions or from open wounds occur most commonly. Aspirin aggravates the bleeding tendency.

Physical Examination: Pallor and tachycardia (after recent hemorrhage). Evidence of local hemorrhage into joints or muscles or subcutaneously, or from skin wounds or surgical sites.

Diagnostic Tests: Anemia and reticulocytosis after hemorrhage. The partial thromboplastin time (PTT) is prolonged, but other standard tests for coagulation defects (platelet count, prothrombin time, fibrinogen level) yield normal results. The plasma level of factor VIII is low, typically less than 5% of normal.

Course: With careful avoidance of trauma and aspirin, and infusions of factor VIII as needed, most patients can lead essentially normal lives. Recurrent hemarthroses may lead to permanent damage to joints. Administration of some blood products can result in transmission of infections such as AIDS and hepatitis B and C. Some patients form antibody to

factor VIII and so fail to derive benefit from infusions of it.

Treatment: Modification of lifestyle so as to reduce the danger of trauma. Avoidance of aspirin. Treatment of severe bleeding and suspicion of bleeding (as in closed head injury) with infusions of factor VIII concentrate. Aminocaproic acid may be used when the response to factor VIII is inadequate. Preoperative administration of desmopressin acetate, which temporarily boosts factor VIII levels.

Disseminated Intravascular Coagulation (DIC)

A disorder of coagulation characterized by both formation of thrombi diffusely in the circulation and a bleeding tendency.

Cause: Excessive thrombin in the circulation, which causes widespread formation of small thrombi; the resulting consumption of fibrinogen and platelets leads to a bleeding tendency; in some cases cleavage of fibrin in clots by plasmin aggravates bleeding. This disorder can be triggered by a variety of factors: severe injury (particularly burns), complications of pregnancy and childbirth (amniotic fluid embolism, puerperal infection), septicemia, malignant disease, and transfusion reaction.

History: Abnormal bleeding, especially from surgical incisions or venipuncture sites. Thrombi may cause ischemia, manifested by gangrene of extremities or signs of renal or adrenal infarction.

Physical Examination: Findings depend on the underlying disorder and the severity and location of thrombosis and hemorrhage.

Diagnostic Tests: Blood studies show depletion of fibrinogen and platelets and prolonged prothrombin time. The blood also contains fibrin degradation products, most significantly D-dimer, which is not found in unaltered fibrinogen. Hemolytic anemia may be present.

Treatment: Management of DIC begins with identification and treatment of the underlying cause, if possible. Fibrinogen and platelets are replaced by intravenous infusion. In addition, heparin may be used to block further thrombin activity, with or without aminocaproic acid to block breakdown of fibrin.

QUESTIONS FOR STUDY AND REVIEW

1. List three hematologic disorders that are genetically induced:

   a. _____

   b. _____

   c. _____

2. List three hematologic disorders that are acquired:

   a. _____

   b. _____

   c. _____

3. List three hematologic disorders that are invariably fatal:

   a. _____

   b. _____

   c. _____

4. Which formed elements of the blood have no nuclei?

   _____

   _____

   _____

   _____

   _____

5. Define or explain these terms:

   a. Bence Jones protein _____

   _____

   b. hemolysis _____

   _____

   c. lymphoblast _____

   _____

   d. Philadelphia chromosome_____

   _____

   e. reticulocyte _____

   _____

   f. thrombocytopenia_____

   _____

6. Which hematologic disorders are treated with splenectomy? Why?

_____

_____

_____

_____

7. Which disorders are sometimes helped by bone marrow transplants?

_____

_____

_____

_____

8. During the 1980s, the mortality of hemophilia among children drastically increased. Why? How was this trend reversed?

_____

_____

_____

_____

_____

_____

_____

_____

CASE STUDY: YOU'RE THE DOCTOR

Beryl Anderton is a 20-year-old exchange student from England. She is brought to your office by Megan Winant, who is one of your regular patients and the mother of the local college student with whom Beryl is rooming during her year in this country. When Ms. Winant phoned the office to make the appointment, she spoke briefly with you to tell you that she was concerned that Beryl might have an eating disorder. The ostensible reason for the visit, however, is recurrent abdominal pain and constipation.

1. How likely do you think it is that Ms. Winant has made a correct diagnosis? How did you come to this conclusion?

_____

_____

_____

_____

_____

2. Will you want Ms. Winant to be present in the room when you interview the patient? Why or why not?

_____

_____

_____

_____

Ms. Anderton is a pleasant, vivacious young woman who makes light of her digestive complaints. She states she is just having difficulty in getting used to American cooking. She describes intermittent periumbilical cramping, excess "wind," and hard stools despite taking over-the-counter laxatives almost daily. She denies nausea, vomiting, sensitivity to particular foods, hematochezia, fever, and weight loss. She does not drink or smoke and takes no medicines. She is a vegetarian. She is not sexually active. Her mother died in an automobile accident when she was 4 and her father, a real estate agent and member of Parliament, is remarried. She feels her mental and physical health are very good. She plans a career in chemical engineering. She runs or swims and works out every day, frequently running 10 or more miles at a stretch. She denies headaches, sleep problems, anxiety, depression, and menstrual irregularity. However, she is vague about the date of her last menstrual period.

3. How do you feel now about the likelihood that Ms. Anderton has an eating disorder? Justify your opinion.

_____

_____

_____

_____

The patient is wearing a loose, baggy sweater and jeans. She declines to remove these completely for examination, but it is evident that under the flapping garments she is extremely thin. Vital signs are normal except for a resting pulse of 54, perhaps normal in a high-performance athlete. Her weight is 92% of her normal weight-for-height. The skin is pale and dry; hair is of normal texture. Head, eyes, ears, nose, and throat are normal. There are no cervical masses and the thyroid is not enlarged. The heart tones are normal, with no murmurs, clicks, or gallop rhythm. Lungs are clear. The abdomen is scaphoid and the lower ribs and iliac crests stand out prominently under the stretched skin. The abdomen shows no surgical scars or striae. On palpation you note no tenderness, guarding, masses, organomegaly, or tympanites, but the patient is so thin that you can feel stool in the sigmoid colon. Bowel sounds are diminished to normal. Rectal examination reveals no pelvic abnormalities but the rectal pouch contains a mass of very hard brown stool, which is negative for occult blood. She declines a pelvic examination.

4. Rank these diagnostic possibilities from 1 to 4, where 1 is the most likely diagnosis and 4 is least likely.

___ thyroiditis

___ carcinoma of the colon

___ pregnancy

___ anorexia nervosa

You advise her that your examination discloses no evidence of serious illness, but that you believe some basic laboratory tests should be done. You prescribe a stool softener and order a complete blood count, chemistry profile, thyroid stimulating hormone level, and urinalysis. These studies are all normal except for the CBC, which shows a microcytic, hypochromic anemia: erythrocyte count 3.9 million/mm^3 (normal 4.2–5.4), hematocrit 30% (normal 37-47), MCV 77 μm^3 (normal 80-96). She denies any recent blood loss or family history of anemia.

5. What is your differential diagnosis at this point?

_____

_____

_____

_____

You make a diagnosis of iron-deficiency anemia, perhaps related to her vegetarian diet. You also advise her that her body weight is considerably lower than it should be and you advise her to increase her caloric intake and perhaps reduce her exercise level. You point out that she is at risk of various physiologic imbalances, including osteoporosis, if she becomes amenorrheic as a result of weight restriction and exercise. You prescribe ferrous sulfate orally and ask her to return in 3 months for re-evaluation.

When next seen she has gained 4^1/$_2$ pounds and admits she feels somewhat better. Her constipation has improved somewhat with the stool softener but she has more flatulence than ever. She had a normal menstrual period about 3 weeks ago. She has been taking ferrous sulfate religiously. Repeat laboratory studies show an erythrocyte count of 4.8 million/mm^3, hematocrit 33%, MCV unchanged at 77.

6. Do you think she has anorexia nervosa? Explain your answer.

_____

_____

_____

_____

_____

7. Why do you suppose she still has a microcytosis and hypochromasia, or do you suspect a laboratory error? What will you do now?

_____

_____

_____

_____

_____

You order additional laboratory studies: serum ferritin, serum iron and iron binding capacity, and reticulocyte count. These all yield normal results. A stained blood smear shows some basophilic stippling of erythrocytes and a few target cells.

8. What is your interpretation of this result?

_____

_____

_____

_____

9. Do you believe she has been taking her iron as regularly as she says? Why or why not?

_____

_____

_____

_____

10. What further investigations are in order?

_____

_____

_____

_____

You ask what her mother's maiden name was, and learn that it was Pappageotes. Since this raises the likelihood that her microcytic anemia, with normal serum iron level, is due to a Mediterranean hemoglobinopathy, you order hemoglobin electrophoresis. This confirms that Ms. Anderton has beta thalassemia minor. When first seen she probably had iron-deficiency anemia as well; this has been corrected by iron supplementation, but the erythrocyte abnormality remains. You advise her that this is generally an asymptomatic condition for which no treatment is needed, but that she should continue to take iron and to strive for a healthy balance of diet and exercise.

11. Summarize the characteristic features of thalassemia minor:

_____

_____

_____

_____

_____

SUGGESTIONS FOR ADDITIONAL LEARNING ACTIVITIES

1. Play the traditional pen and paper game "hangman," but instead of guessing letters, guess the answers to questions you've prepared from this chapter. Write questions on the fronts of index cards and fill in the answers on the backs. Play alone, or play with someone else, taking turns drawing cards. If you answer the question correctly, draw another card. If you can't come up with the right answer, begin drawing the stick figure on the gallows.

2. You are a health reporter for CNN preparing a feature presentation on advances in leukemia (or choose another disease discussed in this chapter). Your time in front of the camera will be limited to 2 minutes, but your career depends upon the accuracy of your reporting and the audience's interest in your story. Utilize medical journals at your school or local hospital library or the Internet to find the latest information. Make your presentation factual and exciting. If you have access to a video camera, record your presentation.

3. Make drawings of normal and diseased red blood cells and white blood cells, using an anatomy textbook, encyclopedia, or on-line resources as a guide. Use color markers, crayons, or watercolor paints to enhance your illustrations. Label the key features of your drawings.

Musculoskeletal Disorders

(Outline continued on next page)

LEARNING OBJECTIVES

Upon completion of this chapter, you should
be able to

- describe the basic anatomy and physiology
  of the musculoskeletal system;

- explain common signs, symptoms, and
  diagnostic measures pertaining to disorders
  of the musculoskeletal system;

- classify common diseases affecting the
  musculoskeletal system by their cause,
  diagnosis, and treatment.

MUSCULOSKELETAL DISORDERS
(continued)

DISORDERS OF BONE
Osteoporosis
Paget Disease
Osteomyelitis

DISORDERS OF JOINTS
Arthritis
Degenerative Joint Disease (DJD;
        Osteoarthritis)
Gout

QUESTIONS FOR STUDY AND REVIEW

MUSCULOSKELETAL DISORDERS

ANATOMY AND PHYSIOLOGY OF THE MUSCULOSKELETAL SYSTEM

The musculoskeletal system comprises those structures that lend support and mobility to the body and that enable us to perform voluntary actions: bones, cartilage, muscles, and associated connective tissue structures (tendons, ligaments).

Bone is a type of tissue in which a framework or matrix of organic (protein) fibers is reinforced by deposits of calcium and phosphorus salts, which provide strength and rigidity. Bone is not inert material. It has a rich blood supply, it can heal after severe injury, and its calcium content is in equilibrium with the calcium level of the blood. Most bones are covered by a dense sheet of connective tissue called periosteum. Each of the long bones of the extremities is divided into a diaphysis (shaft), an epiphysis (enlarged, knobby end) and a metaphysis (transitional zone between the diaphysis and the epiphysis). Long bones, and some others, are hollow and contain bone marrow in their cavities. Bone marrow is the site of production of red blood cells, polymorphonuclear leukocytes, monocytes, and platelets.

Cartilage is a noncalcified connective tissue similar to bone. In most joints, the contacting surfaces of the bones are covered by protective layers of cartilage. Some weightbearing joints (intervertebral joints, knees) contain thick cushions of tougher cartilage (fibrocartilage). Cartilage also provides semirigid support for the nose, the external ear, the larynx, and the trachea and bronchi.

Muscle is a unique type of tissue that has the property of contracting (shortening) under appropriate stimulation, usually neural. The respiratory, digestive, and urinary tracts contain smooth muscle, which is innervated by (receives its nerve supply from) the autonomic nervous system (discussed in Chapter 19) and is not subject to voluntary control. The muscle of the heart is also not subject to voluntary control.

The anatomic description of each voluntary muscle includes mention of its shape and position, its origin (bone or other structure that serves to anchor it), insertion (bone or other structure that is moved or stabilized by the muscle), action, blood supply, and innervation. Each muscle is supplied by a nerve containing motor fibers (to transmit impulses from the brain and spinal cord) and sensory fibers (for proprioception, that is, perception of position and movement). Each motor nerve is attached to its muscle at a motor end-plate, where nerve impulses trigger contraction of muscle fibers.

While some muscles are attached directly to the periosteum of the bones that serve as their origin and insertion, most muscles are modified at one or both ends and equipped with connective tissue bands that serve for attachment to muscle. A narrow, cordlike band is called a tendon; a broad, sheetlike connection is called an aponeurosis. Some tendons (for example, those at the wrist and ankle) pass through tubular sheaths that act somewhat like pulleys to control direction of pull and reduce local friction. The subcutaneous tissue overlying some bony prominences (shoulder, heel) contains one or more bursas (purselike cushions containing a little fluid to protect underlying surfaces and reduce friction).

A joint is the site at which two bones articulate (connect, generally in an arrangement whereby one or both can move with respect to the other). As mentioned above, the ends of bones forming a joint are usually protected by articular cartilage and sometimes by heavier fibrocartilage cushions (intervertebral disks, menisci of knees). The entire joint is surrounded by a capsule of synovial membrane, a delicate, highly vascular connective tissue that secretes a lubricating fluid in small amounts. A ligament is a band of inelastic connective tissue extending across the joint from one bone to the other to limit both the direction and the extent of motion at the joint. Most joints have several ligaments (the knee has twelve).

MUSCULOSKELETAL DISORDERS

The musculoskeletal system is subject to numerous hereditary, developmental, traumatic, inflammatory, and degenerative disorders. The cardinal symptoms of most of these are pain, tenderness, stiffness, muscle weakness, other disabilities related to impairment of structure or function, or any combination of these. Diagnosis is based chiefly on the history and physical examination, although x-ray and other imaging techniques and (in selected cases) blood and other laboratory studies, including electromyography, may be required. Treatment relies heavily on analgesics, muscle relaxants, rest, and physical therapy.

A few of the more common musculoskeletal disorders are discussed below. Musculoskeletal injuries are dealt with in Chapter 6. However, many of the conditions described below are due, at least sometimes, to trauma, often of the chronic, repetitive type.

HEREDITARY AND DEVELOPMENTAL DISORDERS

Muscular Dystrophy

This term includes a number of inherited disorders of voluntary muscle tissue having various clinical features. Some begin in infancy and others in middle age; some cause death within a few years and others progress slowly and have little impact on lifestyle or life expectancy. Progressive muscular weakness and wasting of muscle tissue are features of most types of muscular dystrophy. In some types, enlargement of affected muscles (pseudohypertrophy) occurs. Some are associated with mental retardation or other defects. Diagnosis is made by history (including family history), physical examination, electromyography, muscle biopsy, and detection of elevated serum creatine kinase. Prenatal diagnosis is possible. Treatment is purely supportive, and consists of physical therapy and regular exercise.

Scoliosis

Lateral curvature of the spine in the erect position, due to malalignment of vertebrae. Two types are recognized. Structural scoliosis affects the vertebrae primarily. It may be caused by bone, nerve, or muscle disease, but in 90% of cases the cause is unknown. In most of these cases a genetic cause is likely. This type of scoliosis is both commoner and more severe in women. Onset is around the age of puberty. Nonstructural scoliosis occurs as a result of abnormality or disease other than in the affected vertebrae. Many cases are due to significant discrepancy in leg length, which brings about a compensatory curve in the upper spine to keep the head and shoulders level.

In both types of scoliosis, there is usually some rotational deformity of the spine in addition to lateral curvature. Generally there are no symptoms at first, and detection is made on routine physical examination, chest x-ray, or school screening. Direct inspection of the back often fails to disclose mild scoliosis, especially in overweight patients. When a person with scoliosis bends forward from the waist, one side of the thorax appears more prominent than the other because of the rotatory component of the deformity. X-ray examination and measurement of the curvature is needed for precise diagnosis.

A curvature of more than 20° is considered significant, particularly because it is likely to progress. When significant scoliosis is detected before the mid-teens, vigorous efforts are made to correct it before spinal growth ceases. Correction is by bracing or casting. In severe or neglected cases, surgical fusion of the spine may be indicated. Untreated scoliosis may lead to severe deformity and disability, even compromise of cardiac and pulmonary function.

Osgood-Schlatter Disease

During fetal development, long bones are formed by deposition of calcium in a cartilage matrix. Until long bone growth is complete, in the mid to late teens, growth centers at the epiphyses remain soft to allow for continuing longitudinal growth. Undue stress on some of these growth centers, due to physical and especially athletic activity, may cause local inflammation and pain. Osgood-Schlatter disease affects the tibial tubercle, where the tendon running down from the patella inserts on the front of the upper end of the tibia. The condition is commoner in boys and is usually bilateral. Symptoms are pain at the site, particularly after exertion, and limping. A firm tender mass can be felt. Spontaneous resolution occurs within a few months to two years. Treatment is with rest, analgesics, and occasionally splinting.

Legg-Calvé-Perthes Disease

Avascular necrosis (death of tissue due to loss of blood supply) of the head of the femur, occurring in children near the middle or end of the first decade of life. Symptoms are hip pain and limping. Imaging studies including radionuclide scan can show altered physical and chemical properties of the affected part of the femur. Spontaneous healing occurs after two or three years, but may leave the child with a badly deformed femoral head and serious hip joint malfunction. Treatment is by splinting or casting to keep the hip in abduction during weightbearing, and occasionally surgery.

DISORDERS OF MUSCLES, TENDONS, LIGAMENTS, AND BURSAS

Tendinitis (Tenosynovitis)

Inflammation of a tendon or, more precisely, of a tendon sheath. The cause is usually repetitive or extreme strain on the tendon, as in an occupational or athletic setting. The symptoms are pain on active or passive movement of the part, localized tenderness over the tendon, and sometimes swelling and crepitus (rubbing or grating sound) with movement. Disability may be severe but spontaneous resolution usually occurs if the inciting activity can be stopped. Treatment is with analgesics and anti-inflammatory agents, wrapping or splinting, and local heat. Injection of adrenal corticosteroid into the site of inflammation often yields prompt if temporary relief, but repeated injections may lead to complications, including rupture of the tendon.

Bursitis

Inflammation of a bursa, usually due to local trauma, often repetitive (kneeling on concrete, working overhead). Inflammation can also result from local infection or as an extension from an inflamed joint. Onset is typically sudden; initial symptoms are sharply localized pain and tenderness and often pronounced swelling, with fluctuancy (the sensation of contained fluid on palpation) due to accumulation of inflammatory fluid within the affected bursa. The diagnosis is usually evident from the history and physical examination. If infection is suspected, the bursa must be aspirated and the fluid examined by smear and culture for pathogenic microorganisms. Treatment options include rest, immobilization if necessary, local heat, nonsteroidal anti-inflammatory drugs, local corticosteroid injections, and antibiotics for infection if present. Common sites of bursitis are subdeltoid (near the point of the shoulder), olecranon (near the point of the elbow), prepatellar (overlying the patella), popliteal (Baker cyst; fluctuant swelling of the bursa behind the knee joint, which communicates with the joint space, as a result of local trauma or disease), and calcaneal (near the point of the heel).

Fibromyalgia Syndrome

A syndrome of chronic musculoskeletal pain accompanied by weakness, fatigue, and sleep disorders.

Cause: Unknown. The condition occurs almost exclusively in adult women with onset before age 50. Depression and viral infection have been proposed as underlying causes in some cases. The disorder sometimes occurs in hypothyroidism.

History: Chronic widespread aching and stiffness, typically bilaterally symmetrical and involving particularly the neck, shoulders, back, and hips, which is aggravated by use of the affected muscles. Usually there are associated fatigue, a sense of weakness or inability to perform certain movements, paresthesia, difficulty sleeping, and headaches.

Physical Examination: Trigger points: sharply localized and extremely tender points, particularly in the neck and back, and often bilaterally symmetric. Some of these points may correspond to sites of pain and others may be painless until palpated. Otherwise examination is normal. There is no fever or local swelling or redness, and joints are not involved.

Diagnostic Tests: Complete blood count, erythrocyte sedimentation rate, and imaging studies yield uniformly normal results.

Course: The condition tends to be chronic, with moderate to severe disability, but symptoms can usually be mitigated by treatment. Symptoms do not progress, and objective signs of disease never develop.

Treatment: Education, exercise, physical therapy. Psychoactive medicines such as amitriptyline and chlorpromazine occasionally help.

DISORDERS OF CARTILAGE

Herniated Disk (Herniated Nucleus Pulposus, HNP; Slipped Disk)

Extrusion of the soft center of an intervertebral disk, with symptoms due to pressure on adjacent spinal nerves.

Cause: Predisposing cause: Degeneration of the intervertebral disk due to aging or other pathologic process. Precipitating cause: Lifting or straining that puts unusual force on the disk.

History: Pain in the back or extremities, often of sudden onset and associated with lifting or straining. The pain may radiate along the course of an extremity like an electric shock, and may be associated with paresthesia and hypesthesia. Movement or coughing may aggravate pain. Bowel or bladder function may be affected.

Physical Examination: There may be tenderness at the site of herniation. Neurologic examination may show impairment of deep tendon reflexes due to compression of dorsal nerve roots (afferent component of reflex arc; see Chapter 19).

Diagnostic Tests: CT and myelography (x-ray of spine with contrast medium injected into the subarachnoid space) may show bulging or displacement of a disk. MRI is a more sensitive technique for showing herniation.

Course: Prolonged disability may occur if the condition is left untreated, although milder cases may often be asymptomatic.

Treatment: Bed rest, analgesics, and muscle relaxants usually provide symptomatic relief. With radiologic evidence of severe or progressive disease or significant neurologic impairment, laminectomy (cutting through the posterior arch of one or more vertebrae) and removal of herniated disk material are indicated.

Torn Meniscus

The menisci are crescent- or C-shaped pads of fibrocartilage within the knee joint, one medial and one lateral, that cushion shocks between the femur and the tibia. Injury to a meniscus is common and usually results from twisting the knee joint with the foot planted, often in an athletic setting. The patient hears a pop and feels sudden severe pain. Swelling develops soon, and the knee may lock or buckle with weight-bearing. The medial meniscus is torn ten times as often as the lateral meniscus. Meniscal tears do not heal. A piece broken off a meniscus remains in the joint as a loose body, and may impair mobility.

Examination shows effusion of fluid into the joint space, crepitus, and a positive McMurray test: extension of the knee from full flexion with the leg and foot externally rotated causes an audible or palpable snap in medial meniscus tear; extension with the leg and foot internally rotated causes a snap in lateral meniscus tear. Treatment is with ice, elevation, a bulky compression dressing, and crutches, with attention to maintaining mobility and muscle strength and tone in the quadriceps muscle (the large, four-headed muscle on the front of the thigh that extends the knee joint). Mild tears may eventually become asymptomatic. For persistent symptoms, arthroscopic (but occasionally open) surgery is required, with removal of loose fragments and reshaping of remaining cartilage.

Patellofemoral Syndrome

Pain in the knee, occurring most often in active teenagers or young adults, due to abnormal friction between the patella (kneecap) and the groove on the femur in which it slides. Any disturbance in the normal alignment or tracking of the patella in its groove, such as may result from uneven pull by the four heads of the quadriceps femoris muscle (the large muscle on the anterior thigh that extends the knee joint), can cause chronic trauma to the back of the patella, with resultant degenerative changes (roughening, fraying, even complete loss of cartilage), known collectively as chondromalacia patellae. The principal symptom is pain with walking, especially on stairs, and with squatting. Physical examination shows tenderness on manipulation of the patella and sometimes swelling and crepitus. X-rays are negative. Some cases resolve spontaneously with rest and anti-inflammatory medicines. Quadriceps exercises (repeatedly bringing the knee into full extension, with tensing of the muscles of the front of the thigh) often help to correct muscle imbalances. Shaving the roughened posterior surface of the patella arthroscopically may relieve pain. If tracking of the patella in its groove on the anterior femur is grossly deviant, surgical transplantation of the patellar tendon may be needed.

DISORDERS OF BONE

Osteoporosis

A disorder in which the density of bone is inadequate for its normal supporting function; decreased bone mass leads to deformity and increased susceptibility to fractures.

Causes: Resorption of calcium from bone to maintain serum calcium level, a complex phenomenon involving parathyroid hormone, intestinal and renal function, activity level, and dietary intake of calcium, phosphorus, and vitamin D. Postmenopausal deficiency of estrogen increases sensitivity of bone to factors that promote calcium loss; 80% of patients are postmenopausal women. Other causes include genetic disorders (cystic fibrosis, Marfan syndrome, osteogenesis imperfecta), endocrine disorders (diabetes mellitus, Cushing disease, thyrotoxicosis, hyperparathyroidism), prolonged amenorrhea in female athletes, and reduced level of mobility and physical activity because of illness, injury, or lifestyle. Asian or Caucasian race, underweight, dietary calcium deficiency, alcohol use, and cigarette smoking are all risk factors.

History: Backache, reduction of stature, kyphosis (forward hunching of the upper spine), pathologic fractures (fractures for which underlying abnormality of bone are partly responsible).

Physical Examination: Unremarkable except for features noted above.

Diagnostic Tests: X-ray examination shows bone deformity or fractures but does not reliably demonstrate minor degrees of demineralization. Bone density is more accurately assessed by CT scan, single-photon absorptiometry (SPA), dual-energy x-ray absorptiometry (DEXA), or ultrasound.

Course: Osteoporosis is responsible for 50% of fractures occurring in women over age 50. Compression fractures of the vertebrae and traumatic fractures of the wrist and femoral neck are most common. Gradual collapse of vertebrae causes loss of body height and senile kyphosis. The one-year mortality after hip fracture is about 20%.

Treatment: Administration of calcium along with vitamin D and calcitonin (orally or nasally). Bisphosphonates (alendronate, etidronate) and the selective estrogen receptor modulator raloxifene improve resistance of bone to enzymatic breakdown. Estrogen is given to postmenopausal women; men with reduced androgen levels are treated with testosterone. Physical therapy, increased mobility.

Paget Disease

A degenerative disorder of bone occurring most commonly in middle-aged and elderly persons.

Cause: An abnormal process of bone breakdown and erratic repair, of unknown cause, resulting in softening and swelling of bone. The disease shows a familial tendency. Viral infection has been implicated in some cases.

History: There may be no symptoms, but most patients experience bone pain, hunching of the back (kyphosis), bowing of the shins, pathologic fractures, and (with cranial involvement) increase in hat size, cranial nerve palsies, and deafness.

Physical Examination: Warmth over affected bones and typical deformities.

Diagnostic Tests: Serum alkaline phosphatase and often serum calcium are elevated. X-rays and bone scans localize lesions and permit accurate assessment of severity.

Course: Progressive deformity. Abnormal bone occasionally undergoes malignant change.

Treatment: Calcitonin (oral or nasal), bisphosphonates, or pamidronate.

Osteomyelitis

Bacterial infection of bone.

Cause: Infection with staphylococci, streptococci, or other organisms. Bacteria may be introduced directly into bone tissue (gunshot wound, surgery, compound fracture) or migrate there from adjacent soft-tissue infection (sinusitis, deep abscess) or a remote source (systemic infections such as typhoid fever or tuberculosis, bacteremia in IV drug abusers). Osteomyelitis due to *Salmonella* frequently occurs as a complication of sickle cell disease and other inherited hemoglobin abnormalities.

History: Gradual or sudden onset of bone pain, fever, and chills.

Physical Examination: Fever, tenderness of site of infection. In severe infection there may be signs of toxemia.

Diagnostic Tests: The erythrocyte sedimentation rate is elevated. Causative organisms can be cultured from material aspirated from infected bone or from the blood. Serologic studies can identify infection due to *Salmonella*. X-ray or, preferably, CT and MRI studies show local swelling, decalcification, and eventually erosive destruction of bone.

Course: Without prompt treatment, infection may become chronic. Bone destruction can lead to severe deformity and disability.

Treatment: Rest, immobilization, analgesics. Antibiotics based on culture findings. Surgical drainage of the infection site. Severe or advanced disease may require radical surgical excision of infected bone (saucerization). Physical therapy as needed.

DISORDERS OF JOINTS

ARTHRITIS

Inflammation of one or more joints. Arthritis is not just one disease, but a group of many (perhaps over 200) having joint inflammation as a common feature. Rheumatoid arthritis is discussed in Chapter 4. Two other types are described below.

Degenerative Joint Disease (DJD; Osteoarthritis)

A joint disorder characterized by degeneration of articular cartilage.

Cause: Unknown. Familial factors may be operative. Cartilage protecting articular surfaces of bones degenerates, allowing bony surfaces to touch and erode each other. Hypertrophy of bone at the affected site adds to symptoms. Onset of symptoms is typically in early middle-age. Trauma, overweight, and the presence of other orthopedic disorders in the area of the affected joint may precipitate or accelerate symptoms.

History: Gradual onset of pain and stiffness in joints, particularly the intervertebral joints, hips, and knees; pain is aggravated by activity and relieved by rest.

Physical Examination: Stiffness, crepitus, and occasional swelling of affected joints. Heberden nodes (small firm nodules at the distal interphalangeal joints of the fingers) may be present.

Diagnostic Tests: X-rays show narrowing of joint spaces due to destruction and wearing away of cartilage; increased density (eburnation) of articular ends of bone due to mutual compaction after loss of protective cartilage; and hypertrophy of bone near the joint, with formation of osteophytes (outgrowths of bone from the surface) variously described as beaking, lipping, and bridging (forming a bridge from one bone to the other).

Course: Progressive pain and stiffening of joints, with eventual deformity and disability, may occur.

Treatment: Rest, physical therapy, prescribed exercise programs, correction of underlying causes if possible, weight reduction in overweight patients, mild analgesics (acetaminophen). Surgical replacement of the hip or knee joint reduces pain and improves mobility.

Gout

A systemic disease with joint symptoms due to deposition of urate crystals.

Causes: Elevation of serum uric acid due to overproduction, impaired excretion, or both. Some forms of gout are hereditary. Signs and symptoms of gout can be precipitated by certain drugs (thiazide diuretics, nicotinic acid, low-dose aspirin), malignancies of blood-forming tissues and other disorders characterized by rapid breakdown of cellular nucleic acid, renal disease, hypothyroidism, and lead

> The metal **lead** has been known and used from antiquity. Medieval alchemists considered it one of the "elements" according to their primitive systems. They gave symbolic names to these elements based on the names of the heavenly bodies as then known. Thus, gold was symbolized by the sun, silver by the moon, quicksilver by the planet Mercury (which is still the usual English name of the element), and lead by Saturn. Compounds or effects of lead were therefore labeled "saturnine," a usage that continues to this day in the somewhat uncommonly heard term "saturnine gout," meaning a kind of gout induced by lead poisoning. What is another meaning of saturnine? Where does it come from?

poisoning (saturnine gout; see box). Nearly all patients are men over 40.

History: Recurrent acute episodes of severe pain, tenderness, and swelling, usually affecting a single joint, often occurring at night, and separated by symptom-free intervals. The first metatarsophalangeal joint is most often affected. After the acute episode, itching and scaling of the skin overlying the affected joint. Eventual development of nodules in soft tissues.

Physical Examination: Redness, swelling, and exquisite tenderness of the affected joint. Tophi (nodular deposits of urate crystals with local inflammation) may appear in cartilage (the outer ear), in tissues around joints (subcutaneous tissue, tendons), or at other sites.

Diagnostic Tests: The serum uric acid level is generally elevated, as well as the erythrocyte sedimentation rate. Microscopic examination of material aspirated from affected joints or tophi shows urate crystals. In chronic disease, x-rays may show tophi in bone as punched out (radiolucent) areas.

Course: Without treatment an acute attack can last for days or weeks. Chronic disease may lead to joint destruction, deformity, and disability. Uric acid kidney stones are a common complication. With advanced disease, renal failure may occur.

Treatment: An acute attack of gout is promptly aborted by colchicine, nonsteroidal anti-inflammatory agents, or corticosteroid. Rest and immobilization may also be important in shortening the attack. Options for prophylactic treatment between attacks include drugs that inhibit uric acid production (allopurinol) or increase its excretion (probenecid). Colchicine can also be used. Abstinence from certain foods (liver, sweetbreads, anchovies) and alcohol is usually recommended, but the impact of dietary restrictions is minimal in a patient taking adequate doses of prophylactic medicine.

QUESTIONS FOR STUDY AND REVIEW

1. Name three musculoskeletal disorders that can be inherited:

   a. _____

   b. _____

   c. _____

2. Name three musculoskeletal disorders that can result from repetitive trauma:

   a. _____

   b. _____

   c. _____

3. Name three musculoskeletal disorders that can lead to chronic disease and disability:

   a. _____

   b. _____

   c. _____

4. Consult a reference book and list five types of arthritis not discussed in this book:

   a. _____

   b. _____

   c. _____

   d. _____

   e. _____

5. Define or explain these terms:

   a. aponeurosis _____
   _____

   b. bursa _____
   _____

   c. crepitus _____
   _____

   d. epiphysis _____
   _____

   e. fibromyalgia _____
   _____

f. kyphosis _____

_____

g. laminectomy _____

_____

h. meniscus _____

_____

i. tophus_____

_____

6. Name some musculoskeletal disorders that show a decided preference for persons of one gender. What does this difference in incidence suggest to you?

_____

_____

_____

_____

_____

7. Orthopedists treat sprains, fractures, scoliosis, Legg-Calvé-Perthes disease, and tendinitis. Rheumatologists treat rheumatoid arthritis, fibromyalgia, and lupus erythematosus. How would you distinguish their fields of interest and expertise? In which practice would you expect to find a preponderance of women patients?

_____

_____

_____

_____

_____

CASE STUDY: YOU'RE THE DOCTOR

Leo Penjak is a 38-year-old assembly worker at an automotive parts factory. He is referred to you, an orthopedist, by his primary care physician because of chronic back pain. Mr. Penjak states that his trouble began about 4 years ago when he was transferred to a new job at the factory as a result of a reduction in force. The new job required more physical effort than the one he had been doing. He had to do a lot more bending and stooping to operate machinery, and he spent about 20% of each shift lifting and carrying trays of parts.

1. Placing yourself in this patient's position at the time of his job change, how would you feel about your employer, your supervisor, and your new job?

   _____

   _____

   _____

   _____

Mr. Penjak states that about 2 weeks after the job change, while lifting a heavy load he experienced a sudden severe pain in his lower back, accompanied by radiation of electric shock-like sensations down both legs, as if he had been "struck by lightning." He states that since then he has never been entirely free of pain. He was initially treated by his primary care physician with a nonsteroidal anti-inflammatory drug, a muscle relaxant, and a narcotic analgesic to be taken as needed at night. He was off work for 2 weeks and returned with restrictions on lifting and bending, but had to take another 2 weeks off before he was able to work a full day even with these restrictions.

2. Limiting yourself strictly to these historical points, how strongly would you suspect that, consciously or unconsciously, Mr. Penjak may have been exaggerating his pain and disability? Outline the reasons for your concerns.

   _____

   _____

   _____

   _____

   _____

   _____

   _____

   _____

He has had numerous medical absences from work since then, including two 3-month periods of total disability leave. On both occasions he was eventually ordered back to work by the state industrial commission after a commission doctor found him able to work. Spine films have shown very early osteoarthritic changes in the lumbar spine but no spondylolysis or spondylolisthesis. Magnetic resonance imaging (MRI) of the back performed on two occasions in the past 15 months has been interpreted as showing equivocal bulging of the thecal sac at the L4-5 and L5-S1 disk spaces, compatible with mild herniation of the nuclei pulposi. Electromyography has not confirmed radicular compression. Mr. Penjak has had several courses of physical therapy and went through a program of "back training" mandated by the industrial commission. He has also attended a chronic pain clinic and has had chiropractic manipulation. None of these measures have afforded more than partial or temporary relief. He is presently working full-time but states he is in constant pain. His physician has declined to prescribe more narcotics for him, but Mr. Penjak states that he has been "popping Naprosyns and Vioxxes like peanuts" for months. His application for total and permanent disability under Social Security is currently pending.

3. What features of Mr. Penjak's history, if any, suggest an organic origin for his pain?

_____

_____

_____

_____

_____

_____

4. What features suggest that he is malingering or exaggerating his problem?

_____

_____

_____

_____

He describes his pain as a steady stinging or burning sensation in the lower back, at the beltline and below, which radiates down the right buttock and posterior thigh as far as the knee. Almost any movement aggravates the pain and causes shock-like sensations to shoot down both thighs and legs as far as the heels. The pain extends all the way across the back but is always more pronounced on the right side. There is some numbness in the right posterior thigh, always more marked when he first awakens in the morning. He can't get comfortable in bed at night and often sleeps on the floor. His general health is good except for allergic rhinitis, for which he uses prescribed medicines with good control. He drinks 1-4 beers daily but stopped smoking cigarettes 14 years ago.

5. What procedures will you use to assess Mr. Penjak's condition?

_____

_____

_____

_____

The patient has good muscular development but also displays truncal obesity. His height is 6'1" and he weighs 234 pounds. Vital signs are normal except for a blood pressure of 156/88. He moves slowly and winces in pain in getting on and off the examining table. The back shows no kyphosis, lordosis, or lateral curvature. There is diffuse tenderness of the lower back to palpation, involving the spinous processes of the vertebrae and the paravertebral muscles from L3 down to the coccyx. There is no palpable spasm and no local tenderness of the sacroiliac joints or sacrosciatic notches. Deep tendon reflexes in the lower extremities are 3+ and bilaterally equal. Toe extensor strength is normal and bilaterally equal. Spine flexion from the erect position is limited by pain to about 15° from the vertical. The patient declines to attempt touching his toes or assuming a squatting position. Straight leg raising is positive at 30° on the right and 45° on the left.

6. Discuss the expected benefit of each of the following treatment options:

   a. more potent analgesics _____

   _____

   _____

   b. surgery_____

   _____

   _____

   c. vocational retraining counseling_____

   _____

   _____

   d. a total and permanent disability pension_____

   _____

   _____

   e. acupuncture_____

   _____

   _____

   f. yoga _____

   _____

   _____

7. Which option(s) will you recommend and why?

   _____

   _____

   _____

   _____

   _____

   _____

SUGGESTIONS FOR ADDITIONAL LEARNING ACTIVITIES

1. Read a section from this chapter and then explain what you've read to someone else. Go through the entire chapter, reading and explaining each section. If you are working with a classmate, take turns.

2. Play a version of the TV game show "Concentration." For a group game, use a single color of construction paper or other heavy stock for playing cards. To play by yourself or with one other person, use regular index cards. Write the names of 10 diseases discussed in this chapter on half the cards and write a synopsis of each of these diseases on the remaining cards. In each synopsis, include at least one historical note, physical feature, diagnostic test, and a treatment. Shuffle the cards and lay them out face down in a 4 x 5 grid. Turn over any two cards and determine if there is a match of disease and synopsis. If they match, leave them face up and take another turn. If they don't match, turn them face down again in their original position and the next player takes a turn. Players must concentrate on which diseases and synopses match as well as on the positions of previously revealed cards.

3. Imagine a new drug developed for the treatment of osteoporosis or another condition discussed in this chapter. Give your new drug a generic name and a brand name under which it will be marketed. List the benefits of treatment with this drug and then list the possible side effects and contraindications. Using this information, script a 60-second television commercial to use in your new marketing campaign.

18

Diseases of the Eye

LEARNING OBJECTIVES

Upon completion of this chapter, you should be able to

- describe the basic anatomy and physiology of the eye;

- explain diagnostic procedures and methods of treatment used in ocular diseases;

- classify common diseases affecting the eye by their signs, symptoms, and treatment.

(Outline continued on next page)

DISEASES OF THE EYE
(continued)

DISORDERS OF OCULAR MOVEMENT
Strabismus

VISUAL IMPAIRMENT

QUESTIONS FOR STUDY AND REVIEW

DISEASES OF THE EYE

ANATOMY AND PHYSIOLOGY OF THE EYE

Each eye is a roughly spherical structure protected on all sides except the front by the bones and soft tissues of the orbit. Blood vessels and nerves enter at the back of the eye. The eyeball (bulb, globe) consists of three concentric layers: the outer sclera, a tough coat of connective tissue; the pigment layer or uveal tract, a delicate, spongy, vascular membrane of pigmented cells; and the innermost layer, the light-sensitive retina. (See Figure 21.)

Anteriorly the sclera is modified to form the transparent cornea, through which light rays enter the eye. The uveal tract consists of three parts: the iris, which regulates the amount of light entering the eye; the ciliary body, which adjusts the focus of the eye; and the choroid, which underlies the retina. The retina is a layer of specialized nerve cells that are stimulated by light rays within the visible range. Nerve fibers of these cells unite to form the optic nerve.

The ocular fundus is the rear wall of the eye as viewed through the pupil with an ophthalmoscope (discussed below). The fundus consists of the retina and its arteries and veins and the disk (optic nerve

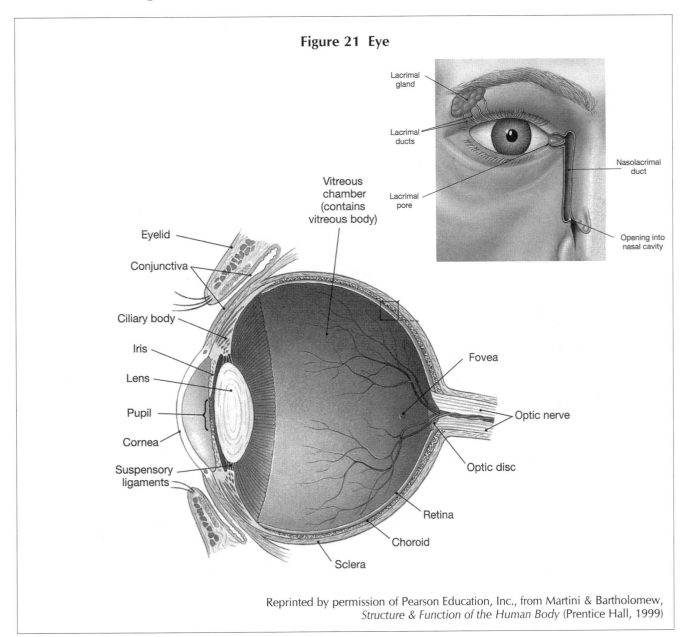

Figure 21 Eye

Lacrimal gland

Lacrimal ducts

Lacrimal pore

Nasolacrimal duct

Opening into nasal cavity

Vitreous chamber (contains vitreous body)

Eyelid

Conjunctiva

Ciliary body

Iris

Lens

Pupil

Cornea

Suspensory ligaments

Fovea

Optic nerve

Optic disc

Retina

Choroid

Sclera

Reprinted by permission of Pearson Education, Inc., from Martini & Bartholomew, *Structure & Function of the Human Body* (Prentice Hall, 1999)

head). The disk appears as a round, ivory-colored plaque raised somewhat from the surrounding retina and having a shallow central depression, the cup. The disk lies on the nasal side of the fundus, not at its center. The central portion of the retina, concerned with central vision and hence the most sensitive, appears as a faint yellow spot, the macula lutea. The retinal vessels (branching arteries, each closely accompanied by a vein) emerge from the center of the disk.

The optic nerve passes back through an aperture in the orbit and crosses the optic nerve of the opposite eye, with which it exchanges some fibers. Behind the crossing, the newly assorted bundles of fibers, called the optic tracts, carry visual impulses into the brain.

On their way to the retina, light rays pass through both the cornea and the lens, a transparent structure suspended just behind the cornea. The shape of the lens can be altered by the pull of muscles originating in the ciliary body, and this alteration adjusts the focal distance of the eye. The iris, the colored part of the eye, lies between the cornea and the lens, and controls the amount of light entering the eye by changing the diameter of the pupil, the black-appearing round aperture in the middle of the iris.

The part of the eye lying anterior to the lens contains a watery fluid, the aqueous humor, which is produced by the ciliary body and drains into small veins in the anterior chamber at the "drainage angle" (the slight angle between cornea and sclera). The space occupied by the aqueous humor is divided into the anterior chamber (between cornea and iris) and the posterior chamber (between iris and lens). Behind the lens, the cavity of the eye is filled with a somewhat denser fluid, the vitreous humor. Both humors are refractive media, participating in the transmission and refraction of light rays.

The eyelids are folds of skin, supplied with oil and sebaceous glands and lash follicles, that shut out light and provide a watertight seal over the eyes. The medial or nasal junction or angle between upper and lower lids is called the inner canthus; the lateral or temporal angle is called the outer canthus. The visible part of the sclera is covered by a delicate vascular membrane, the conjunctiva (bulbar conjunctiva), which is continuous with the lining of the inner surfaces of the eyelids (palpebral conjunctiva). The conjunctiva does not extend over the cornea.

A lacrimal gland is situated near the front of each orbit, above and lateral to the eyeball. This gland produces tears, which moisten, lubricate, and cleanse the eyeball.

Tears flow downward and medially to drain by way of the puncta (minute openings at the inner canthus) and nasolacrimal ducts into the nose.

Each eye is equipped with six extraocular muscles, which produce eye movement and control the direction of gaze. Three cranial nerves (III, oculomotor; IV, trochlear; and VI, abducens) supply these six muscles. In addition, the oculomotor nerve sends motor branches to the upper eyelid, the ciliary body (focus), and the iris (light/dark adaptation). Coordination of the movements and position of the two eyes and fusion of their images into a single three-dimensional one take place in the brain.

SYMPTOMS AND SIGNS OF OCULAR DISEASE

Argyll Robertson pupil: A pupil that constricts when the subject focuses on a near object, but not when the eye is stimulated with light; due to central nervous system disease, most often syphilis.

Blepharospasm: Spasm of the eyelids, usually due to local irritation, photophobia, or both.

Chemosis: Marked watery edema and bulging of the conjunctiva.

Coloboma (iridis): A congenital defect in the iris, in which a wedge-shaped segment is absent, giving a keyhole appearance to the pupil; similar defects are created by certain types of ocular surgery.

Cupping of the disk: As noted above, the normal optic nerve head has a slight central depression (physiologic cupping). Increase in the depth of the cup occurs with increased intraocular pressure (glaucoma) or atrophy of the optic nerve.

Diplopia: Double vision; seeing two overlapping two-dimensional images instead of one three-dimensional image; may result from injury or disease of one or both eyes or from failure of fusion of images in the cerebral cortex, due to alcohol, drugs, fever, infection, neoplasm, or trauma.

Ectropion: Eversion (turning outward) and drooping of the lower eyelid, exposing the conjunctival surface and allowing overflow of tears.

Entropion: Inward turning of the margin of the lower eyelid, often so that the lower lashes touch the eyeball.

Epiphora: Chronic overflow of tears from the lower eyelid onto the cheek; may be due to blockage of the nasolacrimal duct or to deformity of the lower lid (ectropion).

Exophthalmos: Abnormal bulging of the eye between the lids; may be due to local disease (orbital cellulitis or neoplasm) or (when bilateral) to systemic disease (Graves disease).

Hyphema: Presence of blood in the anterior chamber.

Hypopyon: Presence of pus in the anterior chamber.

Itching of the eye or eyelid.

Lacrimation (tearing): Increased flow of tears.

Miosis: Sustained constriction of the pupil, which may be due to ocular or nervous system disease or to the effect of drugs (pilocarpine, morphine).

Mydriasis: Sustained dilatation of the pupil, which may be due to ocular or nervous system disease or to the effect of drugs (atropine, cyclopentolate).

Nyctalopia: Marked reduction of visual acuity at night (that is, under conditions of near-darkness).

Nystagmus: A rhythmic back-and-forth movement of the eyes usually due to congenital abnormality or central nervous system disease.

Ocular discharge: A serous, mucous, or purulent material formed on conjunctival surfaces, often gluing the eyelids together and producing crusting of the eyelashes; usually due to infection or allergy.

Pain in the eye, which may be a superficial irritation or scratchy feeling on the cornea or sclera (as from an abrasion or ulcer) or a deep, throbbing pain within the eyeball (as in acute glaucoma).

Papilledema: Swelling of the optic disk, as observed with an ophthalmoscope (an instrument described below); usually due to increased intracranial pressure ("choked disk") (hemorrhage, neoplasm, disturbance of cerebrospinal fluid circulation) or intrinsic eye disease (optic neuritis). (When disk edema is due to inflammation, the term papillitis is preferred to papilledema.) The disk appears edematous and perhaps injected, and the retinal vessels as they emerge from the swollen disk appear to be kinked ("stepping" of vessels). As a rough measure of the extent of papilledema, the examiner compares the ophthalmoscope setting needed to focus on the disk with that needed to focus on the rest of the retina. Hence a "two diopter choke" means that the setting needed to bring the disk into focus differs by two diopters from the setting that is suitable for examining the rest of the retina.

Photophobia: Aversion to bright light, which causes a sense of pain in the eye, usually because of irritability or spasm of the iris.

Ptosis: Drooping of an upper eyelid that cannot be fully corrected by voluntary effort.

Redness of the eye, due either to local inflammation and hyperemia of the conjunctiva or to hemorrhage in the sclera.

Scotoma (visual field defect): A blind spot; a gap in the visual field of one or both eyes in which objects cannot be seen. A scotoma that appears identical in each eye is always due to a disease or condition of the central nervous system (for example, migraine headache). A scotoma may appear as a black hole or may show flashes or swirls of white or colored light.

Strabismus: A general term for any condition in which the direction of gaze is different in the two eyes, as noted by an observer.

Trichiasis: A growing inward of some eyelash hairs, with resultant irritation of the eye.

Visual impairment, ranging from slight indistinctness of distant objects to complete blindness. Visual impairment may be of gradual or sudden onset, unilateral or bilateral, static or progressive, reversible or permanent.

Xerophthalmia: Abnormal dryness of the eye, usually due to decreased flow of tears.

DIAGNOSTIC PROCEDURES IN OPHTHALMOLOGY

Inspection of the eye and adjacent structures with adequate illumination and often with magnification. For a thorough examination, the eyelids must be retracted and the patient must move each eyeball through a full range of positions.

Fluorescein dye may be applied to the cornea and conjunctiva, and the surface of the eye examined with a cobalt blue light, to detect injuries, ulcerations, or foreign bodies.

Slit lamp examination: A slit lamp is a low-power microscope with built-in illumination projected through a narrow slit. This instrument enables the physician to view a magnified cross-sectional image of the anterior structures of the eye: cornea, anterior chamber, iris, and lens. Significant abnormal findings on slit lamp examination include flare and cells (diminished clarity of the aqueous humor due to protein leakage from the iris; swirls of inflammatory cells in the anterior chamber due to inflammation) and keratic precipitates (KPs) (whitish deposits of inflammatory cells on the posterior surface of the cornea).

Funduscopic examination: Inspection of the fundus (the rear of the interior of the eye, consisting of the retina, its blood vessels, and the optic nerve head). The examination is performed with an ophthalmoscope, an instrument with a light source and a set of changeable lenses to enable the examiner to focus on the fundus regardless of refractive errors in the subject's lens. Possible findings with the ophthalmoscope include swelling or cupping of the disk, vascular and other abnormalities associated with retinopathy (discussed later in this chapter), and retinal detachment.

Vision testing: Usually performed with standard charts containing letters or words of various sizes. For assessment of distant vision, the Snellen chart is placed 20 feet from the subject, and visual acuity is recorded as the smallest line of type in which the subject can read more than half the letters correctly. Each line is designated by the distance at which a person with normal vision can read it. Thus, 20/20 vision is normal, while 20/80 vision means that the subject must be as close as 20 feet to read a type size that a normal person can read at 80 feet. For near vision testing, lines or paragraphs are printed in various sizes of type on a card that can be held in the hand. Testing may involve finding the smallest print that the subject can read at a standard distance, or finding the range of distances through which the subject can read a particular size of type. The eyes are tested both separately and together. For children and illiterates, charts with pictures or symbols are used.

Visual field testing: Use of a black felt sheet or screen mounted on a wall to map areas of impaired or absent vision. An Amsler grid consists of a network of lines, usually white on black, around a central point at which the subject is instructed to gaze while the examiner moves a small object through various parts of the visual field to detect defects.

Perimetry: A means of assessing peripheral vision by testing the subject's ability to discern moving objects or flashing lights at the extreme periphery of the visual fields.

Tests for color-blindness: Usually these are printed figures made up of variously sized dots in various colors and shades. Persons with normal color vision perceive numbers against a background of differently colored dots. Color-blind persons see only a scattering of dots.

Refraction: Determination of near and distant vision more precisely than is possible with vision charts. The instrument used enables the examiner to try a large number of lenses of standard magnification so as to determine the refractive error of each eye and hence the strength of the corrective lens that must be prescribed to correct the error. The instrument is also used in detecting and measuring astigmatism (described later in this chapter).

Tonometry: Determination of the pressure of the aqueous humor, to detect glaucoma. Tonometers of various types are used.

Orbital imaging: X-rays or MRI of the skull with emphasis on the orbit(s) to identify orbital or intraocular foreign body.

Retinal arteriography: Imaging of the retinal arteries with fluorescein injected into an arm vein.

Electroretinography: Instrumental determination of changes in electrical potential of the retina in response to light stimuli; identifies visual abnormalities due to retinal disease.

Ophthalmology is the branch of medicine that is devoted to the prevention, diagnosis, and treatment of eye diseases. This is an exceedingly complex field, which can only be touched on in a book of this scope. The rest of the chapter is devoted to discussions of some of the commoner eye diseases. Numerous terms are defined above and below. If you encounter unfamiliar words, look them up in the Glossary or the Index.

INFLAMMATORY DISEASES OF THE EYE

Conjunctivitis

Inflammation of the conjunctiva.

Causes: Infection, allergy, injury (including injuries due to chemicals, heat, or other radiant energy), or other process affecting the anterior part of the eye. Infection may be due to viruses (particularly certain adenovirus types) or bacteria (including chlamydia and gonococcus). Transmission is generally by hand contact. Neonatal conjunctivitis is acquired from an infected birth canal.

History: Soreness, itching, or irritation of one or both eyes, with redness of the conjunctiva; inability to tolerate contact lenses. Depending on cause and severity, lacrimation or mucopurulent discharge that crusts the lashes and glues the eyelids together, swelling of the eyelids, blurring of vision, or photophobia may also occur.

Physical Examination: Patchy or diffuse injection of the conjunctiva, sometimes with coarsely granular appearance ("cobblestoning," typical of some allergic conjunctivitis). Lid edema, blepharospasm, lacrimation, ocular discharge, photophobia, chemosis (typically allergic), and sometimes blepharitis, keratitis, or enlargement of preauricular lymph nodes (nodes in front of the ear). Slit lamp examination precisely locates areas of inflammation.

Diagnostic Tests: Microscopic examination of conjunctival scrapings can identify infection due to chlamydia. Culture is necessary to confirm gonococcal conjunctivitis.

Course: Most conjunctivitis is benign and self-limited. Untreated gonococcal conjunctivitis can spread to the cornea, causing perforation and blindness. Chlamydial conjunctivitis is of two kinds. *Chlamydia trachomatis* types A-C cause trachoma, a severe conjunctivitis with keratitis, often leading to lid deformity and blindness. Types D-K cause a milder infection, inclusion conjunctivitis, which typically resolves without sequelae. Seasonal or perennial allergic conjunctivitis is typically recurrent or chronic during times of exposure to allergens.

Treatment: Allergic conjunctivitis is treated with topical vasoconstrictors, mast cell stabilizers (cromolyn, lodoxamide), and corticosteroids. Systemic antihistamines and steroids may be required. Bacterial infection is treated with topical sulfonamide or antibiotic drops. Both forms of chlamydial conjunctivitis respond to systemic tetracycline, doxycycline, or erythromycin. Gonococcal conjunctivitis is treated with systemic ceftriaxone.

Hordeolum (Stye)

An acute staphylococcal abscess, typically small, that forms near the margin of an upper or lower eyelid. Treatment is with warm compresses and topical sulfonamide or antibiotic. Incision and drainage may be necessary.

Chalazion

A chronic, nontender fibrotic nodule in an eyelid, resulting from nonresolution of a stye that has developed in a conjunctival gland. The lesion may grow large and become cosmetically objectionable. Treatment is incision and curettage.

Keratitis

Inflammation of the cornea.

Causes: Keratitis may result from injury (chemical, abrasion, erosion, puncture, contact lens wear), infection (bacterial, viral, fungal, or protozoan), or systemic disease. Bacteria causing keratitis include pneumococcus, staphylococcus, *Pseudomonas*, and *Moraxella*. Syphilitic and tuberculous keratitis (due to systemic infection) also occur. Viral keratitis may be due to herpes simplex virus or varicella-zoster virus. Keratitis in contact lens wearers may be due to the protozoan parasite *Acanthamoeba*.

History: Pain in the eye, aggravated by opening and closing the lid; lacrimation, photophobia, visual blurring. There may be a history of corneal trauma (fingernail scratch, cigarette ash, airborne foreign body) or of systemic infection (tuberculosis, syphilis).

Physical Examination: Conjunctival injection, particularly near to the corneal rim. Photophobia, lacrimation, watery or purulent discharge. Staining of the cornea followed by examination with cobalt blue light shows ulceration or other epithelial defects.

Diagnostic Tests: Microscopic examination or culture of scrapings from the cornea may indicate a causative organism.

Course: Certain infections (herpes simplex virus, *Acanthamoeba*) cause progressive and severe damage if untreated, with visual loss due to corneal scarring. Thinning and bulging (descemetocele) of an inflamed zone of cornea may also occur. Corneal infection can extend to the sclera, iris, or optic nerve.

Treatment: Specific antimicrobial treatment, if available, is mandatory. Topical antibiotics usually suffice in bacterial keratitis. Viral infections are treated with topical idoxuridine or trifluridine and systemic acyclovir. Topical steroids are used in selected cases.

Uveitis

Uveitis is inflammation of any part of the uveal tract. Inflammation of the iris is called iritis; of the ciliary body, cyclitis; and of the choroid, choroiditis. Uveitis may occur as a feature of various granulomatous diseases (syphilis, tuberculosis, toxoplasmosis, sarcoidosis) or may appear in various systemic inflammatory diseases (ulcerative colitis, Crohn disease, psoriasis, ankylosing spondylitis, Reiter syndrome, Behçet syndrome). Anterior uveitis (iritis, cyclitis, iridocyclitis) causes unilateral ocular pain, visual blurring, and photophobia.

Examination of the eye shows constriction of the pupil and a flush of redness around the rim of the cornea. Photophobia may be evident. Slit lamp examination shows cells and flare of the aqueous humor, keratic precipitates (KP) of the posterior corneal epithelium, and sometimes hypopyon or distortion of the pupil by adhesions (synechiae; singular synechia). (Anterior synechiae form between the iris and the posterior surface of the cornea; posterior synechiae between the iris and the anterior surface of the lens.) Posterior uveitis (choroiditis) causes gradual loss of vision in one eye, with minimal discomfort. Examination shows cells in the vitreous, and may indicate inflammatory changes in the retina.

The erythrocyte sedimentation rate is elevated. Laboratory studies and chest x-ray may indicate other manifestations of an underlying process and make possible a precise diagnosis. Treatment is with corticosteroids topically or systemically. Mydriatics are given to dilate the pupil and reduce the risk of posterior synechiae. Underlying infection requires specific treatment.

GLAUCOMA

An ocular condition in which the pressure of the aqueous humor is abnormally high. Two types are recognized.

Open Angle Glaucoma

The most common type of glaucoma, consisting of a persistent elevation of intraocular pressure.

Cause: Unknown; apparently related to decreased reabsorption of aqueous humor from the anterior chamber of the eye. However, the drainage angle is not demonstrably narrowed, hence the name (contrast the next condition). Both sexes are about equally affected, and the condition runs in families.

History: Gradual loss of peripheral vision. Appearance of halos around lights, especially at night, when intraocular tension is very high.

Physical Examination: Increased cupping of the optic disk (increased cup:disk ratio).

Diagnostic Tests: Intraocular tension, as determined by tonometry, is elevated (normal 10-21 mmHg). Visual fields are diminished.

Course: Optic atrophy, with partial to complete loss of vision within 15-20 years if untreated.

Treatment: Long-term treatment with miotics: beta-adrenergic blocking agents (timolol, levobunolol, metipranolol), epinephrine, or pilocarpine. Laser surgery (trabeculectomy) may be undertaken in refractory cases to improve drainage.

Narrow Angle Glaucoma

Acute onset of unilateral ocular pain and visual loss due to sudden obstruction of the outflow of aqueous humor.

Cause: Predisposing: A narrow anterior chamber angle (more common in the elderly, in persons with hypermetropia, and in Asians). Precipitating: Prolonged dilatation of the pupil, such as occurs in a darkened theater or after administration of certain drugs (anticholinergic medicines orally, mydriatic drops for eye examination).

History: Sudden onset of pain in one eye, with blurring of vision, halos around lights; often nausea, vomiting, and abdominal pain.

Physical Examination: Redness of the eye, steamy cornea, dilated nonreactive pupil.

Diagnostic Tests: Tonometry shows markedly elevated intraocular pressure.

Course: Severe and permanent visual loss occurs if acute glaucoma is not promptly treated.

Treatment: I.V. acetazoleamide and mannitol are administered to reduce intraocular pressure. Laser iridectomy (destruction of a wedge of iris) permits drainage of the anterior chamber. The unaffected eye is usually operated on prophylactically as well.

CATARACT

An ocular lens that has become cloudy or opaque because of intrinsic physical or chemical change.

Causes: Largely unknown. Infantile cataracts occur after maternal rubella or when the child has galactosemia. Cataract can occur in various systemic diseases (diabetes mellitus, hypoparathyroidism) or as a complication of other ocular disease (uveitis, glaucoma) or injury (penetrating injury of the lens, ionizing radiation). The most common type is senile cataract, occurring as part of aging, with onset after age 50. The risk is increased by cigarette smoking.

History: Gradual painless loss of vision, not improved by glasses, and seeing rings or halos around lights at night.

Physical Examination: Inspection confirms the presence of partial or complete opacity of one or both lenses. A fully developed cataract, with severe impairment of vision, is called "ripe." Slit lamp examination gives more precise information about the type, extent, and location of lenticular opacity.

Course: Without treatment the entire lens eventually becomes opaque and vision is lost. Surgery restores vision at any stage by removing the lens.

Treatment: Surgical removal of the opaque lens by a variety of techniques, leaving the posterior capsule of the lens intact. Surgical extraction is now less frequently used than fragmentation with ultrasound (phacoemulsification). A synthetic lens is usually implanted at the time of cataract extraction.

DISORDERS OF THE RETINA

Retinopathy

A general term for degenerative disorders of the retina, usually accompanied by loss of vision and often due to systemic disease. Two types will be discussed here.

Hypertensive Retinopathy

Degenerative retinal changes due to impairment of blood supply to the retina and choroid in persons with very high, or chronic, hypertension, with variable degrees of visual loss. Chronic hypertension accelerates the development of arteriosclerosis, and many of the physical findings are due to vascular changes. The Keith-Wagener-Barker classification is often used to grade funduscopic observations:

- Grade I: Focal or diffuse narrowing of retinal arterioles, with reduction of the arteriole-venule ratio (AV ratio; normally 4:5) to 3:4 or 1:2; narrowed arterioles may be described as having a copper-wire or silver-wire appearance.
- Grade II: Further narrowing of arterioles, with reduction of the AV ratio to 1:2 or 1:3; crossing phenomena or AV nicking (tapering of a venule where an arteriole crosses it).
- Grade III: All of the above, with "flame" (flame-shaped) hemorrhages and cotton wool spots (exudates); these are fluffy opaque zones of degenerative change following microscopic infarction and hemorrhage in the retina.
- Grade IV: All of the above, with papilledema.

Close observation of the changes of hypertensive retinopathy is of value in judging hypertensive vascular damage elsewhere in the body. There is no treatment.

Diabetic Retinopathy

Degenerative vascular changes in the retina occurring in diabetes mellitus, particularly in poorly controlled diabetes; the principal cause of legal blindness before age 65.

Two forms are recognized. In proliferative retinopathy there is formation of new blood vessels (neovascularization) in the retina, with visual loss and a risk of vitreous hemorrhage and retinal tears. The condition is detected by fluorescein angiography and treated by laser photocoagulation (occasionally, surgery).

In nonproliferative retinopathy, changes are limited to venous dilatation, microaneurysms (appearing as tiny red spots adjacent to vessels), retinal hemorrhages and hard (sharp-bordered) exudates, and retinal edema. Waning, partially resolved retinal edema leaves folds or tucks in the retina, which appear as whitish streaks, often arranged in fanlike configurations. A complete encirclement of the macula by radially disposed streaks constitutes a macular "star figure." Visual impairment correlates poorly with extent of disease. Laser coagulation is the usual treatment. Maintaining good control of diabetes reduces the risk of severe retinopathy.

Macular Degeneration

Age-related loss of central vision due to atrophic or exudative changes in the macula lutea of the retina. Onset is usually after age 50 and the condition typically progresses to complete loss of central vision (legal blindness), with preservation of peripheral vision and the ability to walk and recognize familiar faces and objects. Medical and surgical treatment are ineffectual.

Retinitis Pigmentosa

An inherited degenerative disorder of the retina, causing progressive visual loss beginning usually in childhood. Ophthalmoscopic examination shows edema of the disk and scattered spiderlike patches of pigment in the retina. There is no effective treatment.

Retinal Detachment

Separation of the retina from the choroid as a result of trauma or degenerative changes, particularly in older persons. Myopia and cataract surgery predispose to detachment. The patient experiences visual disturbances (blurring, visual field defects) and may report seeing a curtain floating in the field of the affected eye. The problem tends to be progressive and may lead to complete blindness if the macula becomes separated. Ophthalmoscopic examination shows one or more free margins of retina floating in the vitreous, and sometimes tears in the retina. Treatment is by retinopexy—reattachment with cryotherapy applied to the sclera opposite the site of detachment or laser coagulation applied to free retinal margins. Placement of the detached segment may be facilitated by injection of gas under slight pressure into the cavity of the vitreous humor. Occasionally open surgery is required.

DISORDERS OF OCULAR MOVEMENT

Strabismus

A disorder of ocular motility in which the two eyes do not look in exactly the same direction, and cerebral fusion of their images into a three-dimensional one cannot occur.

Heterophoria is a transient deviation of one eye from the normal position with respect to the other. It may occur as a slight congenital weakness or imbalance of ocular muscles that becomes symptomatic only when the patient is fatigued. Other causes include fever, alcohol, and drug use. Inward deviation of one eye is called esophoria, outward deviation is called exophoria, and normal positioning of both eyes is called orthophoria.

Heterotropia is a persistent deviation of one or both eyes, due to congenital ocular muscle weakness or imbalance. Inward deviation is called esotropia, outward deviation exotropia. If one eye is consistently affected, central suppression of its image eventually occurs, with resulting amblyopia (dulling of vision that cannot be corrected with a lens). Treatment of heterotropia must be carried out before amblyopia has developed. Treatment consists of prismatic lenses that permit images to fuse, occlusion of one eye to preserve the vision of the other, exercises to improve strength and coordination of ocular muscles, and surgery to bring the eyes into line.

Paralytic strabismus results from paralysis of one or more eye muscles due to congenital abnormality, trauma, infection, multiple sclerosis, herpes zoster, neoplasm, or hemorrhage. Surgical treatment may be helpful in selected cases.

Nystagmus refers to involuntary rhythmic movements of the eyes, typically bilateral, due to congenital abnormality, multiple sclerosis, or central nervous system tumor, infection, or hemorrhage, or intoxication (chronic alcoholism). Transitory nystagmus occurs after riding on a merry-go-round or in the presence of vertigo. There is no treatment for nystagmus.

VISUAL IMPAIRMENT

Emmetropia: Normal vision.

Hyperopia (farsightedness): The focus of light rays passing into the eyes lies behind the retina, due to a congenitally short anteroposterior diameter of the eyeball. Treatment is with corrective lenses.

Myopia (nearsightedness): The focus of light rays passing into the eye lies in front of, rather than on, the retina, because of a congenitally long anteroposterior diameter of the eyeball. This condition, much commoner than the preceding, shows a familial tendency and when severe it predisposes to glaucoma. Treatment is with corrective lenses.

Astigmatism: The image falling on the retina is distorted because the curvature of the cornea is not the same in all axes (that is, the cornea is not spherical). Correction is with lenses having a cylindrical curvature to neutralize the effect of corneal distortion.

Presbyopia: Loss of normal accommodation with aging, due to diminished elasticity of the lens, with inability to focus on objects or print near to the eye. Treatment is with corrective lenses for reading. Persons with myopia as well as presbyopia require bifocals or even trifocals to provide a choice of focal distances.

QUESTIONS FOR STUDY AND REVIEW

1. Name and describe four ocular symptoms or signs that are due to intrinsic eye disease:

    a. _____

    b. _____

    c. _____

    d. _____

2. Name and describe four ocular symptoms or signs that are due to neurologic or systemic disease:

    a. _____

    b. _____

    c. _____

    d. _____

3. What is the anatomic boundary between the aqueous humor and the vitreous humor?

    _____

    _____

4. What is the anatomic boundary between the anterior chamber and the posterior chamber?

    _____

    _____

5. Define or explain these terms:

    a. canthus _____

    _____

    b. fundus _____

    _____

    c. keratitis _____

    _____

    d. lacrimation _____

    _____

    e. ptosis_____

    _____

    f. retinopathy _____

    _____

g. scotoma _____

_____

h. slit lamp _____

_____

6. List three disorders limited to the eye that can cause blindness:

a. _____

b. _____

c. _____

7. List three systemic conditions that can cause blindness:

a. _____

b. _____

c. _____

8. Name and describe three abnormalities of vision:

a. _____

_____

b. _____

_____

c. _____

_____

9. Name and describe three malfunctions of extraocular muscles:

a. _____

_____

b. _____

_____

c. _____

_____

CASE STUDY: YOU'RE THE DOCTOR

Emma Townsend is a 57-year-old African-American woman who consults you, her ophthalmologist, about monocular visual impairment of 4-5 days' duration.

About 4 days ago she noted blurred vision in the left eye when reading the evening paper. She attributed this to being tired, but as it continued and became worse during the next 48 hours, she called your office and was advised to come in at once. She denies ocular pain, itching, discharge, flashes of light, and photophobia. She has been seen by you annually for the past 6 years for regular eye checkups. She takes metformin for type 2 diabetes mellitus and lisinopril for mild hypertension. Her blood sugar is under good control and her cholesterol and triglycerides have not been elevated. She has worn glasses, primarily for reading, for the past 10 years but has had no ocular problems except early cataracts. Your examinations in the past have not shown evidence of diabetic retinopathy.

1. What diagnostic considerations does this chief complaint raise?

Ms. Townsend is alert and normally oriented, and seems her usual self. You note nothing unusual in her general appearance. External examination of both eyes shows no conjunctival injection, lid edema, or photophobia. The pupils are round, regular, and symmetrically reactive to light (both directly and consensually) and to accommodation. The anterior chamber is clear. Both lenses show early cataract, as on prior examinations. Funduscopic examination shows slight retinal edema in the inferior nasal quadrant of the left retina, but no vascular changes, pigmentary abnormalities, microaneurysms, hemorrhages, or exudates. The optic disks are normal, without marginal blurring or abnormal cupping. The macular areas appear normal.

2. What additional clues does this additional history give you as to why she is noting visual impairment lately?

Slit lamp examination shows the refractive media to be clear, except for bilateral nuclear cataracts, already noted. A refraction performed earlier by a technician has shown markedly diminished near and distant vision in the left eye that could not be corrected by lenses. A visual field examination shows a significant scotoma in the superior temporal quadrant of the left field.

3. At this point do you begin to suspect that you have missed something in Ms. Townsend's history? Why or why not?

_____

_____

_____

_____

_____

4. Which of the following diagnoses, if any, is/are now highly likely? Rank them in order of likelihood:

___ a. iritis

___ b. detached retina

___ c. acute narrow-angle glaucoma

___ d. intracranial tumor affecting the left occipital cortex

___ e. pituitary tumor affecting the left optic nerve

___ f. hypertensive retinopathy

___ g. proliferative diabetic retinopathy

___ h. migraine equivalent

___ i. toxic effect of lisinopril

___ j. hysterical blindness

5. What are the reasons for your choice(s)?

_____

_____

_____

_____

_____

_____

_____

_____

_____

_____

You advise Ms. Townsend that she has a significant visual defect for which you are unable to find an explanation. You arrange for her to be seen the same afternoon by a retinal specialist. Fluorescein angiography shows chorioretinitis with neovascularization, presumed to be due to histoplasmosis. Laser photocoagulation arrests the process and when you next see Ms. Townsend for a regular examination her visual acuity is essentially the same as it was before her episode of visual blurring.

6. What do you predict for this patient's future?

_____

_____

_____

_____

_____

SUGGESTIONS FOR ADDITIONAL LEARNING ACTIVITIES

1. Compile a list of terms from the sections on the Signs and Symptoms of Ocular Disease, Diagnostic Procedures in Ophthalmology, and Visual Impairment. Add the names of other ocular diseases discussed in this chapter to this list. Have someone else rearrange the letters in each term in order to provide you with a challenging word scramble puzzle.

2. A game of musical chairs is a fun way to add the learning-enhancing effects of music to a study session. Write the questions from the end of this chapter on slips of paper or index cards. You will need at least one question per participant for each game. As music plays, pass questions to your right until the music stops. Then find the answer before the music begins to play again.

3. Arrange a meeting with your regular vision care provider or an optometrist or ophthalmologist in your community. Write down your questions in advance to make the best use of time. Ask about the type of ocular diseases encountered on a regular basis as well as less common conditions, their typical treatment, and information on early diagnosis and prevention. Compare the information you gather in your interview with the material in your textbook. What new information did you learn?

19

Diseases of the Nervous System

(Outline continued on next page)

LEARNING OBJECTIVES

Upon completion of this chapter, you should be able to

- describe the basic anatomy and physiology of the nervous system;

- explain diagnostic procedures and treatments used in neurologic disease;

- classify common diseases affecting the nervous system by their signs, symptoms, and treatment.

DISEASES OF THE NERVOUS SYSTEM
(continued)

INFECTIONS OF THE CENTRAL NERVOUS SYSTEM
Encephalitis
Brain Abscess
Meningitis

NEOPLASMS OF THE CENTRAL NERVOUS SYSTEM
Benign Brain Tumors
Malignant Brain Tumors

HEADACHE
Migraine
Cluster Headache

EPILEPSY

TRANSIENT ISCHEMIC ATTACK AND STROKE
Transient Ischemic Attack (TIA)
Stroke (Brain Attack, Cerebrovascular
Accident, CVA)

ALTERED CONSCIOUSNESS

PERIPHERAL NEUROPATHY
Mononeuritis
Bell Palsy
Polyneuritis

QUESTIONS FOR STUDY AND REVIEW

DISEASES OF THE NERVOUS SYSTEM

ANATOMY AND PHYSIOLOGY OF THE NERVOUS SYSTEM

The nervous system is an exceedingly complex arrangement of nerve cells and their fibers that extends throughout the body and receives, processes, and interprets sensory stimuli; initiates and coordinates voluntary muscular movement; regulates autonomic processes such as heartbeat, vascular constriction and dilatation, bronchiolar caliber, sweating, and gastrointestinal secretion and motility; carries out complex mental functions and operations including memory and recall of past events, recognition of persons and objects, abstract reasoning and practical problem solving, judgment, and language production and comprehension; and is the seat of mood and emotions.

All nerve tissue is made up of nerve cells and their processes. Although nerve cells vary widely in structure and function, all conform to a basic pattern. (See Figure 22.) Each nerve cell (neuron) consists of a cell body containing a nucleus; one or more short treelike processes, called dendrites; and a single long, straight process, the axon. Dendrites conduct nerve impulses toward the cell body, and are therefore called afferent processes; axons conduct impulses away from the cell, and are therefore called efferent processes. The point of contact between processes of two different cells is called a synapse. Chemical substances called neurotransmitters are produced in infinitesimal quantities at nerve endings, and serve to transmit nerve impulses, either stimulating or inhibiting, across the synapse.

The transmission of impulses along a nerve fiber is an electrical event, but it does not occur in the same way as the transmission of electrical current through a wire. The external membrane of a nerve cell is polarized—that is, it is positively charged on the outside and negatively charged on the inside, the voltage difference being in the range of 50-100 mV (millivolts). The passage of a nerve impulse along a nerve fiber is actually a very rapid wave of depolarization, followed immediately by a restoration of the original polarity (repolarization).

The axons of some nerve cells are enveloped in a thin layer of fatty white material called myelin. The myelin sheath serves as an electrical insulator. Nerve tissue consisting of many myelinated fibers is called

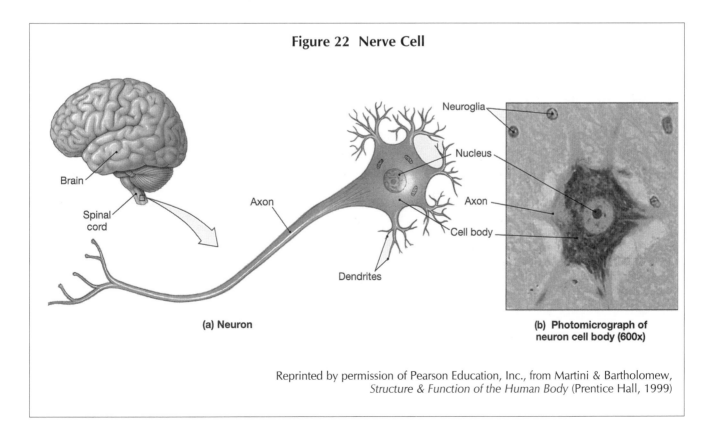

Figure 22 Nerve Cell

(a) Neuron

(b) **Photomicrograph of neuron cell body (600x)**

Reprinted by permission of Pearson Education, Inc., from Martini & Bartholomew, *Structure & Function of the Human Body* (Prentice Hall, 1999)

Figure 23 Cerebrum

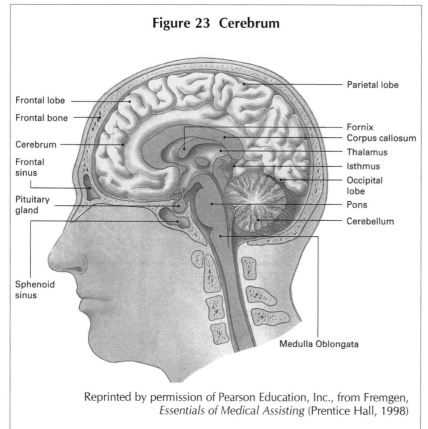

Reprinted by permission of Pearson Education, Inc., from Fremgen, *Essentials of Medical Assisting* (Prentice Hall, 1998)

white matter; tissue consisting chiefly of nerve cell bodies is called gray matter.

The nervous system is divided into two major sections: the central nervous system, consisting of the brain and spinal cord; and the peripheral nervous system, consisting of the peripheral motor and sensory nerves and the autonomic nervous system. The brain, which entirely fills the cranial cavity, is traditionally broken down into major parts on the basis of gross anatomic features:

The **cerebrum**, made up of two symmetric hemispheres and concerned with the higher mental processes; its surface, the cerebral cortex, is thrown into deep convolutions like the kernel of a walnut. The convexities (raised areas) are called gyri, and the grooves between them are called sulci. Deeper grooves (fissures) divide each hemisphere into four lobes: frontal, temporal, parietal, and occipital. (See Figure 23.)

The **cerebellum** lies behind the cerebrum and looks like a smaller version of it, as its name implies. Its principal function is coordination of voluntary motor activity.

Four structures—diencephalon, mesencephalon or midbrain, pons, and medulla oblongata—

compose, from front to back, the ventral surface of the brain; the last two make up the brain stem. The medulla continues below the skull as the spinal cord.

The brain and spinal cord are covered by three protective membranes called meninges. The outer membrane, the dura mater, is in contact with the bony interior of the skull and spinal column. Within the dura is the delicate arachnoid membrane, and within that is the pia mater, which lies on the surface of the brain and spinal cord. (See Figure 24.)

Various types of non-nerve cells, known collectively as neuroglia, serve a supporting and protective function in nervous tissue, particularly in the central nervous system. These include astroglia, oligodendroglia, microglia, and ependyma, some of which are phagocytic and participate in the repair of injury.

Within the cerebrum and the diencephalon is a system of communicating hollow chambers (the two lateral ventricles, the third ventricle, and the fourth ventricle). Cerebrospinal fluid (CSF) is a watery medium that is both formed and reabsorbed within the skull, and serves primarily as a shock absorber. It surrounds the brain and spinal cord in the subarachnoid space and also fills the ventricular system and the hollow central canal of the spinal cord.

Figure 24 Meninges

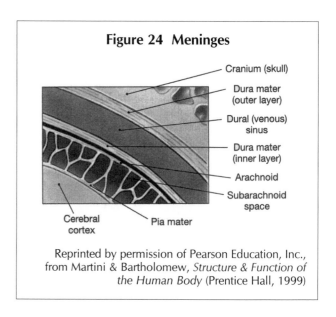

Reprinted by permission of Pearson Education, Inc., from Martini & Bartholomew, *Structure & Function of the Human Body* (Prentice Hall, 1999)

Twelve pairs of **cranial nerves** (traditionally represented by roman numerals) emerge from the ventral surface of the brain and brain stem and serve important sensory and motor functions, chiefly within the head (See Figure 25):

I. **Olfactory**: Sense of smell.

II. **Optic**: Vision.

III. **Oculomotor**: Innervates four of the six extra-ocular muscles and also the ciliary body, the iris, and the upper eyelid.

IV. **Trochlear**: Innervates the superior oblique muscle of the eye.

V. **Trigeminal**: Sensory nerve supply to the face, nose, and mouth; motor supply to the muscles of mastication.

VI. **Abducens**: Innervates lateral rectus muscle of eye.

VII. **Facial**: Motor supply to the muscles of facial expression; also stimulation of tear and salivary glands; some sensory functions, including taste on the anterior two-thirds of the tongue.

VIII. **Vestibulocochlear**: Hearing and equilibrium.

IX. **Glossopharyngeal**: Motor and sensory branches to the ear, tongue, and throat; taste sensation from the posterior third of the tongue.

X. **Vagus**: Sensory fibers to the ear, tongue, and throat; motor fibers to thoracic and abdominal viscera.

XI. **Accessory (spinal accessory)**: Motor innervation of two voluntary muscles of the neck: trapezius and sternocleidomastoid.

XII. **Hypoglossal**: Motor innervation of the tongue.

The **spinal cord** is made up largely of axons of nerve cells, some with cell bodies in the brain (carrying motor impulses to various spinal segments) and others with cell bodies in the cord itself (carrying sensory impulses from spinal segments to various brain centers). Whereas the visible surface of the cerebral cortex is made up of gray matter (cell bodies), with white matter inside, in the spinal cord the white matter, consisting of ascending and descending myelinated nerve fibers, is on the outside, and the gray matter is within. (See Figure 26.)

The peripheral nervous system comprises all nerve tissue outside the brain and spinal cord. Its two major divisions are the spinal nerves and the autonomic nervous system. Spinal nerves are those that originate in the spinal cord and pass between pairs of vertebrae to supply the body with sensation and voluntary motor power. There are 31 sets of spinal nerves, one arising from each spinal segment; these segments correspond closely to the cervical, dorsal, lumbar, and (fused) sacral vertebrae.

Each spinal segment gives off a pair of nerve roots on each side: a dorsal (sensory) root and a ventral (motor) root. Each dorsal root has a visible node or swelling (ganglion) containing cell bodies of sensory nerves. The dorsal and ventral roots fuse to form segmental nerves, which pass forward around the body and give off branches to all external surfaces and internal structures, particularly muscles of the trunk and extremities.

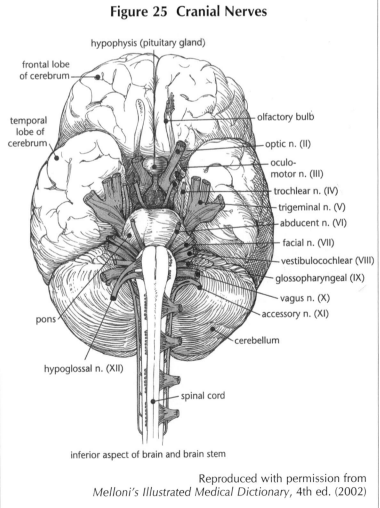

Figure 25 Cranial Nerves

hypophysis (pituitary gland)

frontal lobe of cerebrum

olfactory bulb

optic n. (II)

oculo-motor n. (III)

trochlear n. (IV)

temporal lobe of cerebrum

trigeminal n. (V)

abducent n. (VI)

facial n. (VII)

vestibulocochlear (VIII)

glossopharyngeal (IX)

vagus n. (X)

accessory n. (XI)

cerebellum

pons

hypoglossal n. (XII)

spinal cord

inferior aspect of brain and brain stem

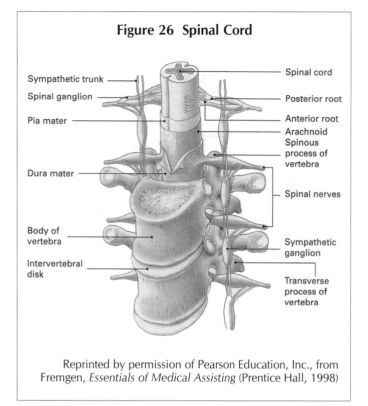

Figure 26 Spinal Cord

Sympathetic trunk
Spinal ganglion
Pia mater
Dura mater
Body of vertebra
Intervertebral disk

Spinal cord
Posterior root
Anterior root
Arachnoid
Spinous process of vertebra
Spinal nerves
Sympathetic ganglion
Transverse process of vertebra

Reprinted by permission of Pearson Education, Inc., from Fremgen, *Essentials of Medical Assisting* (Prentice Hall, 1998)

Each visible and named peripheral nerve is a bundle of thousands of myelinated axons of motor neurons whose cell bodies lie in the brain and spinal cord, and of dendrites of sensory nerves, whose cell bodies are located in the dorsal root ganglia. Motor nerves send signals to voluntary muscles throughout the body. Sensory nerves carry impulses from sensory structures in the skin that respond to pain, pressure, light touch, hot, and cold; from visceral sensors that respond to pressure or stretching and pain; and from proprioceptive sensors in voluntary muscles that signal the brain as to their position, tension, and movement.

The **autonomic nervous system** is a purely motor system concerned with automatic or involuntary activities or processes, such as heart rate and digestion. The bodily effects of emotion (tachycardia, sweating, pallor, sense of constriction in the chest) largely result from the actions of the autonomic nervous system.

Nerves of the sympathetic or thoracolumbar division of the autonomic nervous system arise from a series of ganglia lying along each side of the thoracic and lumbar segments of the spinal cord, but outside the spinal column. These communicate with the spinal cord and with one another by both myelinated and nonmyelinated fibers. The **sympathetic**

nervous system is concerned with the so-called fight or flight response mediated by epinephrine and norepinephrine. Nerves of the sympathetic division are distributed to the eye, where they cause pupillary dilatation; the heart, where they increase the pulse rate; the lungs, where they cause bronchodilatation; and the skin, where they constrict blood vessels, stimulate secretion of sweat, and cause erection of hairs. (See Figure 27.)

The **parasympathetic** or craniosacral division of the autonomic nervous system provides motor innervation to cranial, thoracic, abdominal, and pelvic viscera, generally of an opposite nature to sympathetic innervation. That is, parasympathetic activity occurs chiefly during periods of rest or quiet, and is associated with cardiac rate and with such physiologic processes as gastrointestinal secretion and motility and sexual activity.

Parasympathetic nerves arise only from the brain and from sacral segments of the spinal cord. Three cranial nerves (III, VII, and IX) send parasympathetic fibers to structures in the head (iris, ciliary body, salivary glands; a fourth (X) sends fibers to thoracic, abdominal, and pelvic viscera (heart, lungs, digestive system). Parasympathetic nerves from sacral segments of the spinal cord supply the urinary tract and reproductive system.

SIGNS AND SYMPTOMS OF NEUROLOGIC DISEASE

Altered level of consciousness, varying from slight drowsiness or inattentiveness to confusion and disorientation to deep coma from which the subject cannot be aroused by any stimulus.

Syncope (fainting): Sudden loss of consciousness, usually transitory, due to circulatory or neurologic abnormality, including central nervous system intoxication or injury, but frequently the result of strong emotion in the absence of organic disease.

Amnesia: Loss of memory, recent, remote, or total.

Aphasia: Impairment of the ability to communicate through spoken or written language, or to understand spoken or written language, or both.

Pain: Sensed at or near the body surface, usually burning or stinging (causalgia) or like an electric shock, due to irritation or inflammation of nerves.

Hypesthesia: Partial loss of sensation on one or more parts of the body surface.

Anesthesia: Total loss of sensation on one or more parts of the body surface.

Paresthesia: A sense of tingling or prickling ("pins and needles") on a part of the body surface. The lay term "numbness" may be applied indiscriminately to hypesthesia, anesthesia, and paresthesia.

Headache: Local or generalized, intermittent or constant; can result from infection, neoplasm, or hemorrhage within the cranium, obstruction to the flow of cerebrospinal fluid, trauma, or migraine.

Dysequilibrium: Loss of balance sense; tendency to fall without support.

Vertigo: A subjective sense of spinning. Dysequilibrium and vertigo sometimes occur together, and both may referred to indiscriminately as "dizziness" by the laity.

Muscle weakness (paresis) or complete loss of function (paralysis), local or widespread. Paralysis is divided into flaccid (absence of muscle tone and absence of reflexes) and spastic (muscles tight, with resistance to manipulation and hyperactive reflexes).

Spasm: Sustained contraction, usually painful, of a voluntary muscle.

Tremors: Shaking of parts of the body supplied by voluntary muscles, principally the arms, forearms, and hands. Tremors are divided into resting (occurring only when the affected muscles are not being used for purposeful activity) and intention (occurring only during voluntary movement).

Tic: A rapid involuntary muscle twitch, typically recurrent and stereotyped, affecting one or several body areas.

Chorea: Rapid, jerky, purposeless involuntary movements of one or several muscle groups.

Athetosis: Slow, writhing involuntary movements of the face or limbs.

Figure 27 Autonomic Nervous System

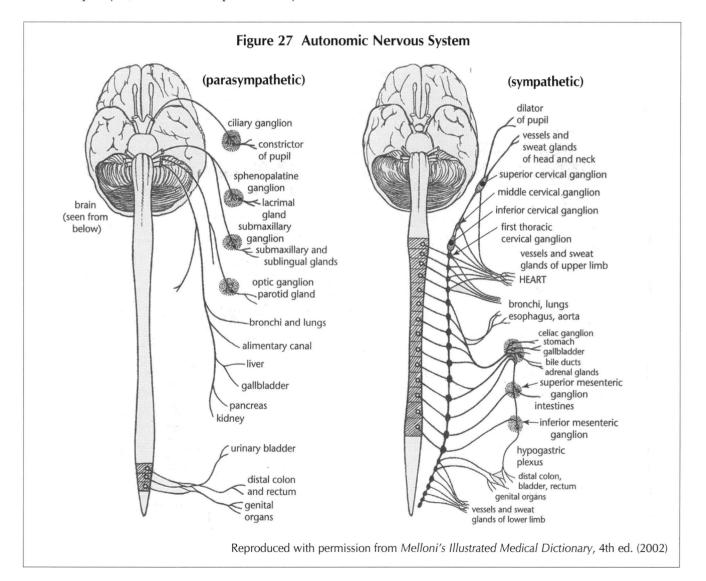

Reproduced with permission from *Melloni's Illustrated Medical Dictionary*, 4th ed. (2002)

Incoordination: Jerkiness and awkwardness in activities requiring smooth coordination of several muscles.

Ataxia: Impairment of complex movements due to loss of proprioceptive impulses from the muscles of the trunk or limbs.

Seizures: Sudden, transitory impairment of central nervous system function, with or without loss of consciousness, and with or without local or generalized contractions of voluntary muscles.

Many other signs and symptoms (visual and hearing impairment, vomiting, disturbance in bowel or bladder function, personality change) often prove to be due to diseases of the central nervous system. Mental disorders are discussed in the next chapter.

DIAGNOSTIC PROCEDURES IN NEUROLOGY

The basic diagnostic procedure in diseases of the nervous system is the neurologic examination, a standardized set of observations and tests performed with the physician's eyes, ears, and hands or with simple instruments. The neurologic examination is modified as dictated by the patient's complaints and condition at the time of examination. (A comatose patient cannot be expected to follow directions or stand and walk.) The following are the essential elements of the basic neurologic examination.

Mental Status Examination: Assessment of the subject's appearance, level of consciousness, mood, orientation, language ability, memory, reasoning capacity, and other elements of mental function. The mental status examination is fully discussed in the next chapter.

Cranial Nerve Examination: A systematic examination of the sensory and motor functions of the **twelve cranial nerves**.

I. **Olfactory**: Testing sense of smell in each nostril with familiar substances such as coffee or cinnamon. This assessment is often omitted, hence the frequent expression, "Cranial nerves II through XII are intact."

II. **Optic**: Testing the subject's vision with standard eye charts. Checking peripheral vision and visual fields by simple techniques. Examination of the ocular fundi with an ophthalmoscope.

III. **Oculomotor**: Testing ocular movements; observing for strabismus, nystagmus, and drooping of eyelids. Testing the ability of the pupil to constrict when stimulated by light and when focused on a near object.

IV. **Trochlear**: (Extraocular movements have already been assessed.)

V. **Trigeminal**: Sensitivity to light touch (wisp of cotton or fine brush) and pain (sterile needle) are tested over the skin of the face. The blink reflex to touching the cornea with cotton is also tested. The integrity of motor branches to the muscles of mastication is tested by having the subject open the mouth wide, and then clench the teeth together.

VI. **Abducens**: (Extraocular movements have already been assessed.)

VII. **Facial**: Testing muscles of facial expression by having the subject wrinkle the forehead, close the eyes tightly, retract the lips so as to show the teeth, and purse the lips as for whistling. Taste on the front part of the tongue may be tested.

VIII. **Vestibulocochlear**: Cold caloric test: when ice-water is poured into the ear canal, a normal vestibular apparatus causes nystagmus with the quick component to the opposite side. Hearing is tested in each ear separately.

IX. **Glossopharyngeal**: With impairment of innervation to one side of the palate, the uvula deviates to the normal side, particularly during the gag reflex. Swallowing is affected by impairment of either the ninth or the tenth cranial nerve.

X. **Vagus**: The subject's ability to speak and to swallow is observed.

XI. **Accessory**: The subject's ability to push against the examiner's hand with each side of the chin indicates integrity of the nerve supply to the sternocleidomastoid and trapezius muscles.

XII. **Hypoglossal**: The examiner notes the symmetry of development of the tongue muscles at rest and the symmetry of movement when the tongue is protruded. Impairment of a hypoglossal nerve causes deviation of the tongue to the affected side.

Spinal Nerve Examination: Sensory innervation of the skin is assessed by testing the subject's ability to recognize light touch (wisp of cotton), pain (sterile needle), hot and cold (test tubes of hot and cold water) on various parts of the body surface. Examination may include tests of stereognosis (ability to recognize the shape of an object by handling it), vibratory sense (ability to sense the vibration of a tuning fork when the stem is placed on a bone near the surface, such as the elbow or the shin), two-point discrimination (ability to distinguish two points close together on the skin). Proprioception is tested by having the subject report whether a toe or finger is moved up or down by the examiner, and by observation of stance and gait. The Romberg test (having the subject stand with feet together and eyes open, then eyes closed) assesses position sense in the trunk and legs.

Motor innervation is tested by observation of muscle development, tone, and voluntary movement in the trunk and limbs, with comparison of the two sides. The examiner notes any wasting, paralysis, spasm or rigidity, or involuntary movements (tremors, tics, chorea, athetosis). Coordination is tested by having the subject perform rapidly alternating movements with the hands or feet. The finger-to-nose and heel-to-shin tests and tandem walking are other ways of judging coordination.

Reflexes: A reflex is a muscular contraction occurring in response to a sensory stimulus. All the nerve cells and fibers involved in a reflex are located in a spinal cord segment, and its sensory and motor roots form a so-called reflex arc; the brain is not involved.

Muscle stretch (deep tendon) reflexes occur in response to sudden stretching of a muscle, usually induced by tapping a tendon with a rubber-headed reflex hammer. Tendon reflexes are tested in several muscles of the upper and lower extremities, with comparison of the two sides.

Superficial (cutaneous) reflexes are muscle contractions in response to stroking the skin; those of the abdominal wall are tested as part of a complete neurologic examination.

Pathologic reflexes are present only in neurologic disorders. The Babinski reflex consists of dorsiflexion of the great toe and flaring of the other toes in response to stroking of the sole of the foot toward the toes. The Chaddock reflex is the same response to stroking of the side of the foot toward the toes. These and similar pathologic reflexes, along with spastic paralysis and rigidity, indicate an upper motor neuron lesion—interruption of motor tracts running between the cerebral cortex and the spinal segment involved, without any impairment of the reflex arc. Flaccid paralysis, absence of normal and abnormal reflexes, and muscle wasting indicate a lower motor neuron lesion—interruption of motor tracts running between the spinal cord and one or more muscles.

Other diagnostic procedures: Besides physical examination, the physician may use other diagnostic procedures to gain more detailed or accurate information about nervous system integrity and function.

Lumbar puncture: Withdrawal of a specimen of cerebrospinal fluid from the subarachnoid space by inserting a needle between two vertebrae (usually L4 and L5) at the lower end of the spinal cord. A manometer (graduated glass tube) is used to measure the pressure of the fluid at the beginning of the procedure (opening pressure) and the end (closing pressure). Specimens of fluid are examined microscopically (stained smear) for cells (neutrophils and lymphocytes) and pathogenic microorganisms; chemically for glucose, protein, and other substances; by culture for bacterial pathogens; and, if indicated, serologically for evidence of syphilis, Lyme disease, or other infections and by cytologic techniques for malignant cells. Normal CSF is water-clear. Xanthochromia (yellowness) of the fluid suggests recent but not current hemorrhage. Frank blood in the specimen may indicate subarachnoid hemorrhage but may also be due to local injury by the needle (traumatic tap).

Electroencephalography (EEG): Measurement and recording of electrical activity of the brain. Recording electrodes are attached at standard sites on the scalp and wires from the electrodes conduct detected electrical impulses to a processer that generates a record as a continuous wave on a strip of moving paper. Tracings are usually made after administration of a short-acting sedative (with the subject asleep, if possible). The effects of hyperventilation and of photic stimulation (exposure to a flashing light) are recorded also. The EEG is particularly useful in identifying and classifying seizure disorders and in localizing or monitoring certain other CNS disorders (neoplasms, infarction).

Imaging studies include CT scan (with or without intravenous injection of contrast medium), MRI, and standard x-ray views of the skull. Angiography may be used to show cranial vasculature with injected contrast medium. In digital subtraction angiography, x-ray images of the head with and without contrast medium are processed by a computer, which deletes all shadows common to both films (skull bones, soft tissue profiles and interfaces), leaving only the vascular system visible. Myelography is visualization of the spinal canal (the tubular enclosure of the spinal cord formed collectively by the vertebrae) by x-ray with contrast medium introduced into the subarachnoid space by lumbar puncture. In positron emission tomography (PET) and single positron emission computed tomography (SPECT), injected radioactive (positron-emitting) substances are incorporated in or metabolized by certain brain tissues; scanning of resulting gamma discharges permits formation of an image that conveys information about biochemical function of brain areas.

Electrophysiologic studies: Measurement of electrical activity in nerves and muscles. Electromyography (EMG) involves insertion of fine needle electrodes into voluntary muscles. Nerve conduction velocity (NCV) is measured by timing the passage of nerve impulses between a stimulating and a recording electrode, which are a precisely measured distance apart.

HEREDITARY AND CONGENITAL NEUROLOGIC DISORDERS

Cerebral Palsy
A nonprogressive disorder of voluntary movement and posture control, first noted at or soon after birth. A somewhat vague term for congenital neurologic impairment that is not hereditary. Most cases are due to maternal infection or drug use, difficult labor, or obstetrical complications. Symptoms vary widely in extent and severity. Most patients have spastic paralysis. About half have seizures, about half are mentally retarded, and about half die by the age of 10. Treatment is principally supportive—physical therapy, orthopedic intervention, family counseling, and the use of drugs to control spasticity.

Congenital Hydrocephalus
Enlargement of the head by excessive fluid pressure within the ventricular system, evident at birth or within the first few weeks of life.

Causes: Obstruction to the normal outflow of cerebrospinal fluid from the ventricular system due to a congenital defect, often the result of maternal infection (toxoplasmosis, rubella, cytomegalovirus, syphilis).

Physical Examination: Abnormally large circumference of the head at birth, or disproportionate increase in head size during early infancy.

Diagnostic Tests: CT scan and ultrasonography confirm ventricular enlargement and may indicate the site of obstruction.

Course: Without treatment, progressive enlargement of the ventricular system can be expected, with damage to the cerebral hemispheres and other intracranial structures.

Treatment: Surgical insertion of a shunt from the obstructed ventricular system to the right atrium of the heart or to the peritoneal cavity.

Neural Tube Defects
A group of congenital abnormalities in the development of the central nervous system during the first two months of fetal life. Some of these are associated with defects in the skull or vertebral column. The cause is generally unknown. Some defects are genetically determined, and others may be induced by maternal infection (rubella).

The risk of neural tube defects is increased by maternal deficiency of folic acid, a vitamin of the B complex. Nutritionists currently advise a daily intake of 1 mg or more of folic acid in pregnant women and in those who may become pregnant. Prenatal diagnosis of a neural tube defect can be made by the finding of elevated alpha-fetoprotein in amniotic fluid obtained by amniocentesis at or after 16 weeks of gestation.

Anencephaly: Absence of cerebral hemispheres. This condition is incompatible with life, and babies born with it typically die within hours.

Microcephaly: Abnormally small, maldeveloped cerebral hemispheres, typically associated with mental and motor retardation.

Cranium bifidum with encephalocele: Failure of the developing cranium to close in the midline either anteriorly or posteriorly, with protrusion of part of the brain through the defect. The prognosis is good with early surgical repair of the defect. A shunt procedure may be necessary to treat associated hydrocephalus.

Porencephaly: One or more cysts or cavities in a cerebral hemisphere communicating with the ventricular system. There may be little or no neurologic impairment.

Hydranencephaly: A more severe form of the preceding, with very little cerebral cortex remaining. Neurologic impairment is more severe.

Spina bifida: A failure of closure of one or more vertebrae in the posterior midline, which may be associated with bulging of meninges (meningocele) or of spinal cord and meninges (meningomyelocele). Neurologic impairment depends on the site and extent of the defect. The prognosis is good with early surgery, but paralysis present at birth cannot be reversed.

Huntington Disease (Huntington Chorea)

A genetic disorder (autosomal dominant) characterized by progressive muscle rigidity and dementia accompanied by chorea and often seizures. Onset is by age 40 and may be in childhood. Death occurs in 5-15 years.

Tourette Syndrome (Gilles de la Tourette Syndrome)

A chronic, familial motor disorder, sometimes triggered by drugs, and characterized by tics (repetitive, irregular habit spasms involving particularly the face, sometimes partially repressible) and involuntary vocal utterances, sometimes obscene. Drug therapy with haloperidol or clonidine may help control tics. Supportive counseling with attention to speech and behavior problems is crucial.

DEMYELINATING AND DEGENERATIVE DISEASES

Multiple Sclerosis (MS)

A chronic sensory and motor disorder of variable presentation, due to loss of myelin from nerve cells in the central nervous system.

Cause: Patchy deterioration of the myelin sheaths of nerve tracts in the brain and spinal cord and in the optic nerve leads to deterioration of nerve function. The cause is unknown; genetic, infectious, and autoimmune factors have been suggested. Onset is usually between 20 and 40. The incidence is higher in women and in cooler latitudes. Disease is sometimes apparently precipitated by fatigue, emotional stress, pregnancy, or viral respiratory infection.

History: Irregular, intermittent or progressive impairment of sensory or motor function: hypesthesia, paresthesia, visual disturbances, disorders of equilibrium; muscular weakness, spasticity, or unsteadiness; tremors, nystagmus, diplopia, disturbances of swallowing or bladder function.

Physical Examination: Findings on neurologic examination are typically diffuse and highly variable: hypesthesia or anesthesia, irregularly distributed muscle weakness with spasticity and hyperactive deep tendon reflexes, Babinski reflex, impaired abdominal superficial reflexes, ataxia, uncoordinated (scanning) speech, tremors, nystagmus, temporal pallor of the optic disks followed by optic atrophy, visual field defects, emotional lability.

Diagnostic Tests: The spinal fluid may show moderate lymphocytosis and elevation of immune globulins, including oligoclonal IgG globulins (antibody to myelin) not found in serum. The electroencephalogram may show nonspecific abnormalities. MRI of the brain and spinal cord shows multiple patchy lesions. Visual evoked potential testing may corroborate the diagnosis.

Course: The disease is highly unpredictable. Four patterns are distinguished: relapsing remitting, primary progressive, secondary progressive, and progressive relapsing. Presenting symptoms often remit for months or years. Typically the disease progresses gradually, with remissions and exacerbations, and eventually produces some disability. Relapses may be triggered by excessive fatigue.

Treatment: Increased rest, particularly during periods of heightened symptoms. Adrenocortical steroids often mitigate neurologic impairment, particularly during acute relapses. Physical therapy and muscle relaxants are helpful in dealing with muscle weakness and spasm. Immunotherapy, plasmapheresis, and synthetic myelin protein are among treatments currently being evaluated. Psychotherapy or counseling may be necessary.

Guillain-Barré Syndrome

A chronic inflammation of peripheral nerves, causing muscle weakness or paralysis.

Cause: Formation of autoantibody to myelin, with resultant segmental demyelination of peripheral nerve fibers, usually reversible. Precipitating causes: acute infection (influenza, infectious mononucleosis, varicella-zoster), myocardial infarction, certain vaccines, surgery.

History: Progressive, symmetric muscle weakness in both arms and legs, paresthesias, hypesthesias, and pain, coming on 1-4 weeks after the precipitating event. The cranial nerves may be involved. Loss of bladder control and respiratory paralysis may occur.

Physical Examination: Peripheral sensation is impaired and deep tendon reflexes are diminished or absent. The pulse and blood pressure may be elevated.

Diagnostic Tests: The spinal fluid contains elevated protein but normal cell counts.

Course: The case fatality rate is about 5%. About 65% of patients who recover have minor neurologic impairment and 10% remain severely disabled.

Treatment: Physical therapy; cardiac monitoring and pulse oximetry, with mechanical ventilation as needed. Intravenous immune globulin. Plasmapheresis to remove antibody from serum.

Amyotrophic Lateral Sclerosis (Lou Gehrig Disease)

Progressive paralysis and wasting of muscles due to degeneration of motor neurons.

Cause: Unknown. There is a genetic predisposition, and men are affected more than women by a ratio of 3:1. Viral or autoimmune factors cannot be excluded. Possible precipitating factors include trauma, extreme stress or fatigue, viral respiratory infection, and myocardial infarction.

History: Onset, between the ages of 30 and 50, of weakness and wasting of voluntary muscles, particularly those in the hands and feet. Fasciculations (repeated twitching of small groups of voluntary muscle fibers) may precede any other symptoms.

Eventually, with brain stem involvement, difficulty in speaking, eating, and even breathing. Depression commonly occurs with progressive deterioration.

Physical Examination: Muscle weakness and atrophy, visible fasciculations, evidence of cranial and spinal motor nerve malfunction without sensory impairment. Heightened deep tendon reflexes, spasticity, and rigidity indicate upper motor neuron degeneration.

Diagnostic Tests: Electromyography and muscle biopsy confirm loss of motor nerve supply to affected areas.

Course: Usually the disease is steadily progressive and death occurs in 2-5 years.

Treatment: Purely supportive; physical therapy, muscle relaxants; nasogastric tube or gastrostomy feedings, tracheotomy and respirator as needed.

Myasthenia Gravis

A chronic disorder of neuromuscular conduction.

Cause: Formation of autoantibody to the patient's own cholinergic receptors. The disease sometimes occurs in conjunction with other autoimmune disorders (rheumatoid arthritis, systemic lupus erythematosus), tumor of the thymus, or thyroid disease. It is commoner in women and onset is usually between the ages of 20 and 40. Severe infection or pregnancy may trigger the first evidence of disease.

History: The chief symptom is rapid fatiguing of muscles, particularly ocular, facial, and pharyngeal. Repeated movements lead to progressive weakening of the muscle, which recovers after an interval of rest.

Physical Examination: Patients may have ptosis, diplopia, difficulty in chewing or swallowing, but no muscle wasting, abnormalities of reflexes, or sensory impairment.

Diagnostic Tests: Anticholinesterase agents (intravenous edrophonium or intramuscular neostigmine) dramatically but briefly improve muscle strength and resistance to fatigue. Electromyography demonstrates progressive fatigue of stimulated muscles; serologic studies detect acetylcholine receptor antibody.

Treatment: Anticholinesterase drugs (neostigmine, pyridostigmine) and, if necessary, adrenal corticosteroids. When thymic tumor is present the thymus is surgically removed. Respiratory paralysis may require mechanical ventilation. Plasmapheresis to remove autoantibodies may be effective in severe exacerbations.

Parkinsonism (Parkinson Disease, Paralysis Agitans)

A chronic, progressive neurologic disorder causing muscle tremor and rigidity.

Cause: Unknown. Neurologic symptoms are due to deterioration and dopamine depletion in certain brain nuclei (corpus striatum, globus pallidus, substantia nigra). It is more common in men and onset is usually between 45 and 65. Certain toxic chemicals (carbon disulfide, carbon monoxide), drugs (chlorpromazine, haloperidol, and other neuroleptic drugs), and a history of encephalitis can induce parkinsonian symptoms.

History: Resting tremor, initially in one extremity, that is exacerbated by emotional stress and reduced during voluntary motion. Stiffness, rigidity, and bradykinesia (slowness of movement) commonly occur, with postural instability and gait disorders.

Physical Examination: Immobile, masklike face, with infrequent blinking. Reduced automatic movements such as swinging the arms while walking. Hyperactive deep tendon reflexes and resistance to passive movement of joints, often with "cogwheel" rigidity. A flexed posture, a shuffling and seemingly hurried (festinating) gait, and difficulty in standing from a sitting position are typical. Seborrhea (excessive secretion of sebum) on the scalp and face and excessive drooling are also often seen. The handwriting becomes smaller (micrographia). There may be mild deterioration of mental function.

Course: Typically progressive, with death in about 10 years.

Treatment: Drug treatment is helpful in advanced disease: amantadine, anticholinergics (trihexyphenidyl, ethopropazine), levodopa and carbidopa, bromocriptine, and selegiline. Surgical removal of degenerating brain tissue may be a good choice in younger patients. Physical and speech therapy and counseling are important for most patients.

INFECTIONS OF THE CENTRAL NERVOUS SYSTEM

Encephalitis

Inflammation of the brain due to viral infection.

Cause: Most cases of encephalitis are due to viruses transmitted by mosquitoes (Eastern and Western equine encephalitis, Japanese B encephalitis) or ticks. Numerous other viruses (coxsackievirus, herpes simplex virus, mumps virus, HIV) can cause encephalitis.

History: Abrupt onset of fever and headache, with muscle weakness or paralysis, restlessness, personality or behavioral changes, delirium, seizures, and lethargy that may progress to coma.

Physical Examination: Fever, depressed level of consciousness, signs of meningeal irritation (see *Meningitis* below), evidence of focal or diffuse neurologic damage including tremors, paralysis, hyperreactive reflexes, and pathologic reflexes.

Diagnostic Tests: Serologic studies can identify the causative virus. The CSF shows increase of pressure, protein, and cells. Abnormal findings on EEG are nonspecific.

Course: Most cases resolve without sequelae after a few weeks, but many are followed by residual paralysis, seizures, and parkinsonism.

Treatment: Largely supportive. Physical therapy; attention to nutrition and hydration. Drug therapy as needed to provide sedation, relieve fever and headache, and control convulsions. Herpes simplex encephalitis responds to acyclovir. In severe disease, adrenal corticosteroids may reduce cerebral edema and inflammation.

Brain Abscess

An abscess can be formed in the substance of the brain by pathogens migrating from infections of the ear or nose, or by bloodborne pathogens in patients with systemic infection. The usual agents are staphylococci and streptococci. Headache and drowsiness or delirium are the presenting symptoms, followed by seizures, coma, and focal neurologic abnormality depending on the location of the lesion. CT scan, MRI, and arteriography identify and localize the mass. Treatment is with intravenous antibiotics and, usually, surgical drainage of the abscess.

Meningitis

Infection of the meninges, with neurologic and systemic effects.

Causes: Infection with bacteria (*Staphylococcus*, pneumococcus, meningococcus, *Haemophilus influenzae*, *Escherichia coli*, *Mycobacterium tuberculosis*), viruses (mumps virus, coxsackievirus, herpes simplex virus), fungi, or protozoans. Causative organisms may be introduced by a penetrating head wound, spread locally from infections of the ears or sinuses, or reach the meninges through the bloodstream from remote sites (pneumonia, endocarditis). Symptoms vary considerably with the etiologic agent; signs and symptoms are milder in viral than in bacterial meningitis, and the prognosis more favorable. Meningitis due to meningococcus (*Neisseria meningitidis*) is a rapidly progressive and highly lethal disease, particularly because the meningococcus causes a severe toxemia that can lead to shock and death, even in the absence of signs of meningitis.

History: Abrupt onset of fever, headache, and vomiting. Painful stiffness of the neck and back muscles, visual disturbances, and irritability, twitching, or seizures. Clouding of the sensorium, delirium, and coma may follow rapidly.

Physical Examination: Fever, depressed level of consciousness. Signs of meningeal irritation include nuchal rigidity (stiffness of the neck, with inability to touch the chin to the chest), painful stiffness of other muscles, hyperreflexia, Kernig sign (inability to extend the knee when the thigh is flexed), Brudzinski sign (passive flexion of the neck causes active flexion of the hip and knee). In an infant, bulging of the fontanelles.

Diagnostic Tests: Lumbar puncture shows elevated pressure. The CSF may be purulent. White blood cells and protein are elevated. In bacterial meningitis, CSF glucose is low. Smear and culture of the fluid identify bacterial agents. In viral (aseptic) meningitis the fluid is clear and the glucose is normal; viral culture may identify the cause.

Course: Without treatment, viral meningitis nearly always resolves without sequelae, and bacterial meningitis nearly always proves fatal, particularly in children and the elderly. Meningococcemia, which may occur with or without meningitis, causes a petechial rash and profound and fulminant systemic abnormalities, including widespread hemorrhages and vascular collapse, sometimes due to adrenal hemorrhage (Waterhouse-Friderichsen syndrome). Patients who have recovered from meningitis may have residual mental retardation, paralysis, or seizures.

Treatment: Meningitis is an emergency. Hospitalization and administration of intravenous antibiotics are routine. Antibiotics are started even before reports of CSF studies are available, and discontinued or changed on the basis of these studies. Antibiotics are usually continued for three weeks or longer. Supportive care, including physical therapy, attention to nutrition and hydration, artificial ventilation, and measures to control fever, reverse shock, and reduce intracranial pressure, is vitally important. Asymptomatic persons who have been closely exposed to a patient with meningogoccal meningitis receive prophylactic rifampin or ciprofloxacin to terminate the carrier state. A vaccine active against some strains of meningococcus is available.

NEOPLASMS OF THE CENTRAL NERVOUS SYSTEM

Primary neoplasms in the cranial cavity usually arise from supporting structures and tissues (meninges, neuroglia) rather than from nerve tissue. Even histologically benign neoplasms can cause severe impairment or death by compressing brain centers, particularly when they are inaccessible to surgery. Symptoms of intracranial tumor include headache (unremitting, increasingly severe, often localized), nausea and vomiting, and focal or general neurologic impairment depending on the location of the tumor (paralysis, visual defects, dysequilibrium, hearing loss). Diagnosis is by various imaging techniques, including particularly CT, MRI, and arteriography. Electroencephalography and lumbar puncture may provide important diagnostic and prognostic information. Brain tumors are treated by surgical excision when possible. Small benign tumors may be amenable to treatment with a gamma knife, a minimally invasive radiosurgical system in which a computer focuses gamma rays from a large number of radioactive cobalt sources so that they converge on the lesion. Chemotherapy and radiation are employed in the treatment of malignant tumors. Other agents (antiemetics, anticonvulsants, corticosteroids) may be prescribed for complications.

Benign Brain Tumors

Meningioma is a relatively common benign tumor, derived from meningeal cells, that grows slowly and causes symptoms by compressing adjacent structures. On CT scan it has a homogeneous appearance, and because of its rich blood supply its image is greatly enhanced after injection of contrast material. Prognosis is excellent after surgical removal. Craniopharyngioma arises in the area of the optic chiasm (crossing of optic nerve tracts on undersurface of brain) and the pituitary gland. Hence the presenting symptoms are usually visual field defects and evidence of pituitary functional impairment. Vestibular schwannoma (formerly called acoustic neurinoma) develops from nerve sheath cells of the eighth cranial nerve, and by compressing the nerve causes hearing loss, tinnitus, and vertigo.

Malignant Brain Tumors

Most primary malignancies of the brain arise from neuroglia. Astrocytoma and astroblastoma are less anaplastic than malignant gliomas. The most malignant brain tumor is glioblastoma multiforme, a highly undifferentiated and rapidly growing neoplasm that invades locally, spreads within the brain via the cerebrospinal fluid, and metastasizes outside the cranium, particularly to the cervical lymph nodes and the lungs. Surgical treatment is seldom feasible. Radiation therapy may be temporarily palliative.

Malignancies from outside the cranium that most often metastasize to the brain are those from the lung, thyroid, breast, gastrointestinal tract, and kidney.

HEADACHE

Chronic or recurrent headaches can result from numerous causes, most of them not directly related to the nervous system. The most common type of headache is due to spasm in the muscles of the scalp, brow, and neck (muscle tension headache), most commonly induced by emotional stress or fatigue. Two forms of headache originating in intracranial structures will be described here.

Migraine

Recurring severe unilateral headache with neurologic concomitants.

Cause: Unknown. Head pain is apparently related to constriction, dilatation, and throbbing of meningeal and other vessels. Chemical factors (release of vasodilator substances, depletion of plasma serotonin) probably play a part. The disease runs in families and is more common in young women, affecting about 15% of adult women in the U.S. Oral contraceptives may bring on headaches in susceptible women.

History: Recurring episodes of severe unilateral throbbing headache accompanied by nausea, vomiting, photophobia, intolerance to noise, and sometimes neurologic symptoms (diplopia, transient local anesthesia or paralysis). In migraine with aura, the patient experiences a warning symptom (aura) before the headache begins. Most often this consists of seeing flashes or zigzags of light in both eyes, usually with transitory visual field defects (scintillating scotomas). In migraine without aura, the headache may be less severe and more generalized. Headaches typically last for many hours and may be severely incapacitating. Often complete relief is not obtained until after sleep. In susceptible persons, a migraine headache may be triggered by emotional stress, fatigue, menstruation, skipping a meal, certain foods (chocolate, prepared foods containing nitrates), alcohol.

Physical Examination: Essentially normal during attacks, and entirely so between attacks.

Diagnostic Tests: Chiefly of use in ruling out more serious disorders; no specific findings.

Course: The disorder often begins in childhood and continues for many years. Depending on the presence of triggering factors, headaches may occur daily or at intervals of months or years.

Treatment: Mild analgesics sometimes help; nonsteroidal anti-inflammatory drugs (ibuprofen, naproxen) and metoclopramide are often useful. Selective serotonin receptor agonists (sumatriptan, rizatriptan, zolmitriptan) orally or by injection can abort a headache at any stage of its development. Ergotamine (orally, rectally, by injection or inhalation), with or without caffeine, frequently aborts an attack if taken immediately on the appearance of an aura. For patients who do not experience an aura, cannot take ergotamine or analgesics, or have extremely frequent headaches (one or more a week), prophylactic treatment usually provides good control. Prophylactic drugs include beta-adrenergic blocking agents (propranolol, timolol) and others (amitriptyline).

Cluster Headache

Recurrent, brief episodes of severe unilateral orbital pain, of unknown cause. Attacks may occur once or several times daily for several weeks and then abruptly cease, perhaps recurring after an interval of weeks or months. Individual headaches may be triggered by alcohol or certain foods. The disorder is most often seen in middle-aged men. Headaches often occur at night, and are accompanied by redness and watering of the eye and by nasal congestion or rhinorrhea on the affected side. Each attack lasts about 20 minutes. There are no specific findings on examination or testing. Treatment of an acute attack with ergotamine or oxygen inhalation is sometimes effective. Prophylaxis against recurring headache may be achieved with ergotamine, lithium, adrenocortical steroids, methysergide, or the drugs used for prophylaxis of migraine headache.

EPILEPSY

A neurologic disorder in which the patient experiences recurrent seizures consisting of transient disturbances of cerebral function due to paroxysmal neuronal discharge.

Causes: Seizure disorders, especially those first causing symptoms in childhood, are often idiopathic. Seizures can be induced by cerebral trauma, infection, vascular disease, neoplasms, degenerative diseases (Alzheimer disease), drugs and chemical poisons, metabolic disorders (renal failure, hypoglycemia), and, in children, high fever. In persons with idiopathic epilepsy, seizures may be triggered by physical or emotional stress, lack of sleep, fever, drugs, alcohol, alcohol withdrawal, menstruation, or flashing lights.

History: Seizures are classified on the basis of overt presentation:

Partial (only part of one cerebral cortex is involved).

Simple (no unconsciousness): Local twitching or jerking; perception of flashing lights or other abnormal sensory phenomena.

Complex (impaired alertness or unconsciousness): Sometimes with psychic symptoms or automatisms.

Generalized (entire cerebral cortex is involved).

Absence (petit mal): Brief loss of attention and perception.

Tonic-clonic (grand mal): In the tonic phase the victim becomes rigid, often cries out, loses consciousness, falls, stops breathing. In the clonic phase, the victim has generalized muscular jerking, may bite tongue or lips, may be incontinent of urine or stool. In the postictal state, after awakening, the subject is drowsy and amnesic for a variable period.

Myoclonic seizures: Repeated shocklike, often violent contractions in one or more muscle groups.

Status epilepticus: One or a series of grand mal seizures lasting more than 30 minutes without waking intervals.

Physical Examination: Between seizures there is no detectable abnormality. Signs of neurologic disease may be found in secondary epilepsy.

Diagnostic Tests: The electroencephalogram generally shows focal abnormalities in the rate, rhythm, or relative intensity of cerebral cortical rhythms, allowing diagnosis and classification of epilepsy. Laboratory studies and CT scan or MRI may be performed to rule out treatable causes of epilepsy.

Treatment: In idiopathic epilepsy, long-term treatment with anticonvulsant medicine (phenytoin, carbamazepine, valproic acid, phenobarbital, ethosuximide, and others) provides excellent control for most patients. Blood levels of medicine may require monitoring to ensure optimum dosage. Avoidance of triggering factors is important. For intractable cases, surgical treatment is sometimes successful.

TRANSIENT ISCHEMIC ATTACK AND STROKE

Transient Ischemic Attack (TIA)

Sudden onset of neurologic symptoms that resolve completely within 24 hours.

Cause: Transient interruption of blood supply to some part of the brain. Common causes include arterial blockage by an embolus (from an infected heart valve, mural thrombus, or sloughed arteriosclerotic plaque) and reduction in blood supply due to the combined effects of arterial disease (arteritis, systemic lupus erythematosus) and reduced flow (hypotension; subclavian steal syndrome, in which blockage of a subclavian artery near its origin leads to reversal of blood flow in a vertebral artery to provide collateral flow beyond the obstruction, at the expense of brain tissue normally supplied by the vertebral artery).

History: Sudden onset of focal neurologic symptoms (weakness, numbness, unilateral loss of vision, diplopia, speech disturbances, vertigo, ataxia, falling) depending on site of circulatory impairment, resolving in less than 24 hours (usually in less than 4 hours).

Physical Examination: Flaccid weakness or paralysis, hyperreflexia, Babinski reflex, hypesthesia or anesthesia, depending on site of lesion. A bruit may be heard over a stenotic subclavian artery. All neurologic signs resolve within 24 hours.

Diagnostic Tests: CT scan may be done to rule out hemorrhage. Arteriography, MR angiography, or carotid duplex ultrasonography may be used to assess the cerebral circulation. X-ray, laboratory, and electrocardiography or echocardiography may trace the underlying cause.

Course: By definition a TIA has no complications. Many patients, however, eventually have one or more strokes.

Treatment: No treatment is needed for the acute episode, which has often resolved before the patient is seen by a physician. Depending on the reason for the attacks, treatment directed against future attacks may include carotid endarterectomy, control of cardiac or systemic disease, and use of anticoagulant medicines. Long-term prophylactic administration of drugs that inhibit platelet aggregation (aspirin, ticlopidine) reduces the risk of further attacks. Heparin and coumadin may be needed if there is a major problem with thrombotic disease.

Stroke (Brain Attack, Cerebrovascular Accident, CVA)

Sudden onset of neurologic symptoms due to interruption of blood supply to some part of the brain. Stroke ranks third as a cause of death in the U.S.

Cause: Blockage of a cerebral artery by a clot (thrombosis) or embolus, or local hemorrhage from a cerebral vessel. Most cases are due to underlying vascular disease (arteriosclerosis, cerebral aneurysm, hypertension, diabetes mellitus, valvular heart disease).

History: Sudden onset of weakness, numbness or paralysis, usually on one side of the body, or other neurologic deficit (loss of vision, dizziness, difficulty speaking, confusion, loss of consciousness), depending on part of brain affected. Severe headache, vomiting, or seizures may also occur. Usually there is a history of cardiovascular disease, sometimes of preceding TIAs. Neurologic deficit may progress to coma and death.

Physical Examination: Evidence of neurologic deficit, depending on location and extent of brain tissue involved, and duration of circulatory impairment. Muscle weakness or paralysis, which may initially be flaccid but eventually becomes spastic, with rigidity, hyperreflexia, Babinski and other pathologic reflexes. Aphasia, confusion, delirium, coma.

Diagnostic Tests: CT scan of the head can show areas of hemorrhage or infarction. Magnetic resonance imaging may also be used, without contrast material. Lumbar puncture helps to distinguish hemorrhage (blood in fluid, elevated opening pressure) from thrombosis. Blood studies, electrocardiography, and other diagnostic procedures may be used to identify underlying disease.

Course: Many cases of stroke resolve without any residual symptoms. Paralysis, weakness, or dementia may worsen. Stroke may progress rapidly to a fatal termination when the damage is extensive.

Treatment: If neurologic impairment is progressive and hemorrhage has been ruled out, anticoagulants (IV heparin followed by oral coumadin) are used during the acute phase. In selected cases, tissue plasminogen activator (TPA) is administered to dissolve a freshly formed thrombus. Vigorous supportive treatment (oxygen, parenteral nutrition, prevention of respiratory and urinary tract infection, prevention of bedsores) must be instituted early. Physical therapy is important to maintain mobility and achieve maximum rehabilitation as neurologic function returns. Braces or splints may be necessary to promote mobility despite weakness of certain muscle groups.

ALTERED CONSCIOUSNESS

Depression of the level of consciousness or alertness can result from a wide variety of causes, some intracranial (trauma, hemorrhage, infection, neoplasm, vascular obstruction, increased intracranial pressure) and some systemic (anoxia, hyper-

---

Glasgow Coma Scale

Best motor response (upper extremity)
- 6   Obeys command
- 5   Localizes pain
- 4   Withdraws from stimulus
- 3   Abnormal flexing
- 2   Extensor response
- 1   None

Best verbal response
- 5   Oriented (makes sentences)
- 4   Confused speech (words)
- 3   Gibberish (vocal sounds)
- 2   Incomprehensible sounds
- 1   None

Eye opening
- 4   Spontaneous
- 3   To speech
- 2   To pain
- 1   None

---

capnia, shock, drugs, chemical poisons, electrolyte imbalance, hepatic or renal failure). Various grades of impaired consciousness may be roughly distinguished as clouding or blunting (obtusion) of the sensorium, drowsiness (somnolence), stupor, semicoma, and (deep) coma. Coma demands vigorous diagnostic efforts (thorough history and physical examination with emphasis on neurologic findings, funduscopic examination, blood and urine studies, lumbar puncture, EEG, and head imaging). A widely used measure of the level of consciousness is the Glasgow Coma Scale (see box). Treatment of coma includes attention to airway, respiratory function, and circulation, and vigorous efforts to reverse or eliminate identifiable causes. Delirium and dementia are discussed as mental disorders in the next chapter.

PERIPHERAL NEUROPATHY

Disease or damage affecting one or more peripheral nerves, with resultant impairment of sensory or motor function or both. Mononeuritis is impairment of function in a single peripheral nerve. Polyneuritis is peripheral neuritis involving more than one nerve.

Mononeuritis

Causes: Trauma, local compression or entrapment (carpal tunnel syndrome, Bell palsy, both discussed below), local disease or infection (sarcoidosis, amyloidosis, Lyme disease, leprosy), or systemic disease (see systemic causes under polyneuritis below).

History: Hypesthesia, anesthesia, paresthesia, causalgia, weakness, wasting of muscles.

Physical Examination: Reflexes diminished or absent, muscular atrophy.

Diagnostic Tests: Electromyography and nerve conduction velocity tests confirm neural malfunction. Other studies may be undertaken to find the basic cause.

Treatment: Treatment of the underlying cause, when possible. Surgery, physical therapy.

Two common types of mononeuritis due to nerve entrapment are discussed here in more detail.

Carpal Tunnel Syndrome

Pain, tingling, and hypesthesia or anesthesia in the thenar (the fleshy part of the palm proximal to the thumb and index finger), with weakness and eventual atrophy in muscles of the thenar supplied by the median nerve, as a result of compression of this nerve on the volar aspect of the wrist where it passes through the carpal tunnel, formed by wrist bones and the non-yielding carpal ligament. Many cases are induced by repetitive wrist flexion, as in jobs or hobbies. The incidence is increased during pregnancy and among persons with certain systemic diseases (diabetes mellitus, hyperthyroidism, rheumatoid arthritis).

Pain and tingling sometimes wake the patient at night, and elicit the response of shaking the hand to restore normal feeling. Tinel sign (shocklike pain when the volar aspect of the wrist is tapped) and Phalen sign (reproduction of pain or paresthesia when both wrists are flexed with the hands firmly pressing one another back to back for 60 seconds) are positive. Electromyography and nerve conduction velocity studies can confirm the site of nerve compression. Treatment is by removal of known underlying causes; splinting, at least at night; physical therapy; local injection of corticosteroid; and often surgical division of the carpal ligament.

Bell Palsy

Weakness or paralysis of muscles on one side of the face caused by inflammation or compression of the seventh cranial nerve (facial nerve) as it passes through the bony facial canal and emerges at the stylomastoid foramen behind the ear. The cause is unknown, but exposure to cold and herpes simplex virus infection have been suggested. Onset of symptoms is often accompanied by pain below or behind the ear. Onset of facial weakness is characteristically abrupt, producing a characteristic asymmetry of the face and diminished ability or inability to close the eyes, smile, or purse the lips. Speech and eating may be slightly disturbed. There may be impairment of hearing and of taste on the tip of the tongue. The diagnosis is clinically evident, but electromyography and nerve conduction velocity studies may give indications of prognosis. More than half of cases resolve spontaneously in a few days to a few weeks, but residual weakness and asymmetry of the face, occasionally severe, may be permanent. A systemic corticosteroid is usually prescribed.

Polyneuritis

Causes: Hereditary (Charcot-Marie-Tooth disease, Dejerine-Sottas disease, Friedreich ataxia), metabolic (diabetes mellitus, uremia), vitamin deficiency, alcoholism, drugs (INH, phenytoin), chemical poisons (lead, arsenic), autoimmunity (Guillain-Barré syndrome).

History: Essentially as for mononeuritis (see above), but involving nerves throughout the body, often in an irregular and shifting pattern.

Physical Examination: As in mononeuritis.

Diagnostic Tests: As in mononeuritis. Emphasis is on finding a systemic cause (diabetes mellitus, other metabolic diseases, lead poisoning).

Treatment: Removal or treatment of underlying cause, if possible. Otherwise as for mononeuritis.

QUESTIONS FOR STUDY AND REVIEW

1. Which cranial nerves exert their influence below the level of the head?

   _____

   _____

   _____

   _____

2. List five parts of the cranial nerve examination that cannot be performed on an unconscious patient:

   _____

   _____

   _____

   _____

   _____

   _____

3. List five parts of the spinal nerve examination that cannot be performed on an unconscious patient:

   _____

   _____

   _____

   _____

   _____

   _____

4. Define or explain these terms:

   a. ataxia_____

   _____

   b. axon _____

   _____

   c. Babinski reflex _____

   _____

   d. lumbar puncture _____

   _____

   e. polyneuritis _____

   _____

   f. myelin_____

   _____

g. neuron _____
   _____

h. traumatic tap _____
   _____

5. Distinguish between *upper motor neuron lesions* and *lower motor neuron lesions*:

   _____
   _____
   _____
   _____
   _____
   _____
   _____
   _____

6. Name three neurologic disorders that are inherited:

   a. _____
      _____

   b. _____
      _____

   c. _____
      _____

7. Name three neurologic disorders that are caused by systemic disease:

   a. _____
      _____

   b. _____
      _____

   c. _____
      _____

8. Name three neurologic disorders that are usually lethal:

   a. _____
      _____

   b. _____
      _____

   c. _____
      _____

CASE STUDY: YOU'RE THE DOCTOR

Ivan Starks, a regular patient of yours, is brought to your primary care office by his daughter because of an episode of confusion beginning about 2 hours earlier. Mr. Starks is an 74-year-old widower who underwent a triple coronary bypass graft about 4 months ago with stent placement. He had a long history of Prinzmetal angina and coronary arteriography confirmed three-vessel disease. He has no history of hypertension, myocardial infarction, atrial fibrillation, or congestive heart failure. He made a good recovery from his surgery and completed a cardiac rehabilitation program. He lives by himself in an efficiency apartment. He has remained active, going for walks with his dogs, playing with his grandchildren, and gardening. He is currently taking a beta-blocker, an angiotensin converting enzyme (ACE) inhibitor, and clopidogrel (a platelet aggregation inhibitor).

1. What diagnostic considerations does this history raise?

   _____

   _____

   _____

   _____

On awakening this morning he noted blurring or blockage of vision, numbness in the face, vertigo, and slight nausea. While trying to make coffee he dropped a spoon and a cup. When he phoned his daughter to report that he was feeling strange, she noted that he had hiccups and that his speech was slurred or thick. She went to his apartment immediately and found that he had gone back to bed but seemed to be feeling better. Because he still complained of fuzziness of vision and a spinning sensation in the head, and had hiccups, she called your office and was advised by your receptionist to bring him in for an emergency visit.

2. Does this sound like a significant health problem or just a passing spell such as elderly persons often experience? What is the basis for your opinion?

   _____

   _____

   _____

   _____

You see Mr. Starks at 10:30 a.m., about 2 hours after the onset of his symptoms. He appears his usual self and is in no distress, but he walks unsteadily and has hiccups. His tongue seems thick and he stumbles over certain words. He denies recent falls, headache, diplopia, change in medicine, and consumption of alcohol. His vital signs are normal. There is no evidence of head injury. Pupils are equal and reactive. Ocular examination is rendered somewhat difficult by a lateral nystagmus and by cataracts.

Vision is grossly normal and visual fields are grossly intact. Funduscopic examination is attempted unsuccessfully. Ears, nose, and throat are unremarkable. The tongue protrudes in the midline and the gag reflex is intact. The neck is supple and shows no masses, bruits, jugular venous distention, or abnormal pulsations. The heart is regular without murmurs, S3, or S4 and the lungs are clear to auscultation. Paresthesia of the face, noted earlier by the patient, has disappeared, but on careful examination you identify areas of hypesthesia on the right side of the face and on the left forearm and left thigh. Motor strength in the extremities is normal and symmetrically equal. Deep tendon reflexes are normal, and no pathologic reflexes are noted. On the Romberg examination the patient is unable to remain steadily erect even with his eyes open.

3. What course of action will you now advise?

____ a. Rest at home for 24 hours and re-evaluation in the morning.

____ b. Hospital referral for imaging studies.

____ c. Discontinuance of all medicines and a trial of meclizine to suppress vertigo.

____ d. Emergency psychiatric consultation.

4. Why do you recommend the above?

_____

_____

_____

_____

You explain to Mr. Starks and his daughter that he has apparently had a stroke affecting the vertebrobasilar system. Since abnormal findings are present more than 2 hours after the onset of symptoms, this can't be dismissed as a TIA. You arrange for hospital admission and immediate performance of a CT scan without contrast. This shows a small infarct in the medulla.

5. What treatment is indicated for this condition?

_____

_____

_____

_____

6. How would the treatment differ if the CT scan showed a hemorrhage rather than an infarct?

_____

_____

_____

_____

7. Is there anything in Mr. Starks's history that might have suggested that he had sustained a hemorrhagic stroke rather than an ischemic stroke? Explain.

_____

_____

_____

_____

SUGGESTIONS FOR ADDITIONAL LEARNING ACTIVITIES

1. Obtain a medical journal that addresses diseases of the nervous system from your school, community, or hospital library, or access a medical journal through the Internet. Locate the research articles that appear in the journal and notice in particular the abstract that begins these articles. The abstract summarizes the essential information in the article. Choose a research article that interests you and make a photocopy so you can write on it. Read the abstract and then read through the article looking specifically for the points discussed in the abstract. Use a yellow highlighter to mark sections of the article that are referenced in the abstract. Make sure all the information in the abstract is accounted for within the body of the article.

2. Choose a condition discussed in this chapter and write a one-person skit in which you will play the part of a patient discussing your condition with your doctor. Because the doctor isn't actually in your skit, your dialogue should give your audience enough information that they can guess what the doctor may be saying to you. Produce your skit for your class or your family.

3. You are a teacher for a Human Diseases course and you must prepare a final examination for this chapter. Prepare a 20 question oral or written examination and include a separate answer key. If possible, trade exams with someone else and see how you do.

Mental Disorders

(Outline continued on next page)

LEARNING OBJECTIVES

Upon completion of this chapter, you should be able to

- discuss current concepts as to the nature and causes of mental disorders;

- classify major categories of mental disorders by their distinguishing features;

- describe the treatment of mental disorders.

MENTAL DISORDERS
(continued)

OTHER PSYCHIATRIC DISORDERS
Attention-Deficit Hyperactivity Disorder
(ADHD)
Schizophrenia

DELIRIUM AND DEMENTIA
Delirium
Dementia

QUESTIONS FOR STUDY AND REVIEW

MENTAL DISORDERS

INTRODUCTORY REMARKS

Disorders of perception, mood, and behavior have always been placed in a separate category from other illnesses, by both physicians and laity. Except for a few conditions obviously caused by organic disease or injury of the central nervous system (alcoholic dementia, inability to speak after head injury or a stroke), mental illnesses were long thought to result from failure of normal personality development, inadequate adaptation to life stresses, acquired distortions of thought processes, and other vague and intangible factors. The specialty of psychiatry came into being as a field concentrating on disturbances of mood and thought for which no organic basis could be found. Within the past few decades, psychiatric theory has undergone remarkable changes in orientation.

With important exceptions, most modern psychologists and psychiatrists believe that all mental disorders are due to structural, chemical, or electrical abnormalities in the brain. This idea is supported by abundant evidence from diverse sources. Genetic studies show that many mental disorders run in families, and some have actually been traced to specific chromosomal abnormalities. Biochemical research has established a correlation between the distribution of neurotransmitters such as serotonin, dopamine, and norepinephrine in the central nervous system and certain disorders of cognition, mood, and behavior. A chemical basis has been found for the way in which many drugs help in mental disorders, and new drugs designed with specific chemical goals have attained their object of providing improved control of anxiety, depression, and other common disorders. Although drug therapy may still be considered an adjunct to counseling and other forms of psychotherapy, for many disorders it is currently the most rapid, effective, and predictable mode of treatment.

Mental illnesses have been precisely defined and classified by the American Psychiatric Association in a publication called the *Diagnostic and Statistical Manual of Mental Disorders (DSM)*. The fourth edition of this book (DSM-IV), published in 1994, is based on and correlated with the classification, nomenclature, and code numbering of the *International Classification of Diseases*, ninth edition *(ICD-9)*. It categorizes mental disorders and defines them according to precise and stringent diagnostic criteria. Ideally, all professional use of terminology regarding mental disorders should conform to the standards of DSM-IV. Access to a copy of this book is indispensable for the medical transcriptionist who works with records pertaining to mental illness.

The following definition of **mental disorder** is abridged slightly from DSM-IV: A clinically significant behavioral or psychological syndrome or pattern that occurs in an individual and is associated with present distress or disability, or with a significant risk of suffering, death, pain, disability, or loss of freedom.

TERMS PERTAINING TO NORMAL AND ABNORMAL MENTAL FUNCTION

Affect: One's prevailing mood or emotional state, pleasant or unpleasant, particularly as perceived by the examiner.

Amnesia: Loss of memory.

Compensation (overcompensation): A mechanism by which one covers up a defect or weakness by exaggerating or overdeveloping some other property or faculty.

Confabulation: Invention of stories about one's past, often bizarre and complex, to fill in gaps left by amnesia; a typical feature of Korsakoff syndrome in chronic alcoholics.

Cyclothymia: Abnormal lability (instability, changeableness) of mood, which varies between excitement and depression without becoming severe enough to be called bipolar disorder.

Delusion: A distorted belief or perception, such as thinking that one is a famous historical figure (Jesus, Napoleon) or that one is the object of persecution.

Denial: A mechanism by which one refuses to believe, remember, or accept an unpleasant fact or circumstance, such as a painful past experience or the fact of being ill.

Dysphoria: A general feeling of mental or emotional discomfort.

Dysthymia: A depressed mood, usually chronic or recurrent, that is not severe enough to be called major depression.

Encephalopathy: Any organic disease or damage of the brain, particularly the cerebral cortex, that causes impairment of mental or physical functioning; often due to degenerative diseases (Alzheimer disease, Creutzfeldt-Jakob disease) or chemical intoxications (alcohol, lead).

Guilt: A sense of having done wrong, of having failed to meet one's own or others' expectations or standards, or of being inferior or inadequate; as used in psychiatry and psychoanalysis, guilt is a distinct concept from legal or moral guilt, which arises from deliberate violation of moral or civil rules.

Hallucination: A sensory experience, usually auditory or visual, without any physical basis—for example, seeing snakes floating in the air, or hearing voices urging one to do something.

Identification: A mental process whereby one takes on the properties or actions of another with whom an emotional tie exists (a boy walking and talking like his father; a woman dressing and behaving like a movie idol).

Libido: Sexual desire or drive; often, more generally, the totality of pleasure-directed energy or activity.

Mechanism (also **defense mechanism, ego-defensive mechanism, mental mechanism, unconscious mechanism**): An automatic, unconscious mental process whereby repressed emotions (painful feelings, sexual urges) generate new beliefs or attitudes to protect the ego from a sense of guilt, inadequacy, or other negative feelings; see compensation, identification, projection, rationalization, repression, sublimation.

Narcissism: Extreme self-love; excessive preoccupation with oneself and one's own concerns and needs, to the exclusion of normal emotional ties with others.

Neurosis: A mental disorder in which the patient experiences, and gives evidence of, emotional distress, but remains in touch with reality at all times.

Neurotransmitter: A normal chemical substance produced in minute quantities by nerve tissue and involved in the transmission of electrical impulses from one nerve cell to another; the effect of a neurotransmitter may be to stimulate or inhibit the nerve cell on which it acts; well-known neurotransmitters include acetylcholine, dopamine, epinephrine, gamma-aminobutyric acid (GABA), norepinephrine, and serotonin.

Projection: A mechanism whereby one unconsciously attributes one's own thoughts and attitudes (usually negative or unpleasant) to others as a means of dealing with a sense of guilt or inadequacy.

Psyche: A vague term roughly equivalent to "mind."

Psychosis: A mental disorder in which, in addition to emotional distress, the patient experiences a break with reality, manifested by delusions, hallucinations, and grossly bizarre or socially inappropriate behavior.

Rationalization: A mental process of justifying some act or omission through logical reasoning or argumentation, usually as a means of reducing feelings of guilt or inadequacy.

Reality testing: The ability of an individual to perceive reality as it is, not as distorted by abnormal thought processes, disorders of perception, delusions, or hallucinations.

Repression: The mental process of thrusting out of consciousness impulses or desires that are perceived as incompatible with one's own standards or sense of fitness, and that therefore generate unpleasant emotions; repressed material occupies a large part of the subconscious.

Subconscious (mind): Elements of one's personality (feelings, attitudes, prejudices, desires, behavior patterns) of which one is unaware; a general and somewhat vague term including but not always identical to what Freud called the unconscious (*Unbewußtsein*).

Suicidal ideation: Thoughts of committing suicide as a relief from mental distress, without actual attempts at suicide.

Sublimation: Diversion of sexual energy or impulses into higher or more socially acceptable activities.

Transference: The development, on the part of the client, of an emotional bond (positive or negative) toward the therapist.

DIAGNOSIS OF MENTAL DISORDERS

The principal diagnostic method used by psychiatrists in identifying or classifying mental illness is the formal mental status examination. This is a group of diagnostic assessments based on the history as related by the patient and others, and on analysis of data gathered by observing and interviewing the patient. The mental status examination may be performed in a single session, or may be gradually completed through several sessions. Some parts may not be able to be completed at all if the patient is entirely out of touch with reality, or is unable to respond to questions or commands.

The formal **mental status examination** consists of the following parts:

Appearance: dress, grooming, makeup, hair care, jewelry or other adornments. Slovenly, unkempt? Bizarre, mismatched, or incongruous garments or adornments?

Sensorium: Responsiveness to visual, auditory, and tactile stimuli; alertness, attention span; ability to recognize and classify objects.

Activity and behavior: Gait, posture, level of motor activity, speech; bizarre or compulsive actions, mannerisms, posturings, automatisms, mimicry.

Mood (affect): Basic emotional state, and emotional content of responses to examiner (apathetic, blunted, depressed, elated, euphoric, flat, inappropriate, labile).

Thought content: Unconventional thoughts, fantasies, phobias, obsessive ideas, delusions, hallucinations, poverty of imagination.

Intellectual function: Speed, coherence, and relevance of abstract reasoning; mental arithmetic, interpretation of idioms ("time on your hands") and proverbs ("a rolling stone gathers no moss").

Orientation: Awareness of time ("What day, month, year is it?"), place ("Where are we? What city is this?"), person (ability to identify self, relatives, friends).

Memory: Recall of recent and remote events; general information ("How many cents in a quarter? Who is the president?"); confabulation.

Judgment: Competence in analyzing situations, solving problems, taking practical action ("What would you do if the house across the street caught fire?").

Insight: The patient's awareness of being ill or impaired, and awareness of the nature of the problem.

There is a certain overlapping of material between parts of the mental status examination. Some of the observations pertain to the field of neurology rather than psychiatry. In addition to the mental status examination outlined above, the patient may be asked to complete one or more formal, standardized tests of intelligence and personality.

The patient with symptoms of mental disease is also subjected to neurologic examination and may undergo special testing (blood and urine tests to rule out metabolic disease and drug intoxication, imaging studies of the central nervous system, electroencephalography) to sharpen the diagnostic focus.

TERMS PERTAINING TO THE TREATMENT OF MENTAL DISORDERS

Aversion therapy: A form of behavior therapy that associates an objectionable or undesirable pattern of behavior with an unpleasant experience or consequence, so as to reduce or extinguish the behavior.

Behavior (behavioral) therapy: Any type of psychotherapy that focuses on the alteration or correction of undesirable behavior, including such responses to external stimuli as anxiety, depression, and physical symptoms of emotion (tachycardia, muscle tension, sweating). Behavior therapy uses conditioning, muscle relaxation techniques, meditation, breathing retraining, biofeedback, guided learning, and other methods.

Client: The recipient of psychotherapy; a term preferred to "patient" when the therapist is not a physician.

Client-centered therapy: A form of psychotherapy in which the client is encouraged, with a minimum of direction by the therapist, to discover the sources of distressing mental symptoms and means of resolving them.

Cognitive therapy: A form of psychotherapy based on promoting the client's rational understanding of the source of distressing emotions, thought patterns, and undesirable behaviors, and correction of these by adoption of more mature, balanced, and realistic attitudes.

Electroconvulsive (electroshock) therapy: Delivery of controlled electric shocks to the brain to alter electrochemical function, primarily in depression. The treatment, administered only by a physician, causes convulsions and loss of consciousness; the patient awakens in a state of disorientation. Several treatment sessions may be necessary before improvement is noted.

Family therapy: Psychotherapy that treats the family as an organic unit and seeks to promote understanding and correction of pathologic attitudes and relationships among members of the unit.

Group therapy: Psychotherapy administered to several persons at once, making use of shared perceptions, experiences, and feelings, group dynamics, and mutual understanding and support.

Hypnosis: A technique in which the therapist places the client into a sleeplike trance, in which outside stimuli are reduced to a minimum, the subconscious is more directly accessible, and the client is more susceptible to the influence of the therapist's suggestions and advice.

Pharmacotherapy: Treatment with drugs, generally prescription drugs; only physicians (but not necessarily physicians specializing in psychiatry) are permitted by law to prescribe drugs.

Play therapy: A form of psychotherapy used with children, in which structured or unstructured play settings with dolls and other toys enable the therapist to identify and correct false attitudes or unhealthy behavior patterns.

Psychiatry: The branch of medicine concerned with the diagnosis and treatment of mental disorders; all psychiatrists are physicians.

Psychoanalysis: A school of clinical psychology founded by Sigmund Freud (see box) and based on lengthy, searching analysis of the patient's mental life, including particularly the content of the subconscious, which can be made manifest by hypnosis, dream interpretation, free association (nondirected reflections voiced by the patient), and other methods; many psychiatrists are psychoanalysts, but not all psychoanalysts are psychiatrists (physicians).

Psychodrama: A type of group therapy in which clients resolve conflicts and distressing emotional states by acting out their fantasies and fears in the setting of a dramatic performance, before an audience of fellow clients.

Psychology: Broadly, the study of all mental processes and functions (perception, memory, judgment, learning ability, mood, social interaction, communication, and others). Clinical psychology is a professional discipline concerned with the nonmedical treatment of mental disorders; a clinical psychologist ordinarily does not hold a medical degree.

Psychotherapy: Any method or technique, except the administration of medicines, used in the treatment of mental disorders.

Rational therapy: A form of treatment in which mental disorders, which are thought to result from misinformation, wrong belief systems, and distorted logic, are improved by the therapist's use of direct, positive teaching and advice.

The founder of both psychoanalysis and modern psychiatry was **Sigmund Freud** (1856-1939), a Viennese physician specializing in neurology. Early in his career he became interested in cases of physical impairment (paralysis, blindness) in which there was no evidence of an organic lesion and that sometimes resolved after the correction or resolution of a mental disorder. He went on to formulate the theory, universally accepted today, that much of a person's mental life is subconscious—not accessible to reflection or memory, yet exerting a potent influence on attitudes, behavior, emotional state, mood, and general physical well-being.

Freud used hypnotism, dream interpretation, and prolonged analytic sessions with the patient to unlock hidden sources of mental and physical illness in the subconscious. The system he developed, known as psychoanalysis, was both diagnostic and therapeutic: through interaction with the therapist and gradual attainment of insight into subconscious thoughts, associations, wishes, and fears, the patient gains understanding of the problems and finds ways of solving them.

According to Freud's view, the human personality consists of three parts: the *ego*, each person's conscious view of reality and personal identity; the *id*, an unconscious reservoir of self-preserving and pleasure-seeking, particularly sexual, instincts and drives; and the *superego*, or conscience, a largely unconscious product of both ego and id, which monitors the ego. Freud posited the existence of many ego-defensive mechanisms, including repression, compensation, and rationalization, by which we attempt to preserve equanimity and self-esteem despite personal failings, life stresses, and the rejection or hostility of others.

Freud lived to see his discoveries and theories accepted throughout the world. Many of his disciples went on to found their own schools of psychoanalysis. Although few modern students of mental illness accept all of Freud's original theories, he is universally honored as the discoverer of the subconscious and of ways to identify its ills and heal them.

Therapist: One who treats; in mental health, anyone administering psychotherapy.

ANXIETY DISORDERS

A group of mental disorders characterized by chronic worry or fear. Anxiety disorders are the most common ones seen by psychiatrists; often anxiety accompanies other disorders (depression, schizophrenia).

Cause: Most anxiety disorders probably result from some malfunction in the part of the brain called the reticular formation. This system regulates sleep and wakefulness as well as many autonomic and endocrine functions. Persons with chronic anxiety have abnormal levels of certain neurotransmitters (norepinephrine, serotonin, gamma-aminobutyric acid) in brain tissue.

History: Persisting or recurring feelings of apprehension, uneasiness, worry, or fear (with or without a clearly defined object) that is out of proportion to any actual danger or threat. The sense of dread may become so absorbing as to distract the patient's attention from personal, social, and occupational activities. Anxiety may be triggered by a wide variety of settings and circumstances. Besides the mental condition of constant worry or dread, the patient usually experiences physical signs of autonomic and endocrine response: heightened muscle tension, rapid pulse, hyperventilation, sweating, insomnia, problems with appetite and sexual function. DSM-IV lists specific criteria for fourteen anxiety disorders. Five of these are described here.

Generalized anxiety disorder: An abiding state of excessive, distressing, and disabling worry about a number of issues, associated with restlessness, muscle tension, irritability, abnormal fatigue, and insomnia. The condition is twice as common in women, and often accompanies depression.

Social anxiety disorder (social phobia): The most common anxiety disorder. A phobia is an irrational fear of some object or situation, with resulting efforts to avoid it. While recognizing that the fear is unfounded or out of proportion to any actual danger, the victim of a phobia is unable to overcome it. The victim of social phobia experiences an exaggerated and persistent fear of embarrassment or humiliation in a social setting, or when appearing or performing in public. This can lead to severe social, educational, or occupational disability. Many persons with this disorder also suffer from depression or alcoholism.

Agoraphobia: An intense fear of being alone or being in a public place from which escape might be difficult, or where help might be unavailable, in case of sudden incapacitation (such as passing out or having a heart attack). Victims of agoraphobia avoid open spaces, crowded enclosures such as stores or churches, tunnels, elevators, and public transportation.

Panic disorder: Recurring sudden, spontaneous attacks of intense anxiety, lasting minutes or hours, and accompanied by marked physical symptoms such as chest pain, tachycardia, dyspnea or choking, sweating, faintness, tremors, and tingling in the extremities. Because of the type and severity of physical symptoms, panic disorder is sometimes mistaken for a heart attack or other life-threatening emergency by both the victim and others, including physicians. Although either agoraphobia or panic disorder can occur by itself, the two are often associated in the same patient.

Obsessive-compulsive disorder (OCD): A chronic anxiety disorder in which the patient suffers from both obsessions and compulsions. An obsession is a recurring or persisting idea, thought, or image that is perceived as intrusive, distracting, and repugnant, but that the victim is unable to ignore or suppress. Examples are recurring thoughts of harming oneself or others; fear of contamination or infection; and worry about losing or throwing away something that is or may later become important. A compulsion is an urge to repeat a ritualistic or stereotyped form of behavior that is recognized by the victim as irrational but that cannot be omitted without an increase of anxiety. Examples include excessive, repetitive handwashing; rigid attention to order or symmetry; repeated checking of locks, switches, or clocks; and performance of everyday actions in a ritualized fashion.

Treatment: The treatment of an anxiety disorder depends on the exact nature of the disorder, its source, and its symptoms. Individual or group psychotherapy can provide emotional support, help the patient to gain insight into the nature of the problem, encourage psychic growth and maturation, and teach positive attitudes and goal-directed behavior. Most anxiety disorders respond well to short-term or long-term drug treatment. Agents that reduce the level of uneasiness and worry are called anxiolytics. Most of the anxiolytics in current use belong to the benzodiazepine class (alprazolam, oxazepam). Certain drugs used in the treatment of depression (fluoxetine, fluvoxamine) are useful in obsessive-compulsive disorder. Paroxetine is beneficial in social anxiety disorder and panic disorder. Beta-adrenergic blocking agents such as propranolol can control the autonomic component of performance anxiety, social anxiety disorder, and panic disorder (tachycardia, sweaty palms, tremors).

MOOD DISORDERS

Mood disorders include all emotional problems in which extreme deviation from a normal sense of emotional comfort and well-being (varying from depression to mania) is the principal symptom. Major depression and bipolar disorder, the chief clinical presentations of mood disorder, are discussed in this section.

Major Depression (Clinical Depression)
Sustained or recurring periods of sadness and hopelessness

Cause: Probably electrochemical malfunction in the limbic system of the brain, which is the principal focus of emotional activity and is intimately associated with memory areas and those concerned with autonomic and endocrine function. Disturbances in the levels, distribution, and metabolism of the neurotransmitters serotonin and dopamine appear to be responsible for emotional symptoms. In the form of depression known as seasonal affective disorder (SAD), patients experience low mood, increased desire for food and sleep, and a reduction in activity level as a consequence of the weather (colder, darker, shorter days of winter, with limited opportunities for recreation, especially outdoors). Depression in its various forms is second only to anxiety in incidence, and it often occurs in conjunction with anxiety. It is 2-3 times more common in women and tends to run in families. There is strong evidence of a genetic predisposition to depressive illness. It is more common in persons who have problems with drugs or alcohol, chronic physical illness, stressful life events, social isolation, or a history of being sexually abused. The first episode typically occurs before age 40. Recurrences are common.

History: Depressed, dejected, or blue mood accompanied by marked reduction of interest or pleasure in virtually all activities; gain or loss of weight, increased or decreased sleep, increased or decreased level of psychomotor activity, fatigue, feelings of guilt or worthlessness, diminished ability to concentrate, hopelessness, and recurring thoughts of death or suicide.

Treatment: A number of highly effective drugs are available to treat depression. These include the older tricyclic compounds (amitriptyline, imipramine), the selective serotonin reuptake inhibitors (SSRIs) (citalopram, fluoxetine, sertraline), monoamine oxidase inhibitors (pargyline, phenelzine), and other agents (bupropion, nefazodone, trazodone, venlafaxine). Many patients experience troublesome side effects (drowsiness, headaches, dry mouth, disturbances of gastrointestinal or sexual function), but some of these tend to diminish or disappear with continued use. Typically it takes 4-6 weeks for full control of depression to be achieved. Antidepressant therapy is ordinarily continued for one year or more. Counseling and other forms of psychotherapy may be useful in hastening remission and reducing the risk of relapse. Seasonal affective disorder often responds to exposure to bright light several hours a day during the winter. For severe depression that does not respond to drug therapy, electroshock therapy is sometimes beneficial.

Bipolar Disorder (Manic-Depressive Disorder)
A type of depressive illness in which the patient's mood oscillates between depression and mania

Cause: Apparently a malfunction of the limbic system. Susceptibility to this disorder has been traced to a gene on chromosome 18. Half of patients have at least one parent with an affective disorder.

History: Alternations of mood between mania and clinical depression, with variable intervals of normal mood in between. A manic episode is a period of abnormal elevation of mood, irritability, or restlessness that lasts at least one week and is accompanied by some or all of the following: inflated self-esteem, hyperactivity, flight of ideas, abnormal talkativeness or pressured speech (rapid, strained speech as if the subject's mouth can't keep up with the flow of thoughts), reduced need for sleep, short attention span, and reckless behavior. Unlike anxiety and simple depression, bipolar disorder may include a loss of touch with reality; that is, it may be a true psychosis. During either the manic or the depressive phase, the patient may experience delusions or hallucinations, or may display grossly bizarre behavior.

Treatment: Drug therapy with lithium salts, carbamazepine, or valproic acid usually controls the manic phase of bipolar disorder and helps to prevent recurrences of mania. Tranquilizers and antidepressants may also be used. Mania generally causes severe impairment of social and occupational functioning and may require hospitalization.

EATING DISORDERS

Anorexia Nervosa

Compulsive pursuit of thinness at the expense of health.

Cause: Unknown. Ninety percent of patients are women, most of them young white women from upper-class families that assign high value to personal drive and achievement. Patients tend to be perfectionistic, obsessional, and control-oriented. Relationships with family members and friends are often superficial and detached.

History: Steady weight loss due to rigorous dieting, often supplemented by strenuous exercise, self-induced vomiting, and use of diuretics or laxatives. Onset is usually during or just after adolescence. Body image is distorted, a normal habitus being perceived as obese. The gain of even half a pound can generate extreme anxiety and depression. Patients tend to deny their dietary practices, to shun encounters with healthcare professionals, and to favor clothing styles that conceal their thinness. They may experience exaggerated sensitivity to cold, constipation, and weakness. Women patients become amenorrheic.

Physical Examination: Emaciation, with wasting of muscle and loss of subcutaneous fat; body weight at least 15% below expected normal weight for height. The skin may become dry and scaly, with increased growth of fine body hair (lanugo). Bradycardia (very slow pulse) and hypotension are common.

Diagnostic Tests: Blood studies may show anemia or electrolyte abnormalities. Levels of some hormones (LH, FSH) may be low.

Course: The mortality rate is about 5%, most deaths being due to nutritional deficiency or suicide. At least 50% of patients have persistent psychiatric

problems throughout life, particularly with eating and sexuality.

Treatment: Counseling, psychotherapy, drug treatment with antidepressants, lithium, or other agents. In severe cases, hospitalization. Acute nutritional and electrolyte deficiency may require intravenous replacement therapy.

Bulimia Nervosa

A behavioral disorder characterized by recurrent episodes of binge eating.

Cause: Unknown. Most patients are women. Personality and family background may be similar to those noted for anorexia nervosa. The prevalence of this disorder in women of college age may exceed 10%.

History: Repeated episodes of uncontrolled binge eating of high-carbohydrate foods, occurring several times a week to several times a day. Usually a binge is followed by feelings of guilt and intense anxiety about possible weight gain; efforts to avert weight gain include self-induced vomiting or use of laxatives or diuretics. Amenorrhea does not usually occur, and most patients are not underweight; some are obese. There is usually some distortion of body image. When compulsive binge eating is combined with irrational anxiety about becoming obese, the term bulimarexia is sometimes used.

Physical Examination: Usually unremarkable. Repeated vomiting may result in erosion of teeth by acid gastric juice, or in chronic pharyngitis. Fingers used by the patient to induce vomiting may show calluses from repeated injury by teeth.

Diagnostic Tests: Electrolyte imbalance may result from repeated vomiting.

Course: The prognosis is fairly good, but many patients retain bizarre eating habits and attitudes throughout life. Vomiting can lead to peptic esophagitis or esophageal rupture.

Treatment: Counseling, psychotherapy, group therapy. Drug treatment with antidepressants and other agents.

ALCOHOLISM AND DRUG ADDICTION

Alcoholism

Chronic excessive drinking of alcoholic beverages, with adverse effects on health and social functioning.

Cause: Unknown. The condition tends to run in families, but personal history and environmental factors are thought to play an important part. In this country, 10% of men and 3-5% of women have drinking problems. Alcoholism is more common in men and in persons under 35. Family members often foster pathologic drinking behavior by making excuses for the patient instead of providing or reinforcing motivation for abstinence.

History: The alcoholic experiences recurrent craving for alcohol; is unable to control or limit drinking on any given occasion; and develops both physical dependence (so that abstinence results in withdrawal symptoms such as nausea, sweating, anxiety, tremors, and delirium) and tolerance (the need to increase the amount of alcohol consumed in order to achieve the desired effect). Excessive drinking may occur daily or only during binges separated by sober intervals lasting days to months. Historical clues to alcoholism include drinking alone, drinking in the morning, drinking to "feel better" or to fortify oneself for unpleasant experiences or encounters, lying about one's drinking behavior, hiding liquor where it will be instantly accessible, blackouts or amnesic episodes associated with drinking, and arrests for public intoxication or driving under the influence of alcohol.

Physical Examination: May be normal except when the patient is intoxicated or experiencing withdrawal symptoms. Examination may show signs of nutritional deficiency (muscle wasting, dermatitis) or hepatic disease (jaundice, enlarged or hard liver) or stigmata of damage to the cardiovascular or central nervous system.

Course: Alcoholism is a chronic, progressive disease, involving a strong need to drink despite negative consequences such as serious social, occupational, or health problems. Alcoholics are more likely to be involved in automobile accidents and to commit violent crimes, including spousal and child abuse and homicide. Organic complications include cardiac arrhythmias, hypertension and stroke, nutritional deficiencies, liver disease (alcoholic hepatitis, cirrhosis), gastritis, and neurologic damage (blackouts, amnesia, personality change, mood disorders). Alcohol abuse during pregnancy can cause fetal damage, including fetal alcohol syndrome (low birth weight, facial deformities, cardiac anomalies, and mental retardation). Chronic alcoholism decreases life expectancy by about 15 years.

Treatment: For acute alcoholism, detoxification (immediate withdrawal from alcohol, with nutritional, psychologic, and pharmacologic support). Counseling, group therapy, support groups (Alcoholics Anonymous). Benzodiazepines, naltrexone. Disulfiram, if taken regularly, reduces the risk of relapse by causing symptoms like a severe hangover if alcohol is consumed.

Drug Abuse and Addiction

Many substances, including natural and synthetic chemicals (marijuana, cocaine, industrial solvents, LSD), legitimate prescription drugs (opiates, synthetic narcotic analgesics, barbiturates, amphetamines, and benzodiazepine tranquilizers), and drugs not legally procurable in the United States even by prescription (gammahydroxybutyrate, heroin) temporarily induce pleasant emotional states, varying from carefree serenity to euphoria and exhilaration. These feelings can lead to **habituation**—that is, the user craves another dose as soon as the effect of the previous dose begin wears off. The nature of habituation is not fully understood. There appears to be a genetic tendency to alcoholism and perhaps to some other types of drug habituation. Some habituating drugs also produce physical **dependence**: after repeated dosing, the body adapts neurologically or biochemically in such a way that withdrawal of the drug can induce physical symptoms such as sweating, restlessness, dysphoria, and even seizures. Drug habituation can be further complicated by the development of **tolerance**—that is, the need to increase dosage continually in order to achieve the desired effect. **Addiction** is variously defined. Usually it means a severe, disabling preoccupation with the use of a drug, involving habituation, dependence, and tolerance. Drug addicts often drop out of the work force and out of society, and some are driven to crime in order to feed their habits.

Drugs of abuse can be chewed, swallowed, smoked, sniffed up the nose, inhaled, injected intramuscularly or intravenously, or inserted into the rectum. Drug abusers are at risk of accidental overdose, toxic effects of impure or adulterated drugs, infection (hepatitis B and C, AIDS) from contaminated needles, and injury to themselves and others. Commonly abused psychoactive drugs can cause anxiety, depression, and psychoses as well as health problems not directly related to the central nervous system, such as hypertension, asthma, pneumonitis, and ischemic heart disease. Acute drug intoxication may require detoxification and emergency medical support. Addiction is treated with aggressive counseling, group therapy, and use of pharmacologic agents to combat withdrawal symptoms. Methadone maintenance (regular administration of methadone, a synthetic narcotic, under controlled conditions) reduces the medical, legal, and infectious risks associated with heroin use.

OTHER PSYCHIATRIC DISORDERS

Attention-Deficit Hyperactivity Disorder (ADHD)

A chronic behavioral disorder, most striking in children, involving hyperactivity, short attention-span, and impulsiveness

Cause: The disease runs in families, and about 25% of patients have at least one parent who is similarly affected. It is 3-8 times commoner in boys. Magnetic resonance imaging has shown abnormalities in the corpus callosum, the band of fibers connecting the two cerebral hemispheres. The theory that sugar and food colorings or other additives trigger hyperactivity is entirely without scientific support.

History: Often there is evidence of behavioral disturbance in infancy, and the full-blown disorder is typically recognizable by the age of 6. The three cardinal features of ADHD are inattentiveness (short attention span, distractability, inability to complete tasks undertaken, difficulty in following directions, tendency to lose personal articles, disregard for personal safety), impulsiveness (blurting out one's thoughts without adequate reflection, butting in front of others in waiting lines), and hyperactivity (restlessness, fidgeting or squirming instead of sitting or standing still, excessive talking). Children with this disorder have a higher incidence of academic failure, conflict with parents, teachers, and law enforcement officials, antisocial behavior, and substance abuse.

Treatment: Central nervous system stimulants (dextroamphetamine, methylphenidate, and pemoline) are usually successful in enhancing learning ability and improving social functioning. These medicines are taken early in the day so as to avoid nighttime insomnia. When improvement in academic achievement is the chief goal of treatment, the patient may be given "drug holidays" on weekends and during school vacations.

Schizophrenia

A chronic or recurring psychosis due to a disorder of thought processes

Cause: Susceptibility to schizophrenia is probably inherited as a complex of variations affecting several genes. Neurophysiologic studies have shown abnormally small size of the part of the brain called the thalamus, and changes in signal intensity in adjacent white matter.

History: Gradual onset, usually before age 40, of cognitive malfunctions—disturbances of perception and thinking characterized by delusions, hallucinations, gross distortion of mental function, or all of these. These basic features of schizophrenia are usually accompanied by reduced energy level, flat or depressed affect, anhedonia (inability to experience pleasure from normally pleasurable activities), and abulia (diminished ability to make decisions). Virtually all patients display impoverished thought content, social withdrawal, and impairment of occupational functioning. Even with intensive psychotherapy and drug treatment, about 25% of persons with schizophrenia require custodial or institutional care. Schizophrenia is divided, on the basis of dominant clinical manifestations, into the following types:

Disorganized (hebephrenic) schizophrenia: Severe breakdown of mental function and incongruous or silly behavior.

Paranoid schizophrenia: Prominent delusions of persecution or grandeur, often reinforced by hallucinations.

Catatonic schizophrenia: Statue-like posturing, rigidity, or stupor.

Undifferentiated schizophrenia: Schizophrenia without defining features.

Residual schizophrenia: History of schizophrenia but only mild, nonpsychotic residual impairment of mental function.

Treatment: Psychotherapy is inconsistently effective in helping patients overcome disordered thinking and improving social functioning. The modern treatment of schizophrenia depends heavily on the use of drugs known as *neuroleptics* or antipsychotics. The older members of this class belong to the group known chemically as phenothiazines (chlorpromazine, fluphenazine, trifluoperazine). Patients treated with these drugs frequently develop parkinsonian symptoms, including tremors, rigidity, and akathisia (extreme restlessness, inability to remain seated). These may be adequately controlled with drugs used to treat parkinsonism (benztropine, trihexyphenidyl). A few persons treated with phenothiazines develop tardive dyskinesia, an irreversible neurologic disorder causing twitching and writhing movements, particularly in the lips and tongue. Neuroleptics in other classes (clozapine, haloperidol, risperidone) are useful alternatives but have their own side effects. Fluphenazine and haloperidol can be given as long-acting injections to patients who have trouble complying with daily oral medicine regimens.

DELIRIUM AND DEMENTIA

Transitory or irreversible impairment of cognitive functions due to organic changes in the cerebral cortex.

Delirium
An acute, often reversible disturbance of brain function characterized by confusion and impairment of consciousness, memory, attention, and mood.

Cause: Usually systemic: intoxication by alcohol or drugs, including prescribed medicines; withdrawal from alcohol (delirium tremens) or drugs; acute infection; endocrine disease (adrenal, pancreatic, pituitary, thyroid); disturbances of electrolyte balance, cardiopulmonary function, or nutrition; degenerative or neoplastic disease of the brain; and head trauma. Deficiency of thiamin in chronic alcoholism can cause either or both of two psychotic disorders: Korsakoff syndrome (amnesia with confabulation) and Wernicke encephalopathy (confusion with neurologic symptoms such as ataxia and ocular paresis).

History: Disorientation and mental confusion, typically of sudden onset, with other evidences of brain malfunction in varying degrees and proportions: impairment of alertness, inability to concentrate, delusions, hallucinations, loss of impulse control, loss of short-term memory, restlessness, and depression.

Treatment: Depends on the cause. Often the only treatment needed is discontinuing medicines with central nervous system side effects. Alcoholic psychoses may respond to intravenous thiamin.

Dementia
Chronic, progressive deterioration of mental function.

Cause: Dementia can be caused by any disease process or agent that destroys or damages cells in the cerebral cortex or association areas of the brain. More than half of all cases of dementia are due to Alzheimer disease, a genetically determined degenerative disease of cortical neurons that typically begins in late middle life. Atherosclerotic obstruction of blood flow to the cerebral cortex (multi-infarct dementia) accounts for another 20%. Among other causes of dementia may be mentioned Huntington chorea, chronic alcoholism, and Creutzeldt-Jakob disease (a rapidly progressive degenerative disease of the brain due to prions, which abnormal proteins that are sometimes inherited but can also be acquired in tissue transplanted from an affected person). Some cases of dementia are due to systemic disease or chemical intoxication, often from prescribed medicines.

History: Usually gradual onset of steady deterioration in certain mental functions: short-term memory loss, inability to understand spoken or written language and to express oneself in speech and writing, diminished or distorted sensory perception, inability to perform purposeful actions, personality changes with irritability and depression, deterioration of impulse control.

Course: Depends on the cause of the disorder. Most dementias are irreversible and progressive. Alzheimer disease and arteriosclerotic dementias typically culminate in death within 5-10 years.

Treatment: Most forms of dementia respond poorly to medical treatment. In some patients with Alzheimer disease, acetylcholinesterase inhibitors (donepezil, galantamine, rivastigmine, tacrine) produce improvement in cognitive function. Anxiolytics, neuroleptics, and antidepressants may be used to control disorders of mood and behavior. Behavioral therapy is sometimes successful in reinforcing acceptable behavior and extinguishing unacceptable behavior. A comfortable, secure environment (preferably home, unless the patient is too disruptive or the burden of care too taxing for the family), with familiar faces and a simple, steady routine, provide a setting in which the patient's impairments are least distressing and disabling. Support and counsel for the family are of major importance in Alzheimer disease and other dementias in which long-term home care is appropriate.

TOPICS FOR STUDY OR DISCUSSION

1. Distinguish between *neurosis* and *psychosis* and give an example of each:

   a. neurosis _____

   _____

   _____

   b. psychosis _____

   _____

   _____

2. Name four types of therapy used in the treatment of mental disorders. Which of these is the most promptly and predictably effective?

   _____

   _____

   _____

   _____

3. Define or explain these terms:

   a. anxiolytic _____

   _____

   b. bulimarexia _____

   _____

   c. compulsion _____

   _____

   d. delusion _____

   _____

   e. hallucination _____

   _____

   f. neuroleptic _____

   _____

   g. obsession _____

   _____

   h. phobia _____

   _____

4. *Insanity* is a legal term referring to the inability of a person (usually an accused criminal) to distinguish between right and wrong and to make appropriate decisions about the rightness of personal actions. Which of the mental disorders discussed in this chapter might make a person legally insane?

_____

_____

_____

_____

_____

_____

5. How might the demonstration of genetic and neurochemical causes for most or even all mental disorders affect philosophy, laws, morality, religion, and other fundamental social institutions in the future?

_____

_____

_____

_____

_____

CASE STUDY: YOU'RE THE DOCTOR

Emily McMurtry, an 81-year-old widow, is brought to the hospital emergency department where you are on duty by her two daughters with the history that she is "mixed up, agitated, and keeps falling." She lives with the daughters, who are unmarried. She has been under the care of a local internist for several years for hypertension and arteriosclerotic heart disease. There have been no recent changes in her medicines, which include estrogen with progesterone, an angiotensin converting enzyme inhibitor, a thiazide diuretic, and donepezil.

1. What diagnostic possibilities does this history suggest?

_____

_____

_____

_____

_____

Ms. McMurtry appears well nourished and her hair and clothing are neat. She is calm and in no apparent distress. However, she avoids making eye contact with you, and your attempts to take a history from her elicit only partial sentences of dubious relevance, with a lot of repetition. ("I was . . . I was . . . I was . . . I was . . . and they they . . . they . . . We were there . . . there in the . . . ") She is afebrile. Her pulse is 68 with frequent premature beats. Blood pressure is 177/93. During your examination the patient is passively cooperative but seems not to understand what is going on. The pupils are equal and react to light. Bilateral cataracts make it impossible to do a good fundus examination. Ears, nose, and throat are normal. There are no cervical masses or bruits. You find no evidence of injuries from falls. Heart tones are normal except for frequent ectopic beats and a grade 1/4 systolic ejection murmur best heard at the aortic area and transmitted to the carotids. The lungs are clear and the abdominal examination shows no tenderness, masses, or organomegaly. Pelvic and rectal examinations are deferred. Cranial nerves II through XII are intact. Neurologic examination shows normal strength, mobility, and sensation in all four extremities. No tremors or pathologic reflexes are noted.

2. Do your findings favor delirium, dementia, a stroke, or some other diagnosis? Give the reasons for your diagnosis.

You order basic blood studies and an electrocardiogram. While these are being done, you talk to Ms. McMurtry's daughters. They are both semi-retired tellers at a savings bank. They stagger their work schedules so that one is always at home with their mother. They tell you that she has been increasingly difficult to manage at home because of her confusion and spells of agitation. They also state that she has balance problems and falls frequently. She has been taking donepezil for about 2 years for Alzheimer dementia. Although at first it seemed to help her stay calm and focused, her condition has been deteriorating recently. They are somewhat vague as to when these problems became acute, but they agree that they are unable to manage their mother at home in her present condition. They have brought all her medicines as well as a suitcase with personal articles and changes of clothing so that she can stay in the hospital until she is "better." They have not looked into the question of custodial or nursing home care.

3. Can you think of any reasons for doubting the accuracy or good faith of Ms. McMurtry's history as related by her daughters?

Laboratory studies show very mild anemia, slight elevation of BUN and creatinine, a normal blood sugar, and normal electrolytes. The electrocardiogram shows only unifocal ventricular premature beats and mild nonspecific ST segment changes consistent with diffuse coronary artery disease but without evidence of acute or old infarction. You call Ms. McMurtry's regular internist to discuss your findings with him. He informs you that she has had mild Alzheimer dementia for the past 3 years, but that when last seen by him about 7 weeks ago she seemed neither better nor worse than she was a year ago.

4. Outline the evidence that would support hospitalization for this patient:

_____

_____

_____

_____

_____

_____

_____

5. Outline the evidence that does not support hospitalization for this patient:

_____

_____

_____

_____

_____

_____

_____

You and he agree that there is no justification for hospitalizing this patient, but that nursing home care should be given strong consideration. When you present the results of your examination and of your consultation with Ms. McMurtry's private physician to her daughters, they become indignant and inform you that they are leaving at 5:30 the next morning on a 12-day cruise. They have had their airline and cruise ship tickets for 2 months and nothing is going to stop them from taking this trip—not even their mother's need for custodial care.

6. What do you do now?

_____

_____

_____

_____

_____

_____

_____

SUGGESTIONS FOR ADDITIONAL LEARNING ACTIVITIES

1. Prepare a scavenger hunt based on the conditions or symptoms discussed in this chapter. Instead of listing these directly on the scavenger list, include only bits of information that the hunter will use when searching the chapter. For example, "It is 2-3 times more common in women and tends to run in families" is a clue that might identify major depression. Trade lists with another student or ask a friend or family member to prepare a scavenger list for you.

2. The parts of a mental status examination are discussed in the section, "Diagnosis of Mental Disorders." Place yourself in the role of the examining physician and write your own list of questions or procedures you would use to perform a complete mental status examination on an imaginary patient.

3. Contact a community mental health services organization or facility and obtain information on resources available in your community. Which resources require a physician referral and which are open to the general public? What types of treatments are available through these resources? Obtain statistics about the usage of these services. Prepare a one-page report detailing your findings.

Glossary

Terms not found in the Glossary should be looked up in the Index.

ablation: total removal of a part, normal or abnormal, by surgical or chemical means.

ACE: angiotensin converting enzyme

acquired: not congenital.

ACTH: adrenocorticotropic hormone

acute: developing relatively suddenly and running its course in a few days or weeks.

adenoma: a benign tumor arising from glandular epithelium.

ADH: antidiuretic hormone.

ADHD: attention-deficit hyperactivity disorder.

affect: one's prevailing mood or emotional state, pleasant or unpleasant, particularly as perceived by an examiner.

agammaglobulinemia: inability to form antibodies, due to inherited B lymphocyte dysfunction.

aggressive: referring to a prompt, energetic program of treatment.

AHG: antihemophilic globulin.

AIDS: acquired immunodeficiency syndrome.

airborne: referring to infections that can be spread through the air, usually by droplets of respiratory secretions but sometimes on particles of moisture or dust, or free-floating.

ALL: acute lymphoblastic leukemia

allele: either of two genes making up the pair that occupy a specific locus on a specific chromosome.

alopecia: loss of scalp hair, due to either genetically determined male-pattern baldness or disease.

amenorrhea: absence of menstruation.

amino acid: any of several simple organic compounds that serve as building blocks of protein.

anastomosis: (1) a normal or abnormal joining together of arteries, veins, or both; (2) surgical joining of two hollow or tubular structures, as blood vessels or sections of intestine.

amnesia: loss of memory, recent, remote, or total.

anaplastic: referring to tumor tissue containing primitive, undifferentiated cells, unlike the structurally differentiated cells of normal tissue.

aneurysm: an abnormal dilatation in an artery.

angiography: x-ray study of an arterial system with injected contrast medium.

anoderm: transitional zone of tissue between skin and anal mucous membrane.

anorexia: loss of appetite.

antecubital: referring to the hollow in front of the elbow.

apex (cardiac): the bluntly pointed lower extremity of the heart.

aphasia: impairment of the ability to communicate through spoken or written language, or to understand spoken or written language, or both.

ARDS: adult respiratory distress syndrome.

arrhythmia: irregular rhythm of the heartbeat, with or without an abnormally slow or fast rate.

arteriovenous fistula: an abnormal communication between an artery and an adjacent vein.

ASA: acetylsalicylic acid (aspirin).

ascites: swelling of the abdomen due to effusion of fluid into the peritoneal cavity.

ASC-US: atypical squamous cells of undetermined significance.

ASO: antistreptolysin O.

asymptomatic: causing no symptoms, often referring to a disease or condition that is discovered during a routine or screening examination, or in the evaluation of another condition.

atelectasis: deflation (collapse) of a segment of lung tissue due to blockage of air passages leading to it.

atherosclerosis: hardening and even calcification of arterial walls, with narrowing of their lumens.

atypical: unusual; not typical, not conforming to expected appearance or function.

auscultation: listening to selected body regions with a stethoscope, principally to assess heart sounds, breath sounds, and bowel sounds.

autosome: any of the 22 chromosomes besides the sex chromosomes X and Y.

avulsion: the ripping or tearing away of a part.

AV: atrioventricular; arteriovenous

bacteria (singular, bacterium): one-celled organisms on the borderline between animals and plants, varying enormously in structure, physical and chemical properties, and disease-causing capabilities. Examples: staphylococci (staph), streptococci (strep), chlamydia.

BAL: bronchoalveolar lavage.

benign neglect: a program of doing essentially nothing when a disease is either beyond hope of cure by even the most radical methods, or is expected to resolve without any specific treatment.

blepharitis: inflammation of one or both eyelids.

bloodborne: referring to infections transmitted by blood transfusion, contaminated surgical or dental instruments, needles shared by intravenous drug abusers, or other means whereby blood is transferred from one person to another.

BMI: body mass index.

BPH: benign prostatic hyperplasia.

bradyarrhythmia: a pulse that is both irregular and abnormally slow.

bradycardia: abnormal slowness of the heartbeat (pulse less than 60/min).

bronchoalveolar lavage (or **washing**): flushing of a bronchus and adjacent lung tissue with fluid to remove cells or other material for laboratory study.

bruit: a humming or buzzing sound, synchronous with the heartbeat, heard by auscultation over a narrowed place in an artery.

bulla (plural, bullae): a blister or bleb.

BUN: blood urea nitrogen

CABG: coronary artery bypass graft.

callus (not callous): a zone of thickened epidermis caused by repeated friction or pressure.

cardiogenic: caused by some abnormality or disorder of the heart.

cardiomegaly: enlargement of the heart.

carrier: a person who has recovered from a communicable disease but still harbors living and virulent organisms and can transmit them to others.

cast: a microscopic mass, usually cylindrical, found in the urine in certain abnormal conditions.

cavitation: formation of one or more abnormal cavities, usually referring to cavities of the lung in pulmonary tuberculosis.

CBC: complete blood count.

CEA: carcinoembryonic antigen.

cellulitis: a bacterial infection that spreads through tissues instead of remaining localized.

chorea (from Greek *choreia* 'dancing'): a clinical disorder manifested by recurring sudden, intricate, well-coordinated but involuntary and purposeless muscle movements, which may affect gait, use of the arms and hands, and even speech.

chronic: pertaining to an illness having a protracted course, often lifelong.

cicatrix (scar): a zone of fibrous tissue occurring at the site of a healed injury or inflammatory or destructive lesion extending into the dermis.

CK: creatine kinase.

clone: a colony or family of cells that are all derived from a single ancestor cell.

clubbing of the digits: a deformity of the tips of all ten fingers in which the distal phalanges are swollen, spongy, and warm to the touch, and the angles between the distal phalanges and the nails are flattened out.

CML: chronic myelogenous leukemia.

CMV: cytomegalovirus.

CNS: central nervous system.

coitus: sexual intercourse.

colostomy: a surgically created opening from the colon to the abdominal wall, through which feces are passed rather than by the rectum; may be temporary or permanent.

comedo (plural, comedones): a papule consisting of a dilated sebaceous duct or gland plugged with keratin debris.

communicable disease: an infection that is capable of being transmitted in any way from one person to another.

comminuted fracture: a fracture resulting in more than two fragments.

comorbidity: the presence of two or more unrelated diseases in the same patient at the same time.

compensation (overcompensation): a mechanism by which one covers up a defect or weakness by exaggerating or overdeveloping some other property or faculty.

complication: a disease or abnormal condition induced by a pre-existing condition, which renders treatment more difficult, recovery more protracted, or death more likely.

compound fracture: a fracture accompanied by an open wound, from which a bone fragment may protrude.

confabulation: invention of stories about one's past, often bizarre and complex, to fill in gaps left by amnesia; a typical feature of Korsakoff syndrome in chronic alcoholics.

congenital: present at birth, though not necessarily inherited.

conservative: a mode of treatment that has a low risk of causing side-effects but less likelihood of effecting a cure than other available methods.

contagious: referring to an infectious disease that can be transmitted to others by close exposure (direct touch, sexual contact, exposure to respiratory, digestive tract, or other secretions).

cor pulmonale: dilatation or hypertrophy of the right side of the heart due to lung disease.

cosmetic: referring to physical appearance; said of surgical procedures designed primarily to improve the patient's appearance, such as breast augmentation, revision of scars, and excision of benign skin lesions.

CREST syndrome: an autoimmune disorder characterized by connective tissue disorders (systemic sclerosis, abnormal calcifications), Raynaud phenomenon, and swallowing difficulties.

crust: a hard, friable, irregular layer of dried blood, serum, pus, tissue debris, or any combination of these adherent to the surface of injured or inflamed skin; a scab.

cryoprobe: a cryosurgical instrument containing a circulating refrigerant, which can be rapidly chilled and can deliver subfreezing temperature to tissues with precision.

cryotherapy: local treatment of neoplasms or other lesions by freezing.

CSF: cerebrospinal fluid.

CT: computed tomography.

culture: the growth of microorganisms from a specimen (blood or other body fluid, secretions, tissue) under controlled laboratory conditions.

cure: complete extinction of a disease, usually by arresting the basic process or removing the cause.

cutaneous: pertaining to skin.

CVA: cerebrovascular accident; costovertebral angle.

CVP: central venous pressure.

cyanosis: bluish color of skin, particularly lips and nail beds, due to presence of excess unoxygenated blood in the circulation.

cyclothymia: abnormal lability (instability, changeableness) of mood, which varies between excitement and depression without becoming severe enough to be called bipolar disorder.

cyst: an abnormal thick-walled structure containing fluid or semisolid material.

cystinuria: an inherited disorder characterized by excessive urinary excretion of cystine and other amino acids.

cytology: microscopic examination of stained cells, chiefly to detect malignant or premalignant changes.

D&C: dilatation and curettage.

decibel: a measure of the loudness of sound; one tenth of a bel (named for Alexander Graham Bell).

deficiency: due to a lack or insufficiency of some essential chemical substance or property.

degenerative: caused by deterioration in the structure or function of cells or tissues.

delusion: a distorted belief or perception, such as thinking that one is a famous historical figure (Jesus, Napoleon) or that one is the object of persecution.

dementia: impairment of intellectual function.

dendritic keratitis: infection of the cornea by herpes simplex virus, causing a shallow, painful ulcer having a branching, treelike (dendritic) pattern.

denial: a mechanism by which one refuses to believe, remember, or accept an unpleasant fact or circumstance, such as a painful past experience or the fact of being ill.

dependent edema: edema of the lower extremities, aggravated by the dependent (downward hanging) position.

dermatitis: inflammation of the skin.

dermatosis: a general term for any abnormal condition of the skin, but usually excluding inflammatory conditions, which are called dermatitis.

dermographism: the property of abnormally sensitive skin by which strokes or writing with a pointed object are reproduced on the skin surface as raised red lines.

developmental: characterized by some abnormality in the development of a tissue, organ, or body part, either before or after birth.

devitalized: deprived, by injury or disease, of adequate blood supply to sustain life.

DEXA: dual energy x-ray absorptiometry.

DIC: disseminated intravascular coagulation.

dilatation: widening or expansion.

disabling: causing impairment of normal functions or capabilities, such as the ability to see, stand, and walk, or earn a living.

discoid: consisting of small flat plaques.

dislocation: a disturbance in the position of two bones with respect to one another, due to application of a deforming force to a joint.

displaced fracture: a fracture in which the relative positions of the fragments are significantly different from what they were before the fracture.

diverticulum (plural, diverticula): a blister- or bubble-like outpouching of a hollow or tubular organ.

DJD: degenerative joint disease.

DM: diabetes mellitus.

DNA: deoxyribonucleic acid.

DOE: dyspnea on exertion.

Down syndrome (trisomy 21, mongolism): genetic aberration producing characteristic physical stigmata and mental retardation.

droplet spread: transmission of respiratory and other infections by fine mists of respiratory secretions expelled into the air by coughing or sneezing.

dysmenorrhea: pain occurring with menstruation, typically felt low in the pelvis and in the low back, and often severe.

dyspareunia: pain in the vulva, vagina, or pelvis with sexual intercourse.

dysphagia: difficulty or pain in swallowing.

dysphoria: a general feeling of mental or emotional discomfort.

dyspnea: shortness of breath.

dysthymia: a depressed mood, usually chronic or recurrent, that is not severe enough to be called major depression.

dysuria: pain in the urethra or vulva with urination.

EBV: Epstein-Barr virus.

ecchymosis: a broad zone of red or purple discoloration (more than 1 cm in diameter) due to hemorrhage under the epidermis.

ECG: electrocardiogram.

ectropion: eversion (turning outward) and drooping of the lower eyelid, exposing the conjunctival surface and allowing overflow of tears.

eczema: dermatitis; an inflammatory disorder of the skin characterized by burning or itching and redness, blistering, weeping, crusting, or scaling.

EDC: expected date of confinement (childbirth).

edema: local or diffuse swelling due to accumulation of fluid in tissues.

EEG: electroencephalogram.

effusion: an abnormal accumulation of fluid in a body cavity, such as the pleural space or pericardium.

elective: referring to a treatment that is not necessary to preserve life or well-being, or one that has been deferred until a more appropriate time.

electrodiagnostic procedures: methods for recording the electrical activity accompanying the function of certain organs or tissues (electrocardiogram, electroencephalogram, electromyogram, and others).

electromyogram: an electrodiagnostic test that measures muscle function.

embolization: release of a clot or other solid body into the blood circulation.

EMG: electromyogram.

encephalitis: inflammation of the brain, usually due to viral infection.

encephalopathy: any organic disease or damage of the brain, particularly the cerebral cortex, that causes impairment of mental or physical functioning; often due to degenerative diseases (Alzheimer disease, Creutzfeldt-Jakob disease) or chemical intoxications (alcohol, lead).

endocarditis: inflammation of the lining of the heart, usually due to bacterial infection and chiefly affecting the valves.

endolymph: the fluid medium contained in the inner ear.

endorectal: inside the rectum; said of diagnostic or therapeutic instruments or procedures.

endoscopy: examination of a hollow or tubular organ or cavity with an instrument inserted through a natural orifice or a small incision.

end-stage: referring to a progressively deteriorating condition that has reached the point of lethal (terminal) functional impairment of an organ or organ system (end-stage renal failure, end-stage lung disease).

ENT: ear, nose, and throat.

enterocolitis: inflammatory disease of both the small and large intestines.

entropion: inward turning of the margin of the lower eyelid, often so that the lower lashes touch the eyeball.

epidemiology: the branch of medicine and public health that deals with patterns of disease causation and spread (not necessarily infectious diseases).

epiphora: chronic overflow of tears from the lower eyelid onto the cheek; may be due to blockage of the nasolacrimal duct or to deformity of the lower lid (ectropion).

ERCP: endoscopic retrograde cholangiopancreatography.

erosion: a surface defect in the epidermis produced by rubbing or scratching.

erysipelas: a spreading streptococcal infection of skin and subcutaneous tissues, with redness, heat, and sometimes blistering or sloughing.

erythema: abnormal redness, usually referring to skin or mucous membrane.

erythematous: having an abnormal red color.

eschar: the crust that forms on a burn.

ESR: erythrocyte sedimentation rate.

essential: of unknown cause; apparently arising spontaneously.

ESWL: extracorporeal shock-wave lithotripsy.

etiology: strictly speaking, the study of the causes of disease; universally used by physicians to mean the cause itself.

exacerbation: an increase in the severity of a disease, particularly when occurring after a period of improvement (remission).

excoriation: abrasion of the epidermal surface by scratching.

exocrine: referring to a gland, such as a salivary gland, that releases its secretion through a duct rather than directly into the blood stream.

exophthalmos: abnormal bulging of the eye between the lids.

extra-articular: affecting or pertaining to structures other than joints.

familial (heredofamilial): due to an inherited abnormality expressed in other members of the patient's family.

fascia: a connective tissue sheath surrounding muscles.

fecal-oral route: the route by which some intestinal and other pathogens are transferred from person to person; contamination of food or water, or direct physical contact, with the infected person's feces leads to ingestion of the pathogen.

fissure: a linear defect or crack in the continuity of the epidermis.

flatulence: excessive air or gas in the digestive system, with bloating and passage of flatus.

flatus: intestinal gas, particularly when excessive.

fomite: any inanimate object that can be the means whereby pathogenic microorganisms are transmitted from an infected person to others.

form: any of several clinical patterns that a disease may manifest (the discoid and systemic forms of lupus erythematosus).

forme fruste: an atypical, prematurely arrested, or incompletely expressed form of a disease.

friable: crumbly; fragmenting or bleeding easily on touch or manipulation; said usually of diseased tissue.

FSH: follicle-stimulating hormone.

FTA-ABS: fluorescent treponemal antibody absorption.

fulminant or **fulminating**: rapidly progressive and severe.

functional: due to a disturbance of function without evidence of structural or chemical abnormality.

fungi: simple microscopic mold- or yeast-like organisms. Examples: ringworm fungus, yeast causing thrush and vaginitis.

GABA: gamma-aminobutyric acid.

GABHS: group A beta-hemolytic streptococcus

GERD: gastroesophageal reflux disease.

globulin: any of several proteins that circulate in the blood; antibodies are globulins.

GnRH: gonadotropin releasing hormone

gonococcus: *Neisseria gonorrhoeae*, the cause of gonorrhea.

grade: a measure of the severity of a disease or abnormal condition, particularly a malignant disease.

gynecomastia: abnormal breast development in a male.

HAART: highly active anti-retroviral therapy.

hairline fracture: a fine crack in a bone, barely visible on x-ray examination.

HAV: hepatitis A virus.

Hb: hemoglobin.

Hbg: hemoglobin.

HBV: hepatitis B virus.

hCG: human chorionic gonadotropin.

Hct: hematocrit.

HCV: hepatitis C virus.

HDL: high-density lipoprotein.

hemoptysis: coughing up blood from the lower respiratory tract.

hepatic: pertaining to the liver.

hereditary: due to an inherited abnormality or tendency.

heroic: referring to radical or extreme therapeutic measures that are only justified by the desperate condition of the patient.

HGSIL: high-grade squamous intraepithelial lesion.

HIDA: hepatobiliary iminodiacetic acid.

histology: microscopic examination of stained, very thin sections of tissue obtained by biopsy or surgical excision, or at autopsy.

HIV: human immunodeficiency virus.

hormone: a chemical messenger produced by glandular tissue and released into the bloodstream to stimulate or inhibit cells or tissues at remote sites.

host: a living organism on or in which another organism, usually a parasite, lives.

HPV: human papillomavirus.

hyperacute: having a very abrupt onset or very brief course.

hyperplasia: an increase in the number of cells in a tissue or organ.

hypertrophic: overgrown, usually as a result of increase in the size of cells.

hypertrophy: overgrowth.

hypesthesia: partial loss of sensation on one or more parts of the body surface.

hyphema: presence of blood in the anterior chamber.

hypotension: abnormally low blood pressure.

Hz: abbreviation for hertz, a measure of the frequency of a vibration, particularly one producing sound; equivalent to one cycle (or double vibration) per second.

idiopathic: of unknown cause; apparently arising spontaneously.

IBD: inflammatory bowel disease.

IBS: irritable bowel syndrome.

IM: infectious mononucleosis; intramuscular.

imaging (diagnostic): any procedure used to study or visualize internal organs or tissues by application of irradiation or other physical energy: x-ray, CT scan, fluoroscopy, ultrasound, magnetic resonance imaging, and others.

immunity: a biological response of the living body to invading microorganisms or other noxious materials.

immunofluorescence: a diagnostic technique involving an antibody that has been tagged with a dye that fluoresces under appropriate lighting.

impacted fracture: a fracture in which the end of a long bone is driven into the body of the bone rather than being broken away from it.

impaction: plugging of an orifice with a dense mass of some material, as cerumen in the external auditory meatus.

impetigo: a spreading bacterial skin infection characterized by pustules and crusted shallow ulcers.

infantile: occurring or becoming evident during infancy.

infarction: death of tissue due to blockage of its blood supply.

infectious (infective): caused by the adverse biologic, chemical, or immunologic effects of the growth of microorganisms in the body.

infectious disease: any disease caused by infection; sometimes used in the narrower sense of transmissible disease.

infectious mononucleosis (IM): a contagious viral infection involving primarily the lymphatic system (spleen, lymph nodes, and liver).

ingestion: swallowing, as food, drink, or medicine.

inoperable: referring to a disease, usually malignant, for which surgical treatment is not an option, because of the extent of the disease or the condition of the patient.

inspection: visual examination of the external body surface and of the mouth and pharynx, the external ear, the nares, and other orifices and cavities accessible to direct examination without a surgical incision.

intermittent: causing symptoms at intervals, with intervening periods without symptoms.

invasive: refers to a procedure requiring the introduction of a needle, catheter, or other instrument into the body through a puncture or incision.

ITP: idiopathic (or immune) thrombocytopenic purpura.

IUD: intrauterine device.

IV: intravenous.

IVP: intravenous pyelogram.

juvenile: occurring in early life.

keloid: a firm, nodular, irregular, often pigmented mass of fibrous tissue, the result of exaggerated or abnormal scarring at a site of injury.

keratitis: inflammation of the cornea of the eye from any cause.

KOH: potassium hydroxide.

KP: keratic precipitate.

KS: Kaposi sarcoma.

KUB: kidneys, ureters, bladder.

lacrimation (tearing): increased flow of tears.

larynx: the voice box, containing the vocal cords and situated between the laryngopharynx (the lowermost part of the throat) and the trachea (windpipe).

LDH: lactic dehydrogenase.

LDL: low-density lipoprotein.

LE: lupus erythematosus.

LES: lower esophageal sphincter.

lesion: any abnormality in tissue due to injury; in a broader sense, any objectively identifiable abnormality due to injury or disease.

leukocytosis: abnormal elevation of white blood cells in the circulation.

LGSIL: low-grade squamous intraepithelial lesion.

LH: luteinizing hormone.

libido: sexual drive; in Freudian psychology, a more general term for the instinct to seek personal gratification and pleasure.

lichenification: thickening, coarsening, and pigment change of skin due to chronic irritation, usually scratching.

life-threatening: referring to a disease or injury that may prove lethal, even with aggressive treatment.

LMP: last menstrual period.

locus: the specific place on a chromosome where a particular gene normally occurs.

LSD: lysergic acid diethylamide.

LVH: left ventricular hypertrophy.

lymphadenopathy: disease of lymph nodes, manifested by swelling, tenderness, or both.

MAC: *Mycobacterium avium* complex.

macular: consisting of flat, abnormally colored spots (macules) on the skin.

macule: a clearly defined zone of skin, less than 1 cm in diameter, differing from surrounding skin in color but not in texture or elevation.

malaise: a general sense of being unwell.

malar: pertaining to or situated on the cheeks.

malignant: tending to cause death.

MAST: military antishock trousers.

masterly inactivity: same as *benign neglect*.

MCH: mean corpuscular hemoglobin.

MCHC: mean corpuscular hemoglobin concentration.

MCV: mean corpuscular volume.

meconium: stool formed in the fetal intestine before birth.

mediastinal: pertaining to the mediastinum, the space between the lungs.

medical: any form of treatment not involving surgery or physical manipulation.

melanoma: a highly malignant tumor arising from pigment cells in the skin.

melena: tarry black stools, due generally to the presence of blood that has been chemically altered by its passage through the intestine.

menometrorrhagia: excessive menstrual bleeding occurring both during menses and at irregular intervals.

menorrhagia: regularly occurring menstrual flow that is excessive in volume and lasts longer than a normal menstrual period.

metrorrhagia: menstrual bleeding occurring at irregular but frequent intervals.

microbiology: the branch of biology and medical laboratory technology concerned with the study of microorganisms (bacteria, fungi), particularly those that are pathogenic for human beings.

microorganism: a living thing, such as a bacterium, that cannot be seen without a microscope.

miosis: sustained constriction of the pupil, which may be due to ocular or nervous system disease or to the effect of drugs (pilocarpine, morphine).

Mohs chemosurgery: stepwise removal of a skin tumor in thin layers with chemical treatment of each layer and microscopic examination of frozen sections

molecular: a disease caused by abnormality in the chemical structure or concentration of a single molecule, usually a protein or enzyme; virtually all molecular diseases are inherited.

monodrug therapy: treatment of a condition such as hypertension or malignancy with a single drug, rather than a combination of drugs.

MRI: magnetic resonance imaging.

MS: multiple sclerosis.

mucosa: a mucous membrane, such as those lining the digestive, respiratory, and urogenital tracts.

multifactorial etiology: indicates that a given disease has more than one cause operating together.

multigravida: a woman who has been pregnant more than once.

multinucleated giant cell: an abnormally large cell, having several nuclei, such as may be detectable in certain viral infections.

multipara: a woman who has given birth more than once.

musculoaponeurotic: consisting of both muscles and aponeuroses (broad, flat sheets of connecting tissue by which some muscles are attached to bone or other muscles).

mydriasis: sustained dilatation of the pupil, which may be due to ocular or nervous system disease or to the effect of drugs (atropine, cyclopentolate).

myeloproliferative: pertaining to abnormal growth of cells in bone marrow

myoglobin: an iron-containing protein in muscle, released into the circulation after extensive injury or infarction of muscle tissue.

NA: Nomina Anatomica.

NCV: nerve conduction velocity.

necrosis: death of tissue due to damage by physical or chemical injury or loss of blood supply.

negative: said of a diagnostic test that reveals no abnormality.

neonatal: affecting newborn infants.

neoplastic: pertaining to an abnormal growth or tumor, benign or malignant.

nephritis: inflammation of the kidney.

neutrophilia: increase in the number of circulating neutrophils

nevus: (1) a mole or other pigmented lesion of the skin; (2) a skin lesion present since birth (birthmark).

nocturia: the need to arise from bed at night to urinate.

nodule: a firm elevation of the skin surface more than 1 cm in diameter.

noninvasive: referring to a diagnostic procedure such as an x-ray examination or electrocardiogram that does not require introduction of instruments into the patient's body.

normal: within the range of expected or healthy sensations or diagnostic findings.

NSAID: nonsteroidal anti-inflammatory drug.

nuchal: pertaining to the back of the neck.

nulligravida: a woman who has never been pregnant.

nullipara: a woman who has never given birth.

nyctalopia: marked reduction of visual acuity at night.

nystagmus: oscillatory (back-and-forth, less often up-and-down) movements of both eyes due to central nervous system disorder.

occult: hidden; not obvious, but sometimes able to be inferred from indirect evidence.

OCD: obsessive-compulsive disorder.

oligomenorrhea: infrequent or scanty menstrual bleeding.

onset: the first appearance of signs or symptoms of a disease.

opportunistic: said of infections to which normal persons are not susceptible, but that can occur in persons with impaired immunity.

orchidectomy: surgical removal of the testicles.

organic: due to some demonstrable abnormality in a bodily structure. osteoporosis: loss of calcium from bone.

orthopnea: shortness of breath in the recumbent position, relieved partly or completely by assuming an upright posture.

OSA: obstructive sleep apnea.

PA: posteroanterior; pulmonary artery.

palliative: directed to the relief of symptoms rather than the elimination of their cause.

palpable: able to be felt (palpated).

palpation: feeling superficial and deep structures with the fingers or palm to detect tenderness, spasm, abnormal masses, abnormal texture of tissues, enlargement of abdominal organs, and other departures from the normal or expected.

palpitation: heart action that is abnormally rapid, abnormally strong, or irregular.

papule: a clearly defined zone of skin, less than 1 cm in diameter, that is raised above surrounding skin, and may differ from it in color or texture.

paraneoplastic syndrome: a group of symptoms caused by hormone-like products of neoplastic tissue.

paresthesia: a sense of tingling or prickling ("pins and needles") on a part of the body surface.

parotid gland: the salivary gland in front of each ear.

paroxysmal: occurring in sudden attacks.

parturient: a woman in labor.

parturition: childbirth.

pathogen: anything capable of causing disease; usually referring to disease-causing microorganisms.

pathogenic: causing disease.

PCP: plasma cell pneumonia (*Pneumocystic carinii* pneumonia).

PCR: polymerase chain reaction.

PCWP: pulmonary capillary wedge pressure.

pectus excavatum: funnel chest, a deformity characterized by depression or hollowness of the sternum.

percussion: tapping with a finger on the body wall, usually with a finger of the other hand interposed, to detect variations in sound quality over abnormal cavities, masses, accumulations of gas or air, or effusions of fluid.

pericarditis: inflammation of the pericardium, the membranous sac surrounding the heart.

period of communicability: the length of time, often beginning before the appearance of symptoms, during which a person with an infectious disease can spread it to others in some way.

peripheral edema: edema of the extremities.

peristalsis: the normal waves of muscular contraction by which the contents of a tubular organ such as the bowel or the ureter are propelled forward.

PET: positron emission tomography.

petechia: a pinhead-sized, round, red or purple macule due to extravasation of blood under the epidermis.

physical therapy: treatment involving application of physical modalities (massage, exercise, heat, cold, ultrasound).

PID: pelvic inflammatory disease.

pit: a small depression in the skin resulting from local atrophy or scarring after trauma or inflammation.

pitting edema: edema that retains the impression of the examiner's fingers after pressure is released.

PKU: phenylketonuria.

plantar (NOT planter): pertaining to the sole of the foot.

plaque: a clearly defined zone of skin, more than 1 cm in diameter, that is raised above surrounding skin, and may differ from it in color or texture; a plaque may consist of many confluent papules.

plasma: the fluid component of blood.

pleural effusion: accumulation of fluid in the pleural space.

pleurisy (pleuritis): inflammation of the pleura.

PMI: point of maximum intensity.

polycythemia: an increase in the number of cells, usually red blood cells, in the circulation.

polymenorrhea: menstrual bleeding that occurs with abnormal frequency.

polyp: a tumor protruding from the surface of a mucous membrane.

polyradiculopathy: inflammation of several spinal nerve roots.

popliteal: referring to the hollow behind the knee.

porphyria (from Greek *porphyra* 'purple'): any disease characterized by elevation of blood levels of porphyrins; the term refers to the color of the urine after standing.

postprandial: after eating a meal.

precordial: in front of the heart.

present [verb, accented on second syllable]: refers to the symptoms or signs that are evident when the patient first seeks medical attention.

primary: said of a disease or condition that does not result from some other disease.

primigravida: a woman who is pregnant for the first time.

primipara: a woman who has given birth once.

prodrome: a period during which (usually nonspecific) symptoms such as fever or malaise precede the appearance of typical signs and symptoms of a disease.

prognosis: expected outcome of a disease.

progressive: characterized by increasingly extensive or severe symptoms or signs.

proteinuria: presence of protein in the urine.

protocol: a therapeutic regimen, usually prescribed for malignant disease, consisting of fixed or proportionate doses of three or more drugs administered concurrently.

pruritus, pruritic: itching.

psychosis: a mental disorder in which, in addition to emotional distress, the patient experiences a break with reality, manifested by delusions, hallucinations, and grossly bizarre or socially inappropriate behavior.

PTC: percutaneous transhepatic cholangiography.

PTH: parathyroid hormone.

PTT: partial thromboplastin time.

puerperal: pertaining to the puerperium.

puerperium: the period between the birth of the child and the return of the uterus to its normal size, with regeneration of endometrium.

pulmonary: pertaining to the lungs or their function.

purpura: an eruption of purple spots on the skin due to local hemorrhages.

purulent: pertaining to the formation of pus.

pustule: a thin-walled sac containing pus.

PUVA: psoralen and ultraviolet A.

RAD: reactive airways disease.

radical: a drastic program of treatment, medical or surgical, with a high risk of adverse effects, justified only by the severity of the patient's condition or the unfavorable prognosis.

radiography: the branch of medical technology concerned with the performance of x-ray and other imaging procedures.

radiology: the branch of medicine concerned with the diagnosis and treatment of disease through the application of x-rays, ultrasound, magnetic resonance imaging, radioactive materials, and related methods.

radon: a radioactive gas, product of the natural breakdown of radium, found in soil and thought to be an important cause of human malignancy.

rape: sexual intercourse, with penetration, that is against the will of the passive participant.

RAST: radioallergosorbent test.

RBC: red blood cell.

reaction, polymerase chain (PCR): a laboratory technique by which very small samples of biological material can be amplified so as to be more readily detected by testing.

recombinant DNA technology: a process whereby nonpathogenic bacteria that have been genetically altered are used to synthesize complex substances such as drugs and hormones.

recurrent: referring to a condition that reappears after symptoms had largely or entirely resolved.

red herring: a misleading diagnostic clue.

regimen: a program or course of treatment, including diet, exercise, and drug therapy.

relapsing: essentially the same as the preceding.

remissive, remittent: referring to a condition of which most or all signs and symptoms have resolved, either naturally or as a result of treatment; remission may be temporary or permanent.

resection: surgical removal of a body part or tumor.

retinitis: inflammation of the retina, the light-sensitive membrane at the back of the eyeball.

rhinitis: inflammation of nasal mucous membranes, usually accompanied by nasal obstruction, excessive secretions, and sneezing.

rhinophyma: enlargement and deformity of the external nose, usually as a result of rosacea.

rhinorrhea: increased flow of mucus from the nose.

rhinoscope: an instrument for examining the interior of the nose.

RPR: rapid plasma reagin.

RTE: renal tubular epithelium.

SA: sinoatrial.

SAD: seasonal affective disorder.

scab: see *crust*.

scale: a flake of epidermis shed from the skin surface.

scar: see *cicatrix*.

SCID: severe combined immune deficiency

scoliosis: lateral curvature of the spine.

secondary: said of a disease or condition that results from some other disease.

self-limiting (-ed): said of a disease such as the common cold that typically runs its course and resolves spontaneously without complications or sequelae, even when left untreated.

senile: occurring as a result of aging.

sensitivity: (1) the ability of a diagnostic test to detect a specific abnormality; (2) susceptibility of a microorganism to inhibition or destruction by an antibiotic or other drug.

sensorium: conscious, alertness, the ability to perceive and process sensory impulses.

sequela [plural, sequelae]: an abnormality or impairment, such as scarring or weakness, that persists after a disease has resolved.

serology: the branch of medical laboratory technology that employs antigen-antibody reactions to diagnose infections and other diseases, particularly autoimmune diseases.

serous gland: one producing a thin, watery secretion, not containing mucus.

sexually transmitted disease (STD): any infection that is transmitted from person to person through sexual activity.

shock: a condition in which the systemic blood pressure is too low to maintain adequate tissue perfusion.

sign: any abnormality of bodily structure or function that is observable by the physician, whether evident to the patient or not.

silent: asymptomatic; referring to a disease or medical event discovered only by chance.

smear: a thin film of fluid or semisolid material (blood, stool, nasal secretions, cells scraped from a surface), usually stained, that is examined microscopically for diagnostic purposes.

SPA: single proton absorptiometry.

specificity: the ability of a diagnostic test to react only in the presence of a specific abnormality and not when that abnormality is absent.

SPECT: single positron emission computed tomography.

speculum: an instrument for inspecting a body cavity or orifice, often equipped with a light source, a magnifying lens, or both.

spirochete: a type of bacterium having a threadlike, spiral-shaped body; spirochetes cause Lyme disease and syphilis.

splenomegaly: enlargement of the spleen.

stage: a measure of the extent to which a disease, particularly a malignant disease, has developed.

status epilepticus: one or a series of grand mal seizures lasting more than 30 minutes without waking intervals.

STD: sexually transmitted disease.

stenosis: abnormal narrowing of a passage or vessel.

stigma: any observable sign or abnormality that is characteristic of a disease or condition, particularly a hereditary one.

stress fracture: a crack in a bone induced by repetitive stress on the same bone (as in jogging or doing step aerobics) rather than by a single violent force.

subacute: lasting somewhat longer than an acute illness.

subclinical: causing no symptoms or signs; essentially the same as *silent*.

supportive: referring to a treatment regimen designed to preserve the patient's comfort, hydration, and nutritional status without affecting the underlying disease.

surgical: a mode of treatment involving physical or mechanical manipulation, usually by cutting into the body to repair or remove diseased or injured organs or tissues.

symptomatic: referring to treatment that is intended to relieve symptoms rather than abolish their cause.

syncope: fainting; sudden loss of consciousness, usually transitory, due to circulatory or neurologic abnormality, including central nervous system intoxication or injury, but frequently the result of strong emotion in the absence of organic disease.

synergism: a positive interaction between two or more drugs in which each boosts the effect of the others.

synthesis: formation of a complex substance, such as a protein or enzyme, from simpler substances.

TA: Terminologia Anatomica.

tachyarrhythmia: a pulse that is both irregular and abnormally rapid.

tachycardia: abnormally rapid heartbeat.

tachypnea: rapid breathing.

TBG: thyroid-binding globulin.

telangiectasis: a permanent dilatation of small blood vessels (capillaries, arterioles, venules), visible through a skin or mucous surface.

telangiectatic: pertaining to telangiectases.

tentative diagnosis: a diagnosis that seems most probable on the basis of available data, but which has yet to be confirmed.

terminal: a disease that is expected to cause death within the near future, regardless of treatment.

therapeutic trial: experimental administration of a drug in an effort not only to relieve symptoms but also to confirm the working diagnosis.

thorax: the chest and its contents.

thrill: an abnormal sensation felt by the examiner over the heart when blood jets through an anomalous orifice or narrowed valve.

TIA: transient ischemic attack.

titer: a term referring to the concentration of a substance such as an antibody detected by quantitative testing of blood.

T-N-M classification: a formal mode of staging that is used for many malignant diseases; T, tumor; N, (lymph) nodes; M, metastases. Arabic numerals are used to indicate the extent of involvement; for example, T1 N2 M0 for a given tumor might mean a tumor that is not locally invasive, with extension to two groups of regional lymph nodes, but no apparent metastases.

topical: referring to a medicine applied directly to skin or mucous membrane.

TPA: tissue plasminogen activator.

transmissible: able to be spread from person to person.

transrectal: said of a diagnostic or surgical procedure that is performed through the rectum.

traumatic: due to injury—physical, chemical, thermal, or psychological.

tropical disease: an infection or infestation that occurs predominantly or exclusively in tropical latitudes.

TSH: thyroid-stimulating hormone.

TUR: transurethral resection.

TVUS: transvaginal ultrasound.

Tzanck smear: a stained smear of material from an ulcer or vesicle, intended to reveal cellular changes due to viral infection.

ulcer: a cutaneous defect extending into the dermis.

UPJ: ureteropelvic junction.

UTI: urinary tract infection.

UVB: ultraviolet B.

UVJ: ureterovesical junction.

Valsalva maneuver: attempt at forced expiration, with the lips and nostrils closed; this drives air into the auditory tubes unless they are obstructed.

vascular: pertaining to vessels, usually blood vessels.

vasculitis: inflammation of blood vessels.

vasoconstrictor: a medicine that constricts blood vessels, either when applied topically or through systemic action.

VDRL: Venereal Disease Research Laboratories.

vector: an animal (for example, a mosquito) that transmits a pathogenic organism from one host to another.

vegetation: an abnormal growth, particularly one formed on a heart valve as a result of endocarditis.

vesicle: a small thin-walled sac containing clear fluid.

VLDL: very low-density lipoprotein.

VMA: vanillylmandelic acid.

VZIG: varicella-zoster immune globulin.

WBC: white blood cell.

wheal: a rapidly appearing and disappearing zone of circumscribed swelling in the skin, usually white with a red halo, due to various types of allergic reaction; the characteristic lesion of hives.

Wood light: an ultraviolet lamp with a filter that selects wavelengths under which certain funguses infecting skin or hair fluoresce brightly.

working diagnosis: a preliminary diagnosis, often very general (fever of unknown origin, seizure disorder) on the basis of which therapy can be started and more specific diagnostic tests chosen.

xerophthalmia: abnormal dryness of the eye, usually due to decreased flow of tears.

Index

psoriasis, 98
psychoanalysis, 320
Pthirus pubis, 95
ptosis, of eyelid, 279
pulmonary embolism, 146
pulmonary infarction, 146
pulmonary tuberculosis, 145
pulse, 109
    jugular venous, 109
pulse pressure, 109
pulsus paradoxus, 118
puncture, lumbar, 299
pupil, Argyll Robertson, 278
purpura, 90
    idiopathic thrombocytopenic,
        251
pus, 28
pustule, 90
pyelogram, intravenous, 176
pyelonephritis, 179
pyoderma, 92

quinsy, 135

radiation injury, 79
radiation sickness, 79
radiation therapy, 61
radio-allergosorbent test (RAST),
    48
rale, 142
rape, 78
rate, 5-year survival, 60
    erythrocyte sedimentation, 245
Raynaud disease, 120
Raynaud phenomenon, 120
reactive airways disease, 144
rebound tenderness, 156
rectovaginal examination, 192
rectum, adenocarcinoma of, 63
red blood cell, 243
red blood cell count, 245
red blood cell indices, 245
reduction of dislocation, 75
    of fracture, 75
reflex, 299
    Babinski, 299
    Chaddock, 299
    pathologic, 299
    hepatojugular, 117
refraction, ocular, 280
reiter syndrome, 184
renal failure, 177
reproductive system, female, 190
reproductive system, male, 180
residual volume of urine, 176

resistance, host, 30
    microbial, 33
respiratory system, anatomy, 142
reticulocyte, 245
retina, 277
retinal detachment, 284
retinitis pigmentosa, 283
retinopathy, diabetic, 283
    hypertensive, 119, 283
Reye syndrome, 35
Rh type, 248
rheumatic fever, 50
rheumatoid arthritis, 49
rheumatoid arthritis factor, 49
rhinitis, allergic, 133
rhinoscopy, 133
rhinosinusitis, 133
rhonchi, sibilant, 144
    sonorous, 144
rhonchus, 142
rhythm, gallop, 109
ringworm, 93
Rinne test, 130
Rochalimaea, 47
Romberg test, 132
rosacea, 97
Roth spots, 114
rub, pericardial friction, 110
    pleural friction, 142
rule, Naegele, 209

Sabouraud medium, 93
Salmonella, 81
salpingitis, 196
sarcoma, Kaposi, 47
Sarcoptes scabiei, 95
scabies, 95
scale, cutaneous, 90
    Glasgow coma, 308
scan, ventilation-perfusion, 147
scarlet fever, 34, 135
Schilling test, 246
schizophrenia, 325
schwannoma, vestibular, 305
sclera, 277
sclerosis, amyotrophic lateral, 302
    multiple, 301
scoliosis, 262
scotoma, 279
screen, strep, 35
screening, cancer, 59
seagull murmur, 116
seasonal affective disorder, 322
sebaceous gland, 89
seborrheic dermatitis, 91

seborrheic keratosis, 98
section, frozen, 59
sed rate, 245
seizure, 306
senile keratosis, 98
sensorium, 319
sentinel pile, 161
septic embolus, 114
sequela, 8
serum sickness, 48
severe combined immuno-
    deficiency disease, 46
sexually transmitted diseases, 182
shaken baby syndrome, 78
sheath, myelin, 293
shingles, 35
shock, 118
    electric, 79
show, bloody, 210
shunt, portacaval, 164
sibilant rhonchi, 144
sickle cell anemia, 247
sickle cell trait, 247
sickness, serum, 48
sign, 6
sign, Brudzinski, 304
    Chadwick, 208
    Grey Turner, 166
    Homans, 121
    Kernig, 304
    Phalen, 308
    Tinel, 308
    Turner, 166
signs of pregnancy, 208
silicosis, 145
simian crease, 22
sinoatrial node, 107
sinus, paranasal, 132
sinusitis, 133
Sjögren syndrome, 50
skin, anatomy, 89
    diseases, 87
slipped disk, 263
slit lamp, 279
smear, Pap (Papanicolaou), 192
    Tzanck, 35, 91, 94
snake venom, 80
social anxiety disorder, 321
social phobia, 321
somatotropin, 227
sonorous rhonchi, 144
sore throat, 134
souffle, funic, 208
    uterine, 208
sounds, heart, 109

The Author

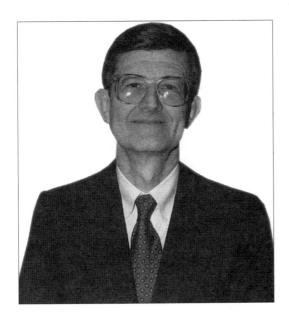

John H. Dirckx, M.D., has been director of the student health center at the University of Dayton in Dayton, Ohio, since 1968. His longstanding interest in classical and modern languages has led to the writing of several books and numerous articles on the language, literature, and history of medicine.

He is the author of *Human Diseases*, first published in 1997 by Health Professions Institute; *H&P: A Nonphysician's Guide to the Medical History and Physical Examination*, 3rd ed. (Health Professions Institute, 2001); *Laboratory Medicine: Essentials of Anatomic and Clinical Pathology*, 2nd ed. (Health Professions Institute, 1995); *The Language of Medicine: Its Evolution, Structure, and Dynamics*, 2nd ed. (New York: Praeger Publishers, 1983), and *Roundsmanship: An Introductory Manual* (Health Professions Institute, 1987).

He is a frequent contributor of educational articles on medicine and medical language to medical transcription periodicals, including *Perspectives on the Medical Transcription Profession* (published by Health Professions Institute) and *Journal of AAMT* (American Association for Medical Transcription), and is medical consultant for *The SUM Program for Medical Transcription Training* developed by Health Professions Institute. He has also served as editor or consultant for several Stedman's publications. In addition, his short fiction appears regularly in national magazines.

His hobbies include book-collecting and music. He and his wife Joyce have five daughters and nine grandchildren.

Answers to Exercises

Questions for Study and Review: These answers appear below. When there is more than one correct response, alternative answer choices are shown. Where a question calls for a response that is more subjective than objective, an example is given.

Case Study: You're the Doctor: The answers to most of these questions are revealed as you proceed to the next shaded box in the scenario. In some instances, a question calls for an opinion and there is no "correct" response. See the author's note in the Preface on page *v* and About the Exercises sections on page *xi* for additional information and suggestions on completing the Case Study questions.

Chapter 1 The Nature of Disease

1. a. acute: developing relatively suddenly and running its course in a few days or weeks.
   b. chronic: having a protracted course, often life-long.
   c. etiology: the study of the causes of disease; universally used by physicians to mean the cause itself.
   d. sign: any abnormality of bodily structure or function that is observable by the physician, whether evident to the patient or not.
   e. symptom: any distress, abnormality, or malfunction experienced by the patient as a result of illness.
   f. syndrome: a combination of symptoms that consistently occur together.
2. a. cystoscopy
   b. biopsy
   Additional answers: endoscopy, colonoscopy, laparoscopy, arthroscopy, surgical excision, and depending upon the collection method, laboratory tests including cultures, cytology, etc.
3. a. electrocardiogram
   b. x-ray
   Additional answers: electrodiagnostics, electroencephalogram, electromyogram, diagnostic imaging, CT scan, fluoroscopy, ultrasound, magnetic resonance imaging, etc.
4. The physician takes into account the patient's history, signs and symptoms of disease, findings on physical exam, negative as well as positive findings, and the results of other tests.

5. Genetic diseases that can be diagnosed by history alone might include cystic fibrosis and acute intermittent porphyria. Those diagnosed by physical exam alone might include Down syndrome and Marfan syndrome. Those diagnosed by lab test alone might include phenylketonuria, Turner syndrome, and Klinefelter syndrome.
6. Example: A wrong diagnosis may be attributed to misleading or incomplete information supplied by the patient, absence of detectable abnormality on physical examination, conflicting laboratory data, examination or testing before the disease was fully manifest, or failure to return to the physician for followup.

Chapter 2 Genetic Disorders

1. a. congenital disorders: present or occurring at birth, regardless of cause, such as maternal infections passed to the infant at birth, congenital herpes simplex or chlamydia, conditions due to maternal drug abuse or toxic exposure, conditions related to lack of oxygen at birth, and chromosomal aberrations such as cleft palate, and Down, Turner, or Klinefelter syndrome.
   b. hereditary disorders: transmitted genetically, regardless of when (if ever) observed, such as cystic fibrosis, phenylketonuria, acute intermittent porphyria, Marfan syndrome, cleft lip and palate (multifactorial), spina bifida (multifactorial), diabetes mellitus, muscular dystrophy, sickle cell anemia.
2. a. karyotype: genetic constitution; also, a photographic representation of a cell's chromosomes, showing the number of chromosomes and readily identifying gross structural aberrations such as deletion and inversion.
   b. gene: functional unit of heredity.
   c. autosomal dominant: a trait or condition that is expressed in a heterozygous individual carried on a gene in an autosome (not sex-linked).
   d. nondisjunction: failure of chromosomes to divide and then pair up correctly during mitosis or meiosis.
   e. trisomy: having three copies of a chromosome instead of two.
3. a. cytogenetics
   b. biochemical genetics
   c. DNA analysis of chromosomes

4. a. Down syndrome, cleft lip and palate.
   b. Marfan syndrome, Turner syndrome, Klinefelter syndrome, cystic fibrosis
5. a. acute intermittent porphyria
   b. phenylketonuria (if treated)
6. Example: The advantage of medical progress is survival of the patient; disadvantages include the costs of lifelong medical care and passing the condition on to the patient's own children (it is autosomal recessive so the patient must have two affected genes).

Chapter 3 Infectious Diseases

1. a. bacteria
   b. fungi
   c. parasites
   d. viruses
2. a. airborne
   b bloodborne
   c. droplet
   d fecal-oral
3. a. disinfectants
   b. antibiotics
   c. chemotherapeutics
   d. antivirals
   Additional answers: sulfonamides, antimalarials, interferons, antimicrobials.
4. Nonspecific symptoms include fever, chills, headache and muscle aches, loss of appetite, nausea, vomiting, and general malaise, any of which may or may not indicate the presence of infection.
5. The identity of the pathogen is the most important piece of information and can be obtained by visually observing the pathogen in the specimen or by detecting antibody to the pathogen in the patient's blood.
6. Lyme disease, streptococcal disease.
7. infectious mononucleosis, varicella, herpes zoster.
8. Example: Most cases of drug resistance in pathogens are due to genetic mutation. Widespread overuse of antibiotics may contribute to premature development of drug resistance. Indiscriminate use of antibiotics should be avoided.

Chapter 4 The Immune System

1. immunity: a set of protective responses in the living body by which infectious and other threats from outside can be repelled or inactivated. Human immunity has three cardinal features: it is stimulus-activated, directed against a specific target, and persisting.
2. a. agammaglobulinemia
   b. Chediak-Higashi disease
   c. DiGeorge syndrome (thymic hypoplasia)

Additional answers: Job syndrome, severe combined immunodeficiency disease (SCID), Wiskott-Aldrich syndrome.
3. a. bacillary angiomatosis
   b. candidosis
   c. cytomegalovirus (CMV) infection (cytomegalic inclusion disease
   Additional answers: herpes simplex, histoplasmosis, Kaposi sarcoma (KS), oral hairy leukoplakia, *Pneumocystis carinii* pneumonia (plasma cell pneumonia, PCP), toxoplasmosis, tuberculosis, varicella-zoster infection.
4. a. allergy: an immunologically mediated sensitivity to a foreign antigen (allergen), with resultant tissue inflammation and organ dysfunction.
   b. anaphylaxis: a life-threatening syndrome of urticaria, swelling of respiratory mucosa, and shock.
   c. antibody: a complex protein that reacts with a specific foreign material or organism by meshing chemically with it.
   d. antigen: any substance that elicits the formation of an antibody.
   e. autoimmunity: results when the body's immune system forms antibodies against some component of itself.
   f. opportunistic infection: infections due to pathogens to which persons with intact immune systems are virtually invulnerable.
5. a. rheumatoid arthritis: a chronic systemic disease causing inflammatory changes in many tissues, particularly joint membranes.
   b. polymyalgia rheumatica: a syndrome of chronic muscle pain and stiffness, fatigue, weight loss, and fever.
   c. lupus erythematosus (LE): a chronic inflammatory disorder of connective tissue due to formation of antibody to nucleoprotein.
6. a. Pro: The immune system protects us from a wide range of pathogens and other threats, defending us over the short term and often leaving us with life-long immunity. We couldn't live without it.
   b. Con: The immune system can malfunction and attack the body it is intended to protect.

Chapter 5 Neoplasia

1. Neoplasia refers to any growth of cells or tissues that is erratic, not in accord with normal bodily needs or patterns of growth and development, and not under the control of normal regulatory mechanisms.
2. a. Malignant neoplasms contain cells that are more primitive, undifferentiated, or anaplastic.

b. Enlarges by infiltrating and invading adjacent tissues.

c. Grows much faster than a benign one arising from the same cell type; also can spread by metastasis.

3. Men are more likely to die of cancer of the lung, prostate, or rectum, while women are more likely to die of lung, breast, or colon and rectal carcinoma.

4. a. carcinogen: chemical toxins leading to neoplasia.

b. debulking: palliative surgery to reduce the volume of a tumor.

c. grading: a measure of a cancer's degree of malignancy, based on histologic evaluation of its cells.

d. oncology: the branch of medicine devoted to the prevention, diagnosis, and treatment of malignant disease.

e. chemotherapy protocol: three or more drugs given according to a precise regimen.

f. staging: a measure of the extent of a malignant disease at the time of evaluation, expressed in Arabic numerals with or without qualifying letters.

5. a. surgery

b. chemotherapy

c. radiation therapy

6. Curative therapy is intended to cure the patient, to completely eradicate the cancer. Palliative therapy is directed to the relief of symptoms rather than the elimination of their cause.

7. Example: Cancer is often a life-threatening condition with considerable effect on the patient's emotional well-being. This can disrupt family and interpersonal relationships. If a cure is not immediately forthcoming, the patient may be unable to return to work. Depending upon the patient's insurance coverage, financial ruin may be inevitable. The cancer itself is physically debilitating but the severe side effects of treatment are often worse than the disease.

Chapter 6 Trauma and Poisoning

1. The physician's first concern is to ensure that the patient has a clear airway, since suffocation is rapidly fatal. Secondly, if the patient is not breathing, artificial ventilation must be started at once. The third priority is heart action and the adequacy of blood flow to tissues.

2. Blunt injury to the chest can fracture ribs and produce severe contusion of heart or lungs, while blunt injury to the abdomen can cause bruising, laceration, or severe hemorrhage of internal organs. In penetrating abdominal injuries, the risk of damage and particularly of hemorrhage is much increased. Puncture of the stomach or intestine releases digestive fluids into the peritoneal cavity and causes chem-ical peritonitis. Penetrating wounds of the chest endanger the heart and great vessels, the lungs, the esophagus, and other structures within the thorax. Puncture of the heart or a main blood vessel can be almost instantly fatal.

3. a. concussion: a violent blow to the skull that causes brief unconsciousness but does no permanent damage to the brain or its supporting structures.

b. contusion: bruising or crushing of cutaneous and subcutaneous tissues, muscles, and other structures, as manifested by local swelling, discoloration due to leakage of blood from the circulation, pain, tenderness, and reduced mobility.

c. laceration: a tearing of tissue due to blunt violence (collision with wall, furniture, or floor; being struck with a hard ball, a bat, or someone's knee) rather than to something sharp.

d. trauma: a general term for an injury of any kind.

e. triage: literally, "sorting"; it means dealing first with those persons who are expected to survive but are most severely injured and in need of immediate treatment, and then with less severely injured persons.

4. Depending upon its severity, virtually every traumatic injury or illness can result in psychological complications. Legal implications are a factor any time a third party might remotely be considered at fault or contributing in some way.

5. a. Chemical poisoning includes strong mineral acids and alkalis, benzene, and carbon monoxide, while biological poisoning examples include insect stings, snake venom, poisonous plants, and contaminated food.

b. Local effects may be erythema, edema, ecchymosis, or pain, while systemic effects include headache, nausea, vomiting, weakness, muscle spasms, hypotension, and shock.

c. General treatment may include emptying the stomach, medications, and oxygen, while specific measures may include an antidote for a particular poison.

Chapter 7 Skin

1. Sweat glands regulate temperature, oil glands protect the skin and retain moisture, hair insulates and protects, and the nails provide protection. They may be a liability in that that they require maintenance and are subject to injury, infection, and other conditions.

2. Dermatitis means inflammation of the skin; e.g., (a) atopic dermatitis; (b) seborrheic dermatitis; (c) contact dermatitis. Dermatosis is a general term for any abnormal condition of the skin, but usually excluding inflammatory conditions, e.g., (a) acne vulgaris; (b) acne rosacea; (c) psoriasis. Also, pityriasis rosea and urticaria.

3. a. alopecia: hair loss leading to temporary or permanent, patchy or diffuse zones of baldness; can result from scarring after trauma or after severe bacterial or fungal infection.

 b. cicatrix: a zone of fibrous tissue occurring at the site of a healed injury or inflammatory or destructive lesion extending into the dermis.

 c. comedo: a papule consisting of a dilated sebaceous duct or gland plugged with keratin debris.

 d. dermographism: abnormally sensitive skin by which strokes or writing with a pointed object are reproduced on the skin surface as raised lines.

 e. macule: a clearly defined zone of skin, less than 1 cm in diameter, differing from surrounding skin in color but not in texture or elevation.

 f. papule: a clearly defined zone of skin, less than 1 cm in diameter, that is raised above surrounding skin, and may differ from it in color or texture.

 g. telangiectasis: dilatation of one or more small blood vessels visible through the skin.

 h. tinea corporis: superficial fungal infection of the skin.

 i. urticaria: an acute, often transitory eruption of intensely itchy papules or wheals.

 j. verruca: virally induced coarse papules of the skin and mucous membranes.

4. Example: If sunburns lead to skin cancer, then one could say that there is such a thing as a "healthy tan," but many people succumb to media images and take this to the extreme, increasing their risk of melanoma.

5. The presence of certain skin conditions can give a picture of the patient's overall physical condition. For example, a bacterial infection like impetigo can occur in situations where hygiene is poor. Skin conditions can also be indicative of systemic disease, such as folliculitis, which may be present in diabetes. Alopecia may indicate systemic lupus erythematosus, iron deficiency, or pituitary deficiency, while hirsutism may indicate polycystic ovary syndrome, congenital adrenal hyperplasia, or functioning (hormone-producing) tumors of ovarian or adrenal tissue.

Chapter 8 Cardiovascular System

1. Blood flows from the aorta throughout the body and returns through the superior and inferior venae cavae into the right atrium, through the tricuspid valve, to the right ventricle, through the pulmonic valve, to the pulmonary artery, to the lungs where it is oxygenated, then to the pulmonary veins, to the left atrium, through the mitral valve, to the left ventricle, through the aortic valve, and back out to the aorta. It passes through four chambers of the heart and four valves.

2. Congestive heart failure (CHF) is a syndrome of impaired hemodynamics due to inability of the heart to maintain normal circulation, while shock is a condition in which the systemic blood pressure is too low to maintain adequate tissue perfusion. The course of CHF is steadily downhill and can lead to death, but shock can lead to death quickly without treatment. Treatment for CHF includes rest, salt restriction, correction of precipitating factors, and medications such as diuretics, ACE inhibitors, and beta blockers, while shock requires vigorous treatment with positioning, volume replacement, compression to maintain circulation, and drugs such as dopamine and adrenal steroids.

3. a. arrhythmia: irregular rhythm of the heartbeat, with or without an abnormally slow or fast rate.

 b. embolism: a clot from its point of origin that travels to a remote site in the circulation where it can obstruct a large capillary zone.

 c. hypertension: sustained elevation of arterial blood pressure above 140 mmHg systolic or 90 mmHg diastolic.

 d. infarction: death of tissue due to blockage of its blood supply.

 e. thrombosis: formation of a clot within the circulatory system.

4. a. cigarette smoking
 b. overweight
 c. sedentary lifestyle
 Additional answers: conditions such as diabetes mellitus and elevated cholesterol inasmuch as they can be controlled.

5. a. family history
 b. male gender
 c. diabetes mellitus
 Additional answers: elevation of total cholesterol, LDL cholesterol, homocysteine, lipoprotein(a), or C-reactive protein.

6. a. coronary artery disease (arteriosclerotic heart disease, ischemic heart disease)
 b. myocardial infarction (heart attack, coronary thrombosis)
 c. hypertension
 d. deep thrombophlebitis
 e. infective endocarditis
 Additional answer: unstable angina pectoris

Chapter 9 Ear, Nose, and Throat

1. (a) conductive hearing loss due to disease or abnormality in the outer or middle ear: cerumen impaction, otitis media with effusion, hardening of the tympanic membrane (otosclerosis), injury or disease of the ossicles; (b) sensory hearing loss due to disease of the cochlea: acoustic trauma, ototoxicity

(aminoglycosides, loop diuretics, cisplatin), aging; and (c) neural hearing loss due to eighth nerve lesions or cerebrovascular disease.

2. Bleeding from the nose may be due to nasal trauma, irritation of the mucosa by dust or dry air, upper respiratory infection or allergic rhinitis, or coagulation defect.

3. a. audiography: a precise measurement of the faintest loudness (in decibels) that the subject can hear, each ear being tested separately at each of several pitches.

   b. auditory tube: the preferred name for what is referred to as the eustachian tube, which connects the middle ear to the pharynx.

   c. cerumen: earwax.

   d. coryza: a common, mild rhinitis caused by viruses, also called "common cold."

   e. epistaxis: bleeding from the nose.

   f. mastoiditis: infection of the mastoid air cells, the epithelium-lined air cells within the skull.

   g. pharyngitis: acute inflammation of the throat due to infection, sore throat.

   h. pinna: the cartilaginous appendage on either side of the head, which collects sound waves like a funnel.

   i. vertigo: a subjective sense of spinning.

4. The ears, nose, and throat are adjacent to one another anatomically, similar in histologic structure, and subject to many of the same diseases. For example, an infection of the throat can produce symptoms in the ears and nose.

5. This question requires a subjective response. Refer to the Case Study in this and previous chapters for additional information on the use/misuse of antibiotic treatment for viral infections.

Chapter 10 Respiratory System

1. a. acute bronchitis
   b. asthma (reactive airways disease, RAD)
   c. spontaneous pneumothorax
   d. pleural effusion
   e. pulmonary embolism and infarction
   Additional answers: adult (or acute) respiratory distress syndrome, chronic bronchitis.

2. a. Significant reduction in measures of air flow, particularly FEV_1 (forced expiratory volume in the first second of exhalation) and peak flow (maximum flow at the beginning of forced expiration).

   b. Arterial oxygen level is depressed.

   c. Reduced vital capacity and flow rates; arterial oxygen level is reduced, and so is arterial carbon dioxide.

3. a. (pulmonary) alveolus (plural, alveoli): microscopic air sac composing lung tissue, through whose extremely thin epithelial walls the respiratory gases can readily diffuse between the air within them and the blood in adjacent pulmonary capillaries.

   b. asthma: chronic or recurrent inflammatory disease of the trachea and bronchi characterized by reversible narrowing of air passages with wheezing, shortness of breath, and cough.

   c. bronchiectasis: irreversible dilatation of large bronchi, due to chronic infection, obstruction, or autoimmune disease.

   d. bronchoalveolar lavage (BAL): obtaining material from lung tissue by washing.

   e. cyanosis: bluish color of skin, particularly lips and nail beds, due to presence of excess unoxygenated blood in the circulation.

   f. hemoptysis: coughing up blood from respiratory passages.

   g. pleura: delicate serous membrane protecting the lungs.

   h. pneumoconiosis: a chronic fibrosis of lung tissue caused by prolonged inhalation of mineral dusts, including coal, silicates, and asbestos.

   i. rhonchus (plural, rhonchi): whistling or honking sound due to passage of air through respiratory passages narrowed by edema, secretions, or neoplasm.

4. Bronchoscopy might be of help in diagnosing pneumonia and pneumonitis as well as other respiratory diseases, especially cases of suspected malignancy.

5. A sputum smear and culture might be helpful in diagnosing acute bronchitis, asthma, bronchiectasis, pulmonary tuberculosis, and to rule out other pathogenic organisms, neoplastic cells, or other abnormal findings.

6. A ventilation-perfusion scan can be of help in diagnosing pulmonary embolism and infarction.

7. Smoking is the single most important preventable cause of respiratory disease and death.

Chapter 11 Digestive System

1. a. gastritis
   b. peptic ulcer disease
   c. gastroenteritis
   Additional answers: cholera, bacillary dysentery, typhoid fever, pseudomembranous enterocolitis, and appendicitis.

2. a. gastroesophageal reflux disease (GERD)
   b. hepatic cirrhosis including hepatitis
   c. acute pancreatitis with resultant esophageal varices

3. a. gastroesophageal reflux disease (GERD)
   b. peptic ulcer disease
   c. gastritis
4. a. peptic ulcer disease
   b. gastritis
   c. diverticulosis
   Additional answer: diverticulitis
5. a. anorexia: loss of appetite (may be accompanied by nausea and vomiting).
   b. Crohn disease: chronic inflammatory disease of the bowel that can lead to intestinal obstruction, abscess and fistula formation, and systemic complications.
   c. dysphagia: difficulty in swallowing.
   d. flatulence: excessive intestinal gas.
   e. GERD: gastroesophageal reflux disease (backflow of gastric juice into the esophagus).
   f. hematochezia: blood in stool.
   g. ileus: failure of normal flow of materials through the digestive tract because of atony or paralysis of the bowel.
   h. melena: black stools, often due to the presence of blood.
   i. pancreas: a flat retroperitoneal organ lying behind and below the stomach, with its right end (head) embraced by the C-shaped curve of the duodenum; it produces enzymes for the digestion of carbohydrate, protein, and fat which are poured into the duodenum and hormones (insulin, glucagon, somatostatin) released directly into the bloodstream.
   j. peritoneum: a delicate serous membrane that lines the abdominal and pelvic cavities (parietal peritoneum) and also covers the stomach, small intestine, and colon (except for the distal part of the rectum), as well as the liver, spleen, uterus, ovaries, ureters, and dome of the bladder (visceral peritoneum).
6. a. cholera
   b. bacillary dysentery
   c. typhoid fever
   Additional answer: pseudomembranous enterocolitis
7. a. *Salmonella*
   b. *Campylobacter*
   c. *Yersinia*
8. a. In Crohn disease, on biopsy, all layers of bowel are seen to be involved, not just mucosa as in ulcerative colitis.
   b. Ulcerative colitis may lead to polyp formation with progression to carcinoma, arthritis, spondylitis, iritis, and oral ulcers.
   c. Other features of ulcerative colitis not mentioned for Crohn disease include the inflammation is primarily limited to the left colon; it is accompanied by fever; mucus and pus may be present in the stool; and hemorrhage may be a complication. Features of Crohn not mentioned for ulcerative colitis include steatorrhea (fat in stool), narrowing of the bowel lumen, and skip areas of normal mucosa on sigmoidoscopy and colonoscopy.
9. a. The mode of transmission for hepatitis A is the fecal-oral route (including contaminated water and food); hepatitis B is transmitted via blood, including shared needles and needlestick injury in healthcare workers with occasional maternal transmission to neonates.
   b. Hepatitis A resolves within 2-3 weeks whereas hepatitis B has an incubation period of 6-12 weeks and may last as long as 16 weeks.
   c. The mortality rate for hepatitis B is somewhat higher than for A and the risk of complications such as carrier status, chronicity, cirrhosis, and hepatocellular carcinoma is greater for hepatitis B.

Chapter 12 Excretory; Male Reproductive

1. a. ureteral stone
   b. prostatic enlargement
   c. pregnancy
   d. urethral stricture
   e. tumor
   Additional answer: inflammation
2. a. prostate disease
   b. pregnancy
   c. ureteral stones
   d. vesicoureteral reflux
   e. other anomalies of the urinary tract
   Additional answers: diabetes mellitus, urethral stones or other obstruction, viral infection, bladder trauma, the presence of a catheter, other pelvic infection
3. a. flank or costovertebral angle (CVA)
   b. ureteral
   c. suprapubic
   d. perineal
   Additional answer: pain with voiding
4. a. anuria: total or nearly total cessation of urine excretion by the kidney.
   b. chancre: mucocutaneous ulcer.
   c. IVP: intravenous pyelogram, an x-ray examination of urinary tract after intravenous injection of radiopaque contrast medium that is quickly excreted in the urine.
   d. microscopic hematuria: blood in the urine that can be detected only by microscopic or chemical examination of the urine.
   e. overflow incontinence: leakage of urine from an over-distended bladder, occurring almost exclusively in men with urinary obstruction due to prostatic disease.

f. Peyronie disease: penile deformity in which fibrotic plaques in the penis can block blood vessels.

g. pollakiuria: increased frequency of urination, without an increase in the total volume of urine.

h. Reiter syndrome: autoimmune disorder consisting of arthritis, conjunctivitis, mucocutaneous lesions.

i. urolithiasis: formation of stonelike concretions (calculi) in the urinary tract, which may obstruct a ureter at a site of natural narrowing such as the ureteropelvic junction (UPJ) and ureterovesical junction (UVJ).

5. Pollakiuria means increased frequency of urination, without an increase in the total volume of urine. Possible causes are acute cystitis, acute pyelonephritis; and chlamydial infection, also benign prostatic hypertrophy, prostatitis, interstitial cystitis, acute urethral syndrome, and pregnancy. Polyuria is an increase in the 24-hour excretion of urine, which can be caused by systemic disease such as diabetes mellitus.

6. Gonorrhea and chlamydial urethritis are both sexually transmitted diseases. They share similar complications and co-infections, and are both treated with antibiotics. Both can be passed from the mother to child at birth. Chlamydial infection is caused by a different gram-negative organism and is more common than gonorrhea, with 10% of asymptomatic women testing positive. It takes longer to show symptoms of a chlamydial infection in men (women can remain asymptomatic in either condition). Although complications are similar, complications from untreated gonorrhea can be much more severe, affecting the joints, cardiac valves, and meninges.

Chapter 13 Female Reproductive

1. a. Stimulates the pituitary to release follicle-stimulating hormone (FSH).
   b. Stimulates the pituitary to release luteinizing hormone (LH).
2. a. Causes the ovary to begin producing estrogen, which is responsible for the development of secondary sexual characteristics (pubic and axillary hair, nipple and breast development, broadening of hips, feminine distribution of body fat).
   b. Stimulates the monthly development or maturation of an ovarian (graafian) follicle, one of hundreds of immature microscopic units, each of which contains an ovum or female sex cell (gamete).
3. A Pap test is done by removing superficial cells from the vagina and cervix for cytologic examination, to judge hormonal effect and to identify abnormal cell changes due to inflammation, infection, dysplasia (cell abnormalities heralding eventual development of malignancy), or actual malignancy. Specimens are taken from three areas: (a) the vaginal vault, with a flat wooden spatula; (b) the squamocolumnar junction (transition line between the squamous epithelium of the vagina and the columnar epithelium of the endocervical canal), with a specially shaped wooden spatula (Ayre spatula); (c) the endocervical canal, with a bristle brush to ensure sampling of columnar epithelial cells.

4. a. anovulation: failure of ovulation to occur at the expected times.
   b. clue cell: epithelial cells heavily studded with bacteria).
   c. dyspareunia: pain in the vulva, vagina, or pelvis with sexual intercourse.
   d. menarche: the first onset of menstruation.
   e. mittelschmerz: German, sharp pain, usually on one side of the pelvis, occurring midway between menstrual cycles.
   f. spinnbarkeit: German, 'ability to be drawn out into a string,' referring to cervical mucus.
   g. *Trichomonas vaginalis*: a sexually transmitted protozoan parasite that causes vulvar itching and vaginal discharge.

5. Breast cancer is the highest incidence cancer in women at 31%, followed by lung cancer at 13% and cancer of the colon and rectum at 11%. Cervical cancer occurs less often. The mortality rate of breast cancer is 25%. The 5-year survival rate for cervical cancer is 60%. Risk factors for cervical carcinoma are smoking, prolonged use of oral contraceptives, sexual contact with many partners, and HIV and HPV infection. Women are at greater risk for breast cancer if they have had no children or if their first pregnancy occurs late in their childbearing years. A family history of breast cancer is also a risk factor.

6. a. dysfunctional uterine bleeding
   b. pelvic inflammatory disease (PID)
   c. salpingitis
   d. endometritis
   e. carcinoma of the cervix
   Additional answers: pregnancy, endometrial carcinoma

7. a. uterine myoma (fibromyoma, fibroid)
   b. dysfunctional uterine bleeding

Chapter 14 Pregnancy and Childbirth

1. a. amenorrhea
   b. nausea and vomiting (morning sickness)
   c. swelling and soreness of the breasts; also uterine enlargement, urinary frequency, varicosities of the vulva and lower limbs, constipation, hemorrhage, heartburn

2. a. enlargement of the uterus
   b. weak and irregular contractions of the uterus
   c. purplish discoloration of the cervix and vagina (Chadwick sign)
   Additional answers: softening of the cervix (Hegar sign), presence of fetus on ultrasound or x-ray, circulatory sounds (funic soufflé, uterine soufflé), fetal movement, skin changes, positive pregnancy test

3. Example: Most reliable is the presence of a fetus on ultrasound or x-ray, as early as 6 weeks' gestation. Fetal heart action can be detected by echocardiography at 6 weeks and by Doppler at 8 weeks.

4. The obstetrician follows the progress of labor primarily by observation, attending to the comfort of the mother and monitoring maternal and fetal well-being.

5. a. chorion: a specialized plate of tissue, the chorion, through which the embryo draws nourishment from the underlying endometrium by way of fingerlike projections (villi).
   b. crowning: encirclement of the largest diameter of the fetal head by the vulva.
   c. eclampsia: a stage characterized by seizures that follows pre-eclampsia, syndrome of hypertension and proteinuria, occurring during the second half of pregnancy.
   d. effacement: the flattening of the cervix from a tubular structure to a ring.
   e. multipara: a woman who has given birth more than once.
   f. presenting part: the part of the fetus that is nearest to, or has entered, the birth canal.
   g. puerperium: the period between the birth of the child and the return of the uterus to its normal size, with regeneration of endometrium.

6. a. 1st stage: from the onset of labor to full dilatation
   b. 2nd stage: from full dilatation of the cervix to delivery of the fetus
   c. 3rd stage: from delivery of the fetus to delivery of the placenta

7. a. evidence of fetal distress
   b. maternal hemorrhage
   c. prolapse of the umbilical cord
   Additional answers: failure of the second stage to progress, inability of the mother to assist or cooperate

8. a. uterine dysfunction
   b. excessive anesthesia
   c. pelvic deformity

9. a. large baby
   b. hydrocephalus
   c. breech presentation

Chapter 15 Metabolism-Embolism

1. a. hypopituitarism as a result of pituitary hormone deficiency
   b. diabetes insipidus caused by a deficiency of antidiuretic hormone (vasopressin)
   c. hypothyroidism resulting from a deficiency of circulating thyroid hormone
   Additional answers: adrenal insufficiency (or Addison disease) resulting from a deficiency of cortisol and related hormones, congenital adrenal hyperplasia related to a cortisol deficiency, diabetes mellitus resulting from insulin deficiency, polyglandular deficiency syndrome.

2. Diseases caused by excessive hormone production:
   a. acromegaly or gigantism caused by excessive growth hormone production (somatotropin).
   b. hyperthyroidism due to excessive circulating thyroid hormone in the blood.
   c. Cushing syndrome (hypoadrencorticism) from production of excessive adrenocortical hormones by a neoplasm of the adrenal cortex; also congenital adrenal hyperplasia mentioned above involves a cortisol deficiency that leads to overproduction of ACTH with excessive androgen production; thus it could be classified as both a deficiency and overproduction disease.

3. a. cretinism
   b. congenital adrenal hyperplasia

4. a. essential amino acids
   b. water
   c. protein, fats, and carbohydrates
   Additional answers: essential dietary minerals (iron, calcium, sodium, potassium, zinc, magnesium, etc.); and vitamins.

5. a. Addison disease: adrenal insufficiency, acute or chronic deficiency of cortisol and related hormones from the adrenal cortex.
   b. carbohydrate: starches and sweets that are chemically degraded in the digestive system to simple sugars, especially glucose.
   c. glucose: a six-carbon sugar that is plentiful in the blood and the principal fuel of cellular energy metabolism.
   d. goiter: a palpable and often visible enlargement of the thyroid gland.
   e. hormone: a chemical messenger or mediator produced by a cell, tissue, or gland.
   f. insulin: a hormone that increases glucose utilization and exerts other complex influences on the metabolism of carbohydrates, proteins, and fats.
   g. metabolism: a general term for the sum of all the chemical and electrical processes that occur in the living body.

h. thyrotoxicosis: hyperthyroidism, a syndrome resulting from excessive thyroid hormone in the circulation.

i. thyroxine: an iodine-containing hormone which circulates in the blood bound to a plasma protein and influences general metabolism, chiefly by regulating gene transcription of body proteins.

j. vasopressin: also known as antidiuretic hormone (ADH), helps to control water balance by promoting reabsorption of water by the kidneys.

6. a. thyroid stimulating hormone (TSH)
   b. adrenocorticotropic hormone (ACTH), which stimulates the adrenal cortex
   c. gonadotropins: follicle-stimulating hormone (FSH) and luteinizing hormone (LH)

7. a. hypopituitarism
   b. acromegaly (gigantism)
   c. diabetes insipidus

8. Example: In hypothyroidism, when the circulating thyroid hormone is low, the pituitary senses this and produces more thyroid stimulating hormone.
   Example: In diabetes mellitus, when blood glucose is elevated due to excessive intake of carbohydrates or insulin resistance in the cells, the pancreas produces more insulin.

Chapter 16 Disorders of Blood

1. a. sickle cell anemia
   b. glucose-6-phosphate dehydrogenase (G-6-PD) deficiency
   c. leukemia
   Additional answers: Glanzmann disease (thrombasthenia), hemophilia, possibly lymphoma

2. a. acquired hemolytic anemia
   b. idiopathic thrombocytopenic purpura (ITP), or immune thrombocytopenic purpura
   c. disseminated intravascular coagulation (DIC)
   Additional answers: erythroblastosis fetalis (hemolytic disease of newborn)

3. a. polycythemia vera
   b. acute lymphocytic leukemia (acute lymphoblastic leukemia, ALL)
   c. chronic lymphocytic leukemia
   Additional answer: multiple myeloma

4. Formed elements in the blood with no nuclei include mature red blood cells and platelets.

5. a. Bence Jones protein: appears in urine in multiple myeloma.
   b. hemolysis: destruction of red blood cells in the body.
   c. lymphoblast: extremely immature lymphocytes.
   d. Philadelphia chromosome: an oncogene present in myelogenous leukemia; a reciprocal translocation of strands of genes between chromosomes 9 and 22.

e. reticulocyte: red blood cells containing fragments of nuclear material that can be detected by staining.

f. thrombocytopenia: deficiency of platelets in the circulation, which can result from diminished production, accelerated destruction, or sequestration in the spleen.

6. Hematologic disorders treated with splenectomy include acquired hemolytic anemia, chronic lymphocytic leukemia, and idiopathic thrombocytopenic purpura (ITP) to control hemolytic anemia.

7. Hematologic disorders sometimes helped by bone marrow transplant include aplastic anemia, chronic myelogenous leukemia, non-Hodgkin lymphoma, multiple myeloma, and Glanzmann disease (thrombasthenia).

8. Example: The AIDS epidemic, which began in the 1980s, tainted the nation's blood supply and led to the infection and death of scores of hemophiliac children who required regular blood transfusions. This trend was reversed when HIV was discovered and tests developed to detect the presence of HIV in donated blood.

Chapter 17 Musculoskeletal Disorders

1. a. muscular dystrophy
   b. scoliosis
   c. Osgood-Schlatter disease
   Additional answers: Legg-Calvé-Perthes disease, some forms of gout

2. a. tendinitis (tenosynovitis)
   b. bursitis
   c. carpal tunnel syndrome

3. a. fibromyalgia syndrome
   b. gout
   c. scoliosis
   Additional answers: fibromyalgia syndrome, osteomyelitis, degenerative joint diseases (osteoarthritis, DJD)

4. a. Bekhterev arthritis (ankylosing spondylitis)
   b. septic arthritis
   c. gonococcal arthritis
   d. psoriatic arthritis
   e. syphilitic arthritis

5. a. aponeurosis: a broad, sheetlike connection.
   b. bursa: purselike cushions containing a little fluid to protect underlying surfaces and reduce friction.
   c. crepitus: rubbing or grating sound.
   d. epiphysis: enlarged, knobby end of a bone.
   e. fibromyalgia: chronic musculoskeletal pain accompanied by weakness, fatigue, and sleep disorders.
   f. kyphosis: forward hunching of the upper spine.
   g. laminectomy: cutting through the posterior arch of one or more vertebrae.

h. meniscus: crescent- or C-shaped pads of fibrocartilage within the knee joint, one medial and one lateral, that cushion shocks between the femur and the tibia.

i. tophus: nodular deposit of urate crystals with local inflammation found in gout.

6. Gender-based musculoskeletal disorders include gout in men and osteoporosis and fibromyalgia in women. This suggests a hereditary component.

7. Orthopedists treat primarily traumatic and developmental structural abnormalities. The musculoskeletal diseases treated by rheumatologists are more systemic, chronic, and debilitating. The rheumatologist is likely to see more women because the systemic-type diseases seem to affect women more than men. Much of an orthopedist's practice is trauma and sports medicine, which involves a predominance of male athletes.

Chapter 18 Eye

1. a. exophthalmos: abnormal bulging of the eye due to local disease (unless bilateral).

   b. xerophthalmia: abnormal dryness of the eye due to decreased flow of tears.

   c. cupping of the disk: a depression in the optic nerve head due to increased intraocular pressure.

   d. hypopyon: pus in the anterior chamber.

2. a. papilledema: swelling of optic disk due to increased intracranial pressure.

   b. nystagmus: rhythmic back and forth eye movements due to central nervous system (CNS) or congenital disease.

   c. scotoma: a blind spot in the visual field due to a CNS condition.

   d. miosis: constriction of the pupil due to CNS disease as well as local disease.

3. Aqueous humor is located anterior to the lens; vitreous humor is located behind it.

4. The anterior chamber is between cornea and iris, while the posterior chamber is between iris and lens. Thus the iris is the boundary between the two chambers.

5. a. canthus: the medial or nasal junction or any angle between upper and lower lids is the inner canthus, and the outer canthus is the lateral or temporal angle.

   b. fundus: the rear wall of the eye as viewed through the pupil with an ophthalmoscope.

   c. keratitis: inflammation of the cornea.

   d. lacrimation: tearing or increased flow of tears.

   e. ptosis: drooping of an upper eyelid that cannot be fully corrected by voluntary effort.

   f. retinopathy: degenerative disorders of the retina, usually accompanied by loss of vision and often due to systemic disease.

   g. scotoma: a blind spot; a gap in the visual field of one or both eyes in which objects cannot be seen.

   h. slit lamp: low-power microscope with built-in illumination projected through a narrow slit.

6. a. retinal detachment

   b. glaucoma

   c. macular degeneration

7. a. diabetes mellitus

   b. hypertension

   c. hypoparathyroidism

   Additional answer: arteriosclerosis

8. a. Hyperopia (farsightedness) is when the focus of light rays passing into the eyes lies behind the retina due to congenitally short AP diameter of the eyeball.

   b. Myopia (nearsightedness) is when the focus of light rays passing into the eyes lies in front of the retina due to congenitally long AP diameter of the eyeball.

   c. Presbyopia is a loss of normal accommodation with aging, due to diminished elasticity of the eyes with inability to focus on objects or print near the eyes.

9. a. Heterophoria is a transient deviation of the eye from the normal position with respect to the other eye.

   b. Heterotropia is a persistent deviation of one or both eyes due to congenital ocular muscle weakness or imbalance.

   c. Paralytic strabismus results from paralysis of one or more eye muscles due to congenital abnormality, trauma, infection, multiple sclerosis, herpes zoster, neoplasm, or hemorrhage.

Chapter 19 Nervous System

1. Cranial nerves exerting their influence below the level of the head include IX, glossopharyngeal (throat); X, vagus (motor fibers to thoracic and abdominal viscera); and XI, accessory (motor innervation of two voluntary muscles of the neck: trapezius and sternocleidomastoid).

2. Five parts of cranial nerve exam that cannot be performed on unconscious patient include I (olfactory), II (optic), V (trigeminal), VII (facial), X (vagus), XI (accessory), and XII (hypoglossal).

3. a. ataxia: impairment of complex movements due to loss of proprioceptive impulses from the muscles of the trunk or limbs.

   b. axon: part of a nerve cell, a single long, straight process.

   c. Babinski reflex: dorsiflexion of the great toe and flaring of the other toes in response to stroking of the sole of the foot toward the toes.

d. lumbar puncture: withdrawal of a specimen of cerebrospinal fluid from the subarachnoid space by inserting a needle between two vertebrae.

e. polyneuritis: disease or damage affecting more than one peripheral nerve.

f. myelin: a thin layer of fatty white material enveloping the axons.

g. neuron: another word for nerve cell.

h. traumatic tap: blood in cerebrospinal fluid due to local injury by the needle during lumbar puncture.

5. Upper motor neuron lesions involve interruption of motor tracts running between the cerebral cortex and the spinal segment, without any impairment of the reflex arc, while lower motor neuron lesions interrupt motor tracts running between the spinal cord and one or more muscles.

6. a. polyneuritis (Charcot-Marie-Tooth disease, Dejerine- Sottas disease, Friedreich ataxia)

b. Huntington disease (Huntington chorea)

c. possibly multiple sclerosis

Additional answer: Amyotrophic lateral sclerosis (Lou Gehrig disease) has a genetic predisposition.

7. a. myasthenia gravis

b. brain abscess

c. transient ischemic attack (TIA); also mononeuritis, polyneuritis

8. a. bacterial meningitis due to meningococcus (*Neisseria meningitidis*)

b. viral meningitis

c. Huntington disease (Huntington chorea)

Additional answers: amyotrophic lateral sclerosis (Lou Gehrig disease), parkinsonism (Parkinson disease, paralysis agitans), stroke (brain attack, cerebrovascular accident, CVA)

Chapter 20 Mental Disorders

1. a. neurosis: a mental disorder in which the patient experiences, and gives evidence of, emotional distress, but remains in touch with reality at all times, such as anxiety, depression, and eating disorders.

b. psychosis: a mental disorder in which, in addition to emotional distress, the patient experiences a break with reality, manifested by delusions, hallucinations, and grossly bizarre or socially inappropriate behavior, such as bipolar disorder, schizophrenia, delirium, and dementia.

2. Types of therapy used in the treatment of mental disorders include pharmacotherapy, currently the most rapid, effective, and predictable mode of treatment; aversion therapy, behavioral therapy, and client-centered therapy; also, cognitive therapy, electroconvulsion therapy, family therapy, group therapy, hypnosis, play therapy, psychodrama, psychotherapy, and rational therapy.

3. a. anxiolytic: agent that reduces the level of uneasiness and worry.

b. bulimarexia: compulsive binge eating is combined with irrational anxiety about becoming obese.

c. compulsion: an urge to repeat a ritualistic or stereotyped form of behavior that is recognized by the victim as irrational but that cannot be omitted without an increase of anxiety.

d. delusion: a distorted belief or perception.

e. hallucination: a sensory experience, usually auditory or visual, without any physical basis.

f. neuroleptic: a class of drugs also known as antipsychotics, used to treat schizophrenia.

g. obsession: a recurring or persisting idea, thought, or image that is perceived as intrusive, distracting, and repugnant, but that the victim is unable to ignore or suppress.

h. phobia: an irrational fear of some object or situation, with resulting efforts to avoid it.

4. Mental disorders that might make a person legally insane include schizophrenia and dementia.

5. This question requires a completely subjective response.